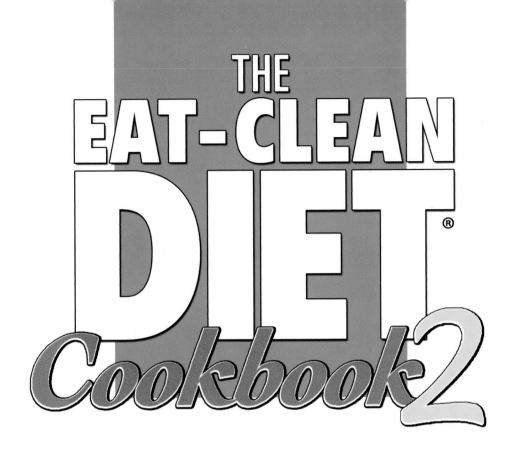

THE EAT-CLEAN DIET® Cookbook 2

Over *150* brand new great-tasting recipes that keep you lean!

W9-CDG-026

FROM *NEW YORK TIMES* BEST-SELLING AUTHOR

TOSCA RENO

RKP ROBERT KENNEDY PUBLISHING

Published by
Robert Kennedy Publishing
400 Matheson Blvd. West
Mississauga, ON
L5R 3M1 Canada

Visit us at **www.eatcleandiet.com**,
www.rkpubs.com and **www.toscareno.com**

Library and Archives Canada Cataloguing
in Publication

Reno, Tosca, 1959-
     The eat-clean diet
cookbook 2 / Tosca Reno.

Includes index.
     ISBN 978-1-55210-089-9

     1. Reducing diets--Recipes.
2. Cooking (Natural foods). I. Title.

RM222.2.R4645 2011   641.5'635
C2010-906762-2

10 9 8 7 6 5 4 3 2 1

Distributed in Canada by
NBN (National Book Network)
67 Mowat Avenue, Suite 241
Toronto, ON
M6K 3E3

Distributed in USA by
NBN (National Book Network)
15200 NBN Way
Blue Ridge Summit, PA
17214

Printed in Canada

Robert Kennedy Publishing
BOOK DEPARTMENT

MANAGING DIRECTOR
Wendy Morley

MANAGING ONLINE EDITOR
Vinita Persaud

PRODUCTION EDITOR
Cali Hoffman

**ONLINE EDITOR & EDITORIAL
ASSISTANT**
Meredith Barrett

ASSOCIATE EDITOR
Rachel Corradetti

ONLINE EDITOR
Kiersten Corradetti

ART DIRECTOR
Gabriella Caruso Marques

ASSISTANT ART DIRECTOR
Jessica Pensabene Hearn

EDITORIAL DESIGNERS
Brian Ross, Ellie Jeon

ART ASSISTANT
Kelsey-Lynn Corradetti

EDITORIAL ASSISTANTS
Tara Kher, Sharlene Liladhar

ONLINE ASSISTANT
Chelsea Kennedy

MARKETING MANAGER
Gail-Jacqueline Beckles

RECIPE DEVELOPER
Kierstin Buchner
www.kierstinbuchner.com

RECIPE PHOTOS
Photographer– **Donna Griffith**
www.donnagriffith.com
Food Stylist– **Claire Stubbs**
Hand Model – **Maya Visnyei**
Props provided by **Laura Branson,
The Prop Room, Robert Kennedy
Publishing, Donna Griffith,
Claire Stubbs**

TOSCA & FAMILY PHOTOS
Photographer– **Paul Buceta**
www.paulbuceta.com
Hair & Make Up– **Valeria Nova**
Stylist– **Rachel Burton and
Nadia Pizzimenti**

INDEXING AND PROOFREADING
James De Medeiros

All other photos **istockphoto.com**

IMPORTANT

The information in this book reflects the author's
experiences and opinions and is not intended to
replace medical advice.

Before beginning this or any nutritional or exercise
regimen, consult your physician to be sure it is
appropriate for you. Ask for a physical stress test.

To my devoted Eat-Clean fans who asked for more and are getting it!

The Eat Clean movement would be nothing without you!

Acknowledgments

As always, a special thank you to the dream team book crew at Robert Kennedy Publishing for making yet another Eat-Clean title come to fruition. There were many ups and downs, but your contributions, edits, designs, and promotions make this book what it is today... a beautiful, consistent, clean read with a powerful message. I couldn't have done this without you.

Thank you also to Kierstin Buchner for developing the most delectable and unique recipes. I am so happy to have found you and your amazing culinary skills in Portland, Oregon. My books are definitely benefiting from your talents.

Thank you to food photographer extraordinaire, Donna Griffith, and talented food stylist, Claire Stubbs. You two are a foody dream duo who make these mouthwateringly delicious recipes jump right off the page and onto the dinner table.

Finally, thank you to my support system at home and around the world. My family, friends and fans motivate me to spread the message of Eating Clean as far as it can go and beyond. Thank you for your guidance, encouragement and love, which lifts me up and reminds me every day why I do what I do.

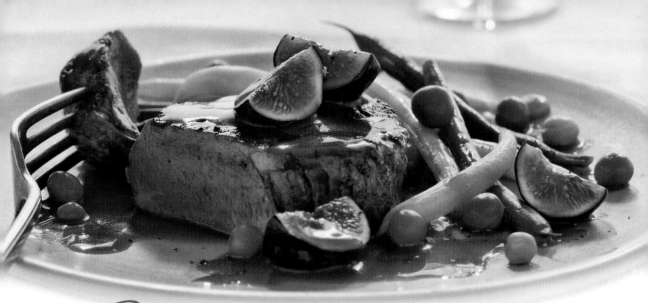

Contents

INTRODUCTION 8

1 BREAKFAST 10

JUMP START GRANOLA 12

HUEVOS RANCHEROS 15

BAKED EGGS 16
with Tomatoes, Turkey Bacon, Chives
and Toasted Breadcrumbs

AÇAI BLUEBERRY BREAKFAST SHAKE . . 19

PAPAYA WITH A KICK 20

HEARTY BLUEBERRY CORN CAKE 23

ORZO FRITTATA 24
with Mushrooms, Peppers and Yellow Squash

SUPER POWER SMOOTHIE 27

SAVORY VEGETABLE WAFFLES 28

CHERRY PROTEIN POP 'EMS 31

CHILI AND SCRAMBLED
EGG BREAKFAST TACOS 32

OAT PORRIDGE 35
with Holiday Spices

STRAWBERRY PEACH KEFIR SMOOTHIE . 36
with Chia Seeds

2 BRUNCH 38

CITRUS SALAD 40
with Mint

MULTIGRAIN WAFFLES 43
with Raspberry Sauce

EGGS SARDOU 44
with Warm Orange Vinaigrette

WHITE PEACH AND BLACK CHERRY
BELLISSIMO 47

SUMMER VEGETABLE PLATTER 48
with Baby Heirloom Tomatoes and Scallion Pistou

SUPER MOIST BANANA WALNUT BREAD . 51

SMOKED SALMON ASPARAGUS BUNDLES . 52

CHEDDAR JALAPEÑO CORN MUFFINS . . 57

TURKEY APPLE BREAKFAST SAUSAGE . . 58

OATMEAL "SCUFFINS" 61
with Currants and Dates

ROASTED PORK TENDERLOIN 62
with Sweet Sage Glaze

PRAWN AND HERBED
YOGURT CHEESE CANAPÉS 65

CRUSTLESS BROCCOLI QUICHE 66
with Caramelized Onions and Blue Cheese

MEXICAN MOCHA CALIENTE 69

SEAFOOD PLATTER 70
*of Crab, Prawns and Oysters on the Half Shell with
Clean Cocktail Sauce and Cucumber Mignonette*

POTATOES O'BRIEN 73

Cheese Please 74

3 SOUP 76

SMOOTH AND HEARTY
BORSCHT-STYLE BEET SOUP 78

CREAMY ARTICHOKE SOUP 81

FRENCH ONION SOUP 82
with Parmesan Croutons

GREEN LENTIL AND VEGETABLE SOUP . 85

JAPANESE VEGETABLE AND TOFU SOUP . 86
(Kenchinjiru)

MEXICALI CABBAGE PATCH SOUP 89

EGG DROP SOUP 90

TOMATO FENNEL SOUP 93
with Lima Beans

GAZPACHO 94

PURÉE OF PARSNIP, CELERIAC
AND APPLE SOUP 97
with Crispy Sage

4 GRAINS & LEGUMES 98

ISRAELI COUSCOUS SALAD 100

OAT GROAT RISOTTO 103
with Mushrooms

FRESH FAVA BEANS 104
with Lemon Anchovy Vinaigrette

GREEK BROWN RICE DOLMAS 107

TABOULI 108
with Quinoa

SPANISH RICE 111

THREE BEAN SALAD 112
with Grilled Corn and Peppers

QUINOA 115
with Sausage and Peppers

5 SAUCES, SPREADS & SALSAS . . . 116

SALSA ROJA 118

CREAMY GUACA-DE-GALLO 121

CLEAN MARINARA SAUCE 122

BABA GHANOUSH 125

BASIL LEMON PESTO 126

NO-COOK FRESH TOMATO SAUCE . . . 129

CHICKEN LIVER PÂTÉ 130

SPICY CLEAN BBQ SAUCE 133

RAPINI PESTO 134

Herbs 136

6 ONE-DISH & EASY MEALS 138

CAMPFIRE SALMON 140
with Fire Roasted Peppers and Eggplant

ITALIAN SAUSAGE 143
with Sloppy Peppers

SHRIMP TACOS 144
with Grilled Pineapple Salsa

GREEK LAMB FLATBREAD PIZZA 147

SAUTÉED SCALLOPS 148
with Four Herb Pesto and Quinoa

PULLED PORK POBLANO VERDE 151

SWEET 'N' SPICY SHRIMP &
CANTALOUPE SALAD 152

ARGENTINE COWBOY STEAK 155
with Grilled Onion Rings, Tomatoes and Chimichurri

SEAFOOD GUMBO 156

KEFIR MARINATED LAMB KEBABS . . . 159
with Vegetables

CHICKEN AND SPINACH LASAGNA . . . 160

BBQ CHICKEN PIZZA 163

LEFTOVER PASTA PIZZA PIE 164

7 VEGETARIAN MEALS 166

VENICE BEACH ROASTED
VEGETABLE AND AVOCADO SUB 168

FRENCH GREEN LENTIL SALAD 171
with Easter Egg Radishes and Mache

PESTO STUFFED PORTOBELLO PIZZAS . 172

PERSIAN COUSCOUS AND CHICKPEAS .. 175
with Kumquats

CURRY SPICED LENTIL FALAFEL 176
with Tahini Sauce

TOFU FAJITAS 179
with Peppers

ROASTED VEGETABLE EGGPLANT
PARMESAN 180

QUINOA RISOTTO 183
with Garlic Herb Creminis

LONG-LIFE VEGETABLE STIR-FRY 184

ROASTED RED POTATOES, ASPARAGUS
AND FRISÉE with Crispy Croutons 187

Vegetarian Done Right 188

8 LUNCH OUTSIDE
THE LUNCHBOX 190

BISON BURGER DOGS 192

SPANISH-STYLE TUNA SANDWICH 195

GARDEN VEGGIE STUFFED
PITA POCKETS 196

QUINOA AND BLACK BEAN
LUNCH BOWL 199

FRESH FIG CANAPÉS 200
with Mint and Balsamic Syrup

VANISHING PARTY NUTS 203

SCATTERED SUSHI BOWL 204
with Ginger Glazed Salmon (Chirashizushi)

SPICY ITALIAN TEMPEH SAUSAGE
AND SPINACH with Rotini 207

EGG SALAD WITH A TWIST 208

GRILLED CHICKEN CAESAR SALAD .. 211
with Spicy Kefir Caesar Dressing and
Grilled Mini Pita Bread

JAMAICAN JERK STEAK 212
with Pineapple Lettuce Wraps

BBQ CHICKEN CHOP CHOP SALAD .. 215

9 PROTEINS 216

HAZELNUT-CRUSTED
VENISON MEDALLIONS 218
with Herb Roasted Carrots and Parsnips

DOVER SOLE WRAPPED ASPARAGUS .. 221
with Dijon Blanc Sauce

BBQ PORK RIBS 222

BAKED CHICKEN TENDERS 225

HALIBUT 226
with Minted Lima Bean Purée

FILET MIGNON 229
with Fig Demi-Glace

MEDITERRANEAN LAMB &
BISON MEATBALLS 230

SPICY AHI POKE 233
with Avocado

OLIVE TAPENADE STUFFED SOLE 234

YELLOWFIN TUNA 237
with Cashew Sauce

BLACKENED SOLE 238

COCONUT SHRIMP 241
with Spicy Orange Dipping Sauce

GRILLED BLUE MARLIN 242
with Strawberry Nectarine Salsa

CRUNCHY BAKED GINGER
DILL SALMON 245

PUERCO PIBIL 246
(Braised Boar in Mexican Achiote Sauce)

CHILI RUBBED GRILLED
OSTRICH TENDERLOIN 249

SALMON 250
with Sun-Dried Tomato Tapenade in Parchment

VENISON BOURGUIGNON 253

A "How-To" for Fish 254

10 SALADS 256

PEACH AND HEIRLOOM
TOMATO CAPRESE SALAD 258

CELERIAC AND FENNEL SALAD 261
with Pomegranate Seeds

COLD SOBA NOODLE SALAD 262
with Cashew Miso Dressing

SUMMER ROOT VEGETABLE SALAD .. 265
with Fresh Cherries

ROASTED SWEET POTATO
AND SPINACH SALAD 266

GRILLED TREVISO AND ENDIVE 269
with Cranberries and Pumpkin Seeds

WARM BRUSSELS SPROUTS SALAD ... 270
with Walnuts and Lemon

ASIAN PEAR, WATERCRESS, PEA
SHOOT AND BLUE CHEESE SALAD ... 273

WINTER GREENS 274
with Cherries and Walnuts

ORZO AND CHICKPEA SALAD ... 277
with Roasted Red Peppers and Dill

BEETS, BLOOD ORANGES
AND ARUGULA *with Feta* 278

11 VEGETABLES 280

BRUSCHETTA 282
with Ricotta, Beet Greens and Walnuts

SUGAR SNAP PEAS AND MORELS ... 285

GRILLED FINGERLING POTATOES ... 286

PATTY PAN SQUASH 289

SAUTÉED FRESH PEPPERONCINI ... 290
with Yogurt Cheese and Baguette

BROCCOLI RAAB (RAPINI) 293
with Sun-Dried Tomatoes

CARAMELIZED CREMINI
MUSHROOMS AND PEARL ONIONS ... 294

BRAISED COLLARD GREENS 297

SMOKY SLATHERED CORN
ON THE COB 298

SESAME MANDARIN SLAW 301

COLCANNON 302
with Kale

GRILLED GARLIC SPEARS 305

BABY YELLOW POTATOES 306
with Parsley

GERMAN-BRAISED BEET TOPS AND
APPLES 309

ROASTED DELICATA SQUASH 310

12 SWEETS & BREADS 312

POACHED PEARS 314

WHITE PEACH SANGRIA 317

MARIONBERRY CRISP 318
with Walnut Oat Topping

WHOLE WHEAT ANGEL FOOD CAKE ... 321
with Fresh Strawberries

PLUM UPSIDE DOWN CAKE 322

CHOCOLATE ALMOND CAKE 325

HOT SPICED APPLE CIDER 326

CRANBERRY PEAR BELLINI 329

SWEET POTATO CUSTARD 330
with Spiced Walnut Clusters

24 CARROT-TINI 333

RHUBARB WALNUT DESSERT TORTA ... 334

EFFERVESCENT DESSERT FRUIT SOUP ... 337

BLUEBERRY BLINTZES 338

BERRY LEMON PARFAIT 341

PAVLOVA 342
with Fresh Summer Berries

Sweeteners 344

SUPPORTIVE RECIPES 346

YOGURT CHEESE 348

EAT-CLEAN COOKING SPRAY 348

CHIPOTLE RANCHERO SAUCE 350

RASPBERRY SAUCE 350

HERBED YOGURT CHEESE 351

CLEAN COCKTAIL SAUCE 351

SCALLION PISTOU 352

TAHINI SAUCE 352

DASHI (ICHIBAN DASHI) 353

PARMESAN CROUTONS 353

CUCUMBER MIGNONETTE 354

CRISPY HERB AND GARLIC CROUTONS ... 354

GRILLED PINEAPPLE SALSA 355

CHIMICHURRI 357

ZESTY HUMMUS 357

JERK SEASONING 358

DIJON BLANC SAUCE 358

FIG DEMI-GLACE 359

SPICY ORANGE DIPPING SAUCE ... 360

OLIVE TAPENADE 360

CASHEW MISO DRESSING 361

INDEX 362

Introduction

When I wrote my first cookbook in 2007 I had no idea what a phenomenon *The Eat-Clean Diet®* series would become. Sure, the original *Eat-Clean Diet* book had been selling well and people were asking for recipes – that's

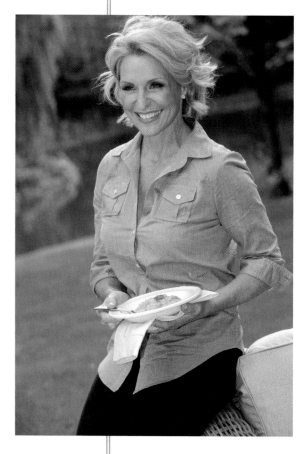

what inspired me to write a cookbook. Little did I know that over four years later, my books would have sold well over a million copies, and many millions of lives would have been transformed by the concept of Eating Clean.

That first cookbook shot to number one on the best-selling cookbook chart its very first week and has been in continuous reprint ever since. In fact, in at least one country it's the top-selling cookbook of the past four years! I am incredibly honored that so many people have put their faith in my words and allowed me into their kitchens. For years now my readers have been begging me for more recipes. In response, I'm thrilled to finally offer you this: *The Eat-Clean Diet Cookbook 2.*

Food has always been important to me. Before my transformation at the age of 40, I was a typical Martha Stewart mom. The food I offered my family was made with love (and, looking back, too much fat!). My love for sharing food has not changed. Great food is one of life's pleasures, and there is no reason to stop enjoying food – or eat food that tastes bad – just because you've chosen a healthier way of life. In fact,

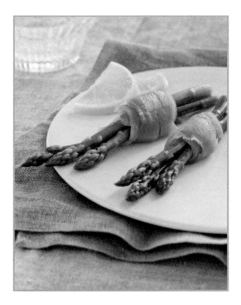

fresh, in-season Clean food in its most natural state is the best-tasting food you can eat. I enjoy experimenting with aromatic spices, subtle herbs and magical combinations of flavors. I learn which foods offer the most nutrition, the highest levels of antioxidants and the most immune-boosting strength, and then I create delicious meals from them.

The Eat-Clean Diet Cookbook 2 contains all-new recipes to suit all tastes and lifestyles. Try the Smoked Salmon Asparagus Bundles for brunch or the Quinoa and Black Bean Lunch Bowl for a refreshing lunch outside the sandwich. Try the Peach and Heirloom Tomato Salad the next time you have guests for dinner or the BBQ Pork Ribs while watching the game.

Nothing is better than seeing my friends and family eat a satisfying meal that I know will keep them healthy, strong and lean. I know I am not just feeding their stomachs, but I'm also providing them with the very best foundation for a healthy, active, long life. When I see them dig in, with smiles on their faces and enjoyment on their tongues, I look around and say: "Life is good."

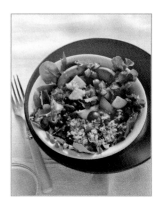

Sincerely,

Tosca Reno

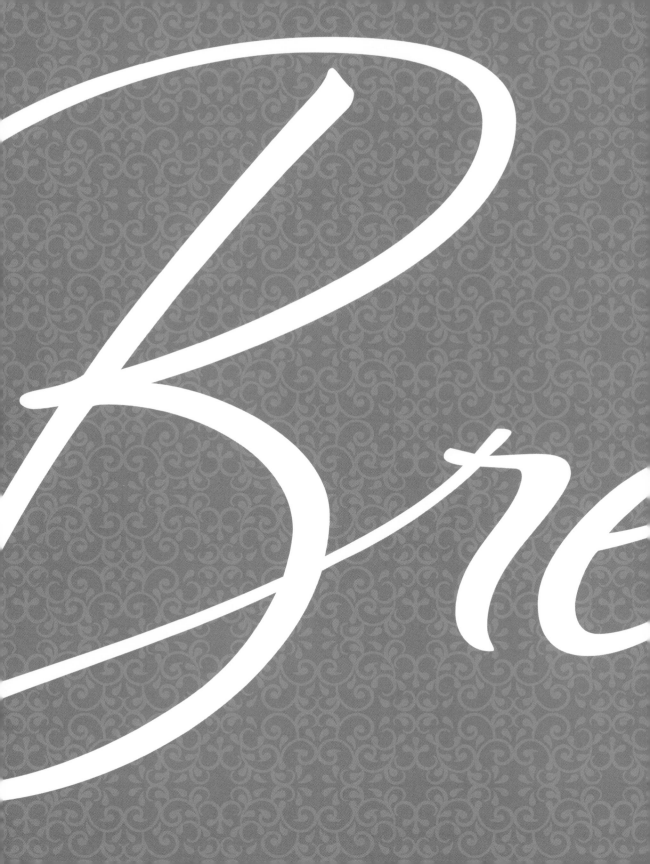

1

Breakfast

12 JUMP START GRANOLA

15 HUEVOS RANCHEROS

16 BAKED EGGS
with Tomatoes, Turkey Bacon, Chives and Toasted Breadcrumbs

19 AÇAI BLUEBERRY BREAKFAST SHAKE

20 PAPAYA WITH A KICK

23 HEARTY BLUEBERRY CORN CAKE

24 ORZO FRITTATA
with Mushrooms, Peppers and Yellow Squash

27 SUPER POWER SMOOTHIE

28 SAVORY VEGETABLE WAFFLES

31 CHERRY PROTEIN POP 'EMS

32 CHILI AND SCRAMBLED EGG BREAKFAST TACOS

35 OAT PORRIDGE
with Holiday Spices

36 STRAWBERRY PEACH KEFIR SMOOTHIE
with Chia Seeds

Servings: 12 x ½ cup
Prep time: 10 minutes
Cooking time:
75-90 minutes

JUMP START GRANOLA

Granola is usually thought of as a "health" food, but typical granola is high in fat, salt, sugar and calories. My version contains unsweetened coconut and dried fruits (they are still sweet, trust me!), natural honey and just a hint of sugar to imitate that sweet, crunchy taste we all know and love.

INGREDIENTS

3 cups / 720 ml old-fashioned rolled oats
1 cup / 240 ml roughly chopped unsalted almonds
¼ cup / 60 ml roughly chopped unsalted cashews
¼ cup / 60 ml raw pumpkin seeds (pepitas)
¼ cup / 60 ml raw sunflower seed kernels
2 Tbsp / 30 ml flaxseed
¼ cup / 60 ml unsweetened coconut flakes
1 heaping Tbsp / 15 ml natural brown sugar
¼ cup / 60 ml honey
¼ cup / 60 ml raw coconut butter or oil, melted
1 tsp / 5 ml real vanilla
¼ tsp / 1.25 ml sea salt
1 cup / 240 ml of your favorite unsweetened dried fruit, such as
    raisins, currants, cranberries, cherries or blueberries

METHOD

1. Preheat oven to 250°F / 120°C. In a large bowl, mix together oats, nuts and seeds, coconut and brown sugar.

2. In a small bowl, combine honey, coconut butter, vanilla and salt. Combine the two mixtures and spread out onto two baking sheets.

3. Bake in the oven 75 to 90 minutes, stirring two or three times so granola browns evenly. Remove from oven and mix in dried fruit. Let cool to room temperature before storing in an airtight container.

NUTRITIONAL VALUE
PER SERVING:
Calories: 324 |
Calories from Fat: 111 |
Protein: 10 g | Carbs: 45 g |
Total Fat: 13 g |
Saturated Fat: 4 g |
Trans Fat: 0 g | Fiber: 7 g |
Sodium: 49 mg |
Cholesterol: 0 mg

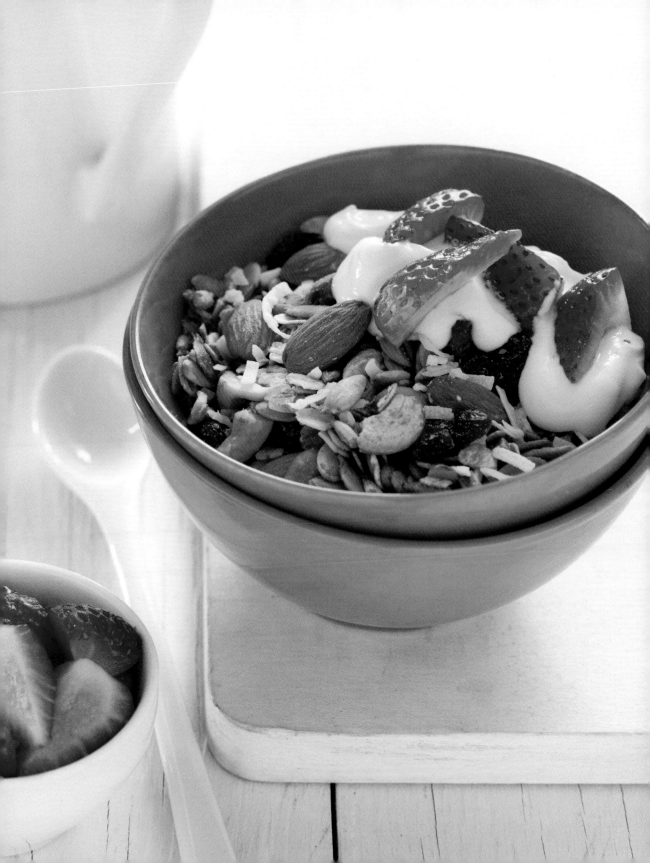

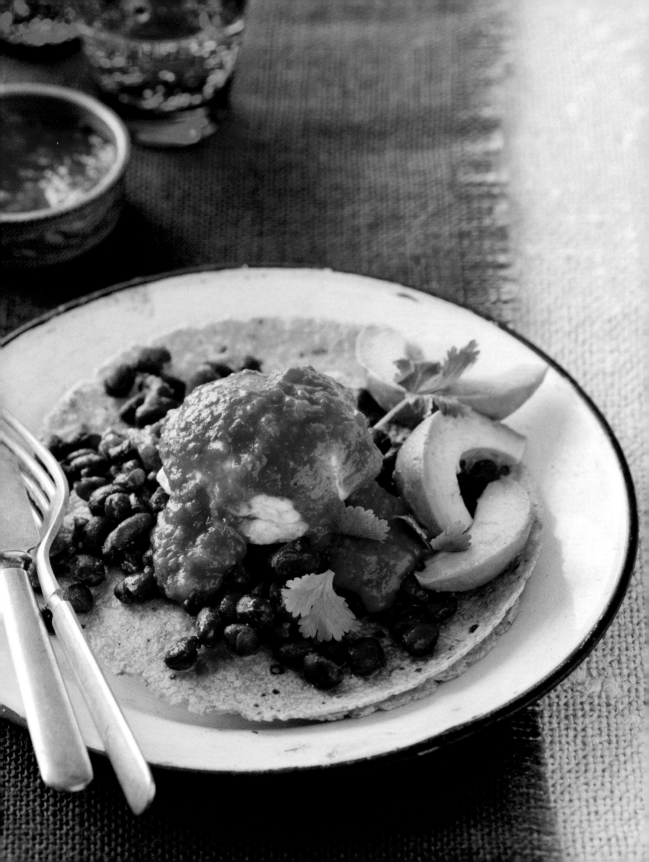

HUEVOS RANCHEROS

Huevos rancheros, which means "ranch eggs" in Spanish, is a classic Mexican breakfast consisting of fried eggs on fried corn tortillas topped with a tomato-chili sauce. That's a lot of frying! I've made my version healthier by poaching the eggs. Less fat, but all the flavor.

INGREDIENTS

1 tsp / 5 ml extra virgin olive oil
2 cups / 480 ml cooked black beans
2 cloves garlic, finely chopped
½ tsp / 2.5 ml ground cumin
½ tsp / 2.5 ml chili powder
½ tsp / 2.5 ml sea salt
¼ tsp / 1.25 ml freshly ground black pepper
Eat-Clean Cooking Spray (see page 348)
8 egg whites
8 sprouted whole grain corn tortillas, 5 to 6 inches in diameter
1 cup / 240 ml Chipotle Ranchero Sauce (see recipe on page 350)
1 avocado, pitted and sliced into 12 slices
Cilantro, to garnish

METHOD

1. Heat olive oil in a large skillet over medium-high heat. Add black beans, garlic, cumin, chili powder, salt and pepper, and cook until heated through, about 3 minutes. Remove from heat and cover to keep warm.

2. Fill an egg-poaching pan with a few inches of water and place the egg poacher on pan, making sure that egg-poaching cups don't touch surface of water. Bring water to a vigorous simmer and spray each cup with Eat-Clean Cooking Spray. Pour two egg whites into each cup, cover, and poach until whites are set and cooked through, about 7 minutes. Remove egg poacher from pan of boiling water and set aside.

3. Place two tortillas, slightly overlapping, on a large plate. Spread ½ cup / 120 ml of black bean mixture over tortillas. Use a sharp knife to loosen edge of egg whites from one poaching cup, invert over beans and unmold. Or, if cups are attached to egg poacher, use a rubber spatula to scoop egg whites out and invert on black bean mixture. Spoon ¼ cup / 60 ml Chipotle Ranchero Sauce (see recipe on page 350) over egg whites, place three slices of avocado next to eggs and garnish with cilantro, if desired. Repeat with remaining tortillas, black beans, egg whites, sauce, avocado and cilantro.

NUTRITIONAL VALUE
PER SERVING
(2 TORTILLAS, ½ CUP /
120 ML BLACK BEAN
MIXTURE, 2 EGG WHITES,
3 SLICES AVOCADO AND
CILANTRO):

Calories: 549 |
Calories from Fat: 145 |
Protein: 28 g | Carbs: 72 g |
Total Fat: 17 g |
Saturated Fat: 1.7 g |
Trans Fat: 0 g | Fiber: 19 g |
Sodium: 632 mg |
Cholesterol: 0 mg

Servings: 2
Prep time: 10 minutes
Cooking time:
22 minutes

BAKED EGGS
with Tomatoes, Turkey Bacon, Chives
and Toasted Breadcrumbs

An often-overlooked way to make your morning eggs is to bake them! This dish is a protein powerhouse, guaranteed to get you out the door with your best foot forward. If you don't have time to make this breakfast before work, try it for dinner!

INGREDIENTS

¼ tsp / 1.25 ml extra virgin olive oil
2 Tbsp / 30 ml whole wheat breadcrumbs
Pinch sea salt
Eat-Clean Cooking Spray (see page 348)
2 pieces cooked natural, nitrite-free, low-fat turkey bacon (about 2 oz), cut into ¼-inch pieces
½ medium tomato, diced
4 tsp / 20 ml chopped chives, divided
8 egg whites
⅛ tsp / 0.625 ml freshly ground black pepper

METHOD

1. Preheat the oven to 350°F / 175°C. Heat oil in a small skillet over medium-high heat. Add breadcrumbs and sea salt. Toast, stirring occasionally, until golden brown, about 2 minutes. Remove and set aside.

2. Place two ramekins on a baking sheet and coat each with Eat-Clean Cooking Spray. Divide bacon, tomato, and half of chives among the ramekins. Pour four egg whites into each ramekin and season with freshly ground black pepper. Sprinkle top of egg whites with half of toasted breadcrumbs. Place baking sheet with ramekins into oven and bake until whites have puffed up and are set, about 20 minutes. Remove, and top with remaining toasted breadcrumbs and chives. Serve immediately.

NUTRITIONAL VALUE
PER SERVING:
Calories: 148 |
Calories from Fat: 47 |
Protein: 20 g | Carbs: 7 g |
Total Fat: 5 g |
Saturated Fat: 1 g |
Trans Fat: 0 g | Fiber: 1 g |
Sodium: 482 mg |
Cholesterol: 10 mg

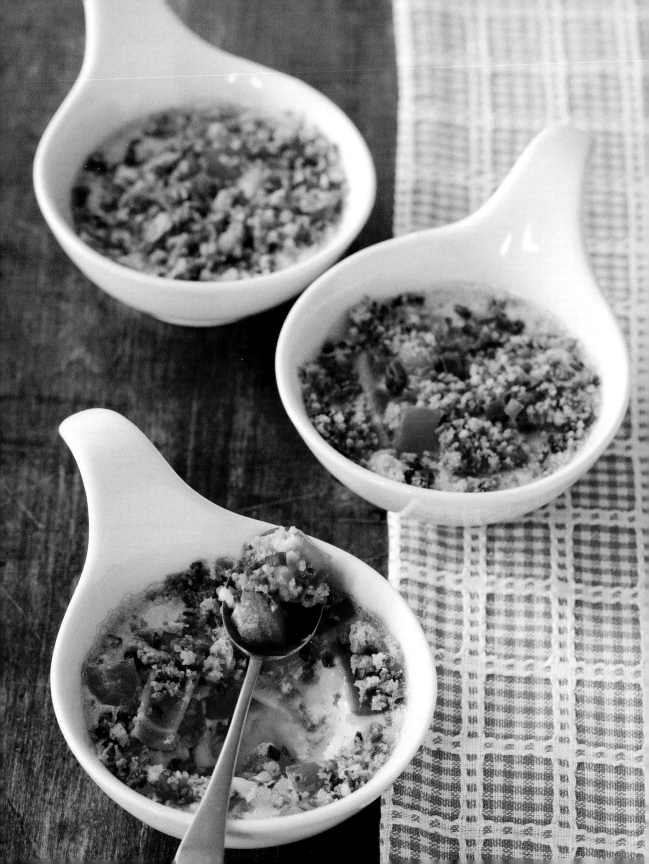

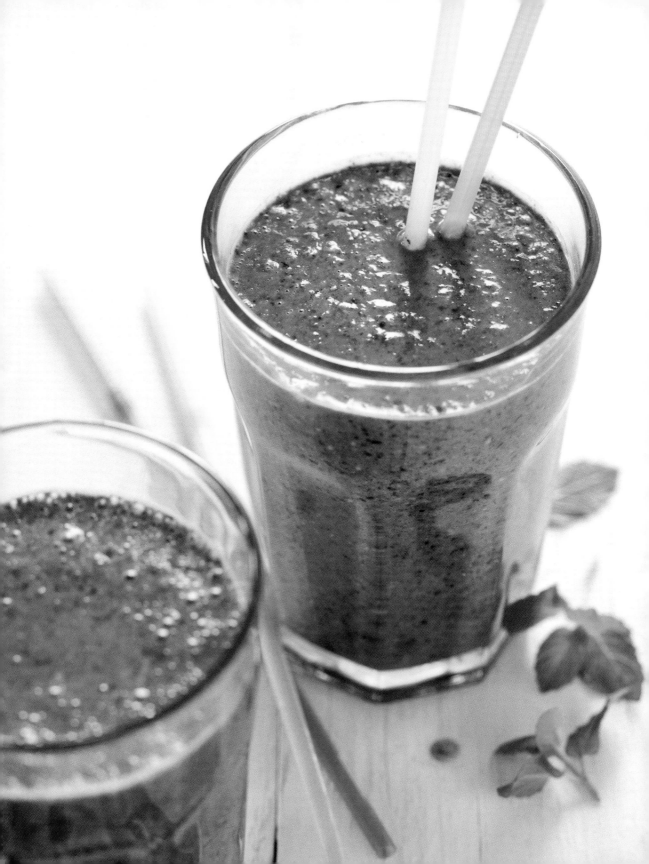

Servings: 2 x 1 cup
Prep time: 5 minutes
Cooking time:
0 minutes

AÇAI BLUEBERRY BREAKFAST SHAKE

A breakfast shake is the perfect start for those who don't have a lot of time in the morning. This one contains oats for staying power, nut butter for brain function and açai berry juice, which is rich in vitamins, minerals and antioxidants. Drink up!

INGREDIENTS

¾ cup / 180 ml plain low-fat kefir or plain low-fat yogurt
½ cup / 120 ml frozen blueberries
½ cup / 120 ml sugar-free açai berry juice
¼ cup / 60 ml plain or vanilla natural protein powder
¼ cup / 60 ml old-fashioned oats
1 Tbsp / 15 ml wheat germ
1 Tbsp / 15 ml chia seeds
1 Tbsp / 15 ml hazelnut butter, or other natural nut butter
1 tsp / 5 ml bee pollen (optional)
¼ cup / 60 ml ice cubes

METHOD

1. Add all ingredients to a blender and blend. Divide mixture between two glasses and serve.

NUTRITIONAL VALUE
PER SERVING:
Calories: 346 |
Calories from Fat: 92 |
Protein: 24 g | Carbs: 38 g |
Total Fat: 11 g |
Saturated Fat: 2 g |
Trans Fat: 0 g | Fiber: 7 g |
Sodium: 244 mg |
Cholesterol: 6 mg

PAPAYA WITH A KICK

Servings: 2 x 2 cups
Prep time: 10 minutes
Cooking time:
0 minutes

No matter what, I always include fruit with my breakfast. Knowing that I'm giving my body healthy vitamins and minerals first thing in the morning always puts me in the right frame of mind to face the rest of the day. Try this papaya dish as a side to your protein – it's the perfect blend of sweet, sour and spicy.

INGREDIENTS

1 ripe papaya
Juice of 1 lime
1 tsp / 5 ml organic raw blue agave nectar
⅛ tsp / 0.625 ml cayenne pepper, or more to taste
Black sesame seeds, to garnish

METHOD

1. Using a sharp vegetable peeler, peel skin from papaya. Cut papaya in half lengthwise and scoop out seeds. Place papaya halves cut side down on a cutting board and cut crosswise into quarter-inch slices (as though you were making half moons).

2. In a small bowl, whisk together the lime juice, agave and cayenne. Divide papaya among two plates and spoon dressing over top. Garnish with black sesame seeds and serve. Can also be chilled before serving.

NUTRITIONAL VALUE
PER SERVING:

Calories: 98 |
Calories from Fat: 8 |
Protein: 1 g | Carbs: 24 g |
Total Fat: 1 g |
Saturated Fat: 0 g |
Trans Fat: 0 g | Fiber: 4 g |
Sodium: 6 mg |
Cholesterol: 0 mg

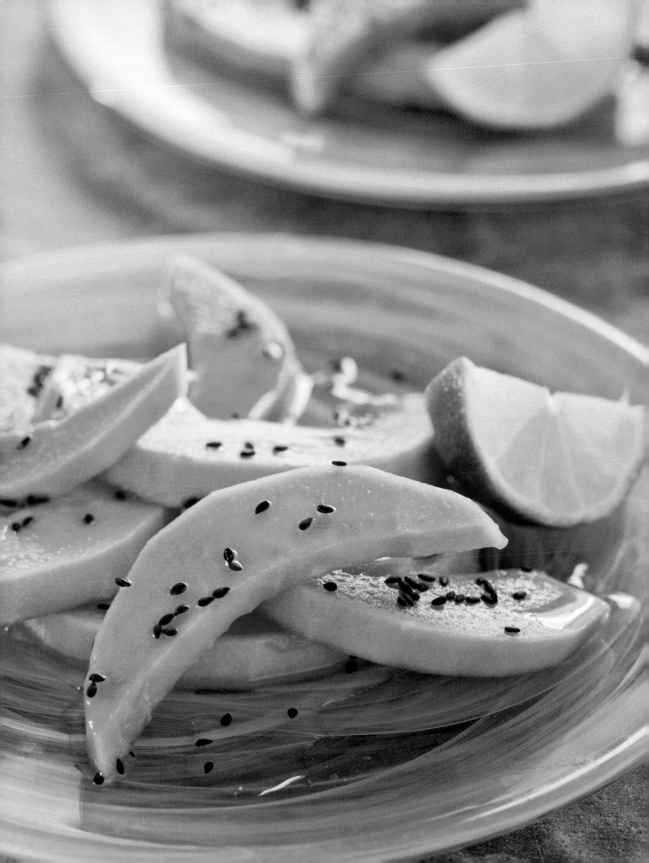

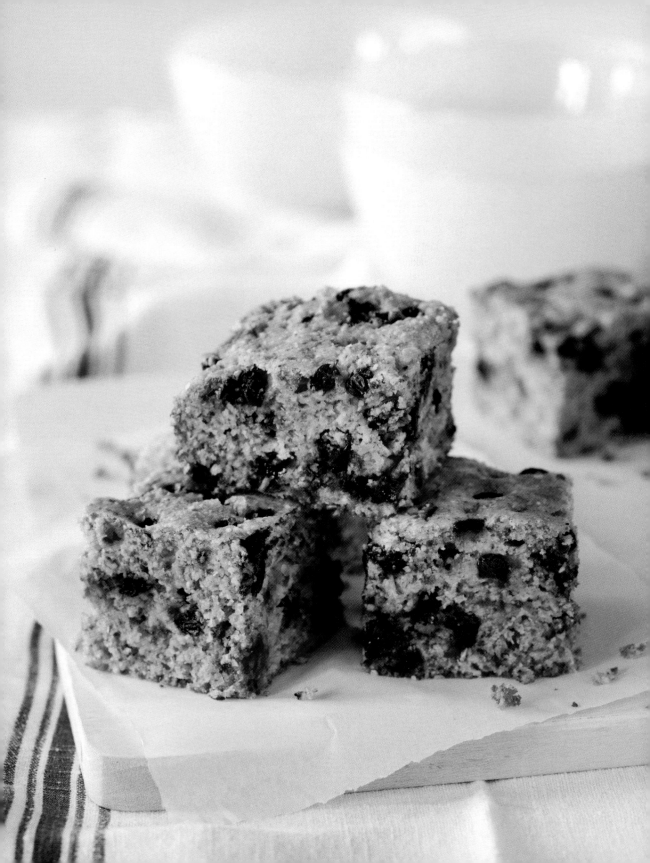

Servings: 16 squares
Prep time: 15 minutes
Cooking time:
20-25 minutes

HEARTY BLUEBERRY CORN CAKE

Cake for breakfast? Sign me up! It seems like a treat, but this cake is hearty, wholesome and filling – exactly what you need to power you through until your next meal. Eat this corn cake alongside several protein-packed egg whites to make it a complete Clean meal.

INGREDIENTS

Eat-Clean Cooking Spray (see page 348)
1 cup / 240 ml stone-ground 100% whole grain cornmeal, medium grind
1 cup / 240 ml whole wheat flour
¼ cup / 60 ml natural unflavored protein powder
2 Tbsp / 30 ml golden toasted flaxseed, cracked
2 tsp / 10 ml baking powder
½ tsp / 2.5 ml baking soda
½ tsp / 2.5 ml sea salt
⅛ tsp / 0.625 ml nutmeg
2 egg whites
1 cup / 240 ml low-fat buttermilk
½ cup / 120 ml finely grated apple
¼ cup / 60 ml honey
8 dates, minced
2 Tbsp / 30 ml virgin unrefined coconut oil, melted
1½ cups / 360 ml fresh or frozen blueberries

METHOD

1. Preheat oven to 425°F / 220°C. Spray a 9 x 9-inch square cake pan with Eat-Clean Cooking Spray.

2. In a large bowl, thoroughly whisk together cornmeal, flour, protein powder, flaxseed, baking powder, baking soda, salt and nutmeg. In a separate bowl, whisk together egg whites, buttermilk, apple, honey, dates and coconut oil until thoroughly mixed. Stir wet ingredients into dry until just combined. Fold in blueberries.

3. Pour mix into pan and spread evenly with a rubber spatula. Bake until a toothpick inserted in center comes out clean, 20 to 25 minutes. Cut into 16 squares. Can be left at room temperature (70°F / 21°C or cooler) for two days, and then refrigerate for up to two additional days.

NUTRITIONAL VALUE
PER 2 ¼ X 2 ¼-INCH
SQUARE:
Calories: 117 |
Calories from Fat: 28 |
Protein: 4 g | Carbs: 19 g |
Total Fat: 3 g |
Saturated Fat: 2 g |
Trans Fat: 0 g | Fiber: 3 g |
Sodium: 141 mg |
Cholesterol: 1 mg

Servings: 4
Prep time: 10 minutes
Cooking time:
10-12 minutes

ORZO FRITTATA
with Mushrooms, Peppers and Yellow Squash

Frittatas are one of my favorite weekend breakfasts. I love that you can throw anything but the kitchen sink in them and they'll still taste great, which is perfect for using up leftover veggies. Here I've added orzo pasta, which adds heft to the dish, making it a well-rounded Clean meal.

INGREDIENTS

2 eggs
5 egg whites
½ tsp / 2.5 ml sea salt
¼ tsp / 1.25 ml freshly ground black pepper
1 tsp / 5 ml extra virgin olive oil
½ cup / 120 ml thinly sliced white button mushrooms
½ cup / 120 ml diced orange or red peppers
½ cup / 120 ml summer squash, quartered lengthwise and thinly sliced
1 clove garlic, minced
1 cup / 240 ml cooked whole wheat orzo pasta
2 Tbsp / 30 ml chopped chives

METHOD

1. Position oven rack on second-from-top position and turn broiler to high. In a medium bowl, beat eggs and eggs whites with salt and pepper. Set aside.

2. Heat olive oil in a 10-inch nonstick ovenproof skillet over medium-high heat. Add mushrooms in a single layer and sauté until they start to brown, about 2 minutes. Add peppers, squash and garlic. Season with a pinch of sea salt and freshly ground pepper, and sauté until soft, about 2 minutes.

3. Reduce heat to medium low. Stir in cooked orzo pasta and chives until all ingredients are well mixed. Pour in beaten eggs, shaking and tilting pan to make sure eggs completely cover and are distributed through orzo and vegetables. Cook until eggs start to set and are lightly browned on bottom, 4 to 5 minutes. Transfer skillet to oven and broil until top is set and lightly browned, and eggs are cooked through, 2 to 3 minutes. Carefully remove the pan – handle will be hot!

4. Use a rubber spatula to loosen edges of frittata and help slide it out of skillet onto a plate. Cut into four wedges and serve.

NUTRITIONAL VALUE
PER SERVING:
Calories: 238 |
Calories from Fat: 52 |
Protein: 14 g | Carbs: 32 g |
Total Fat: 6 g |
Saturated Fat: 1 g |
Trans Fat: 0 g | Fiber: 8 g |
Sodium: 356 mg |
Cholesterol: 109 mg

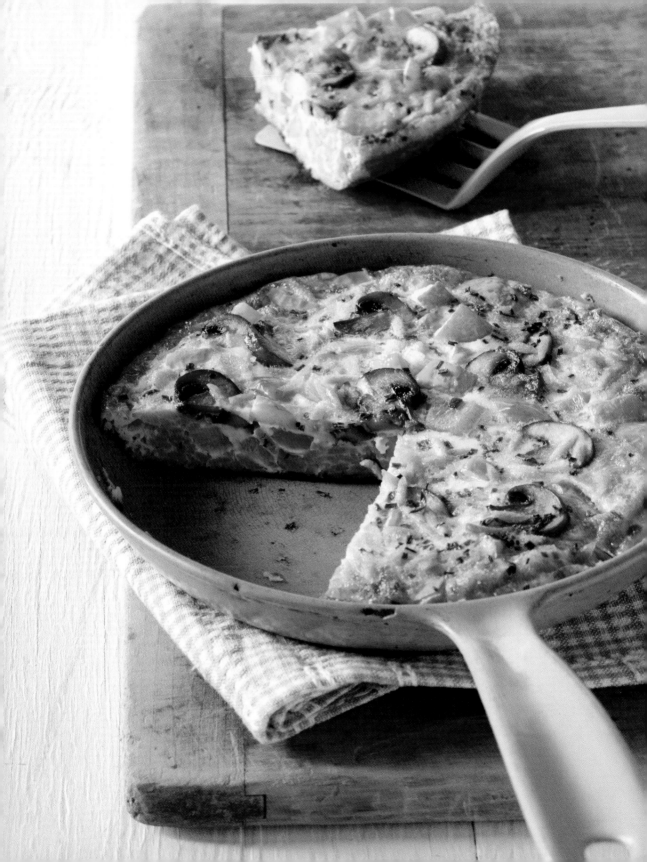

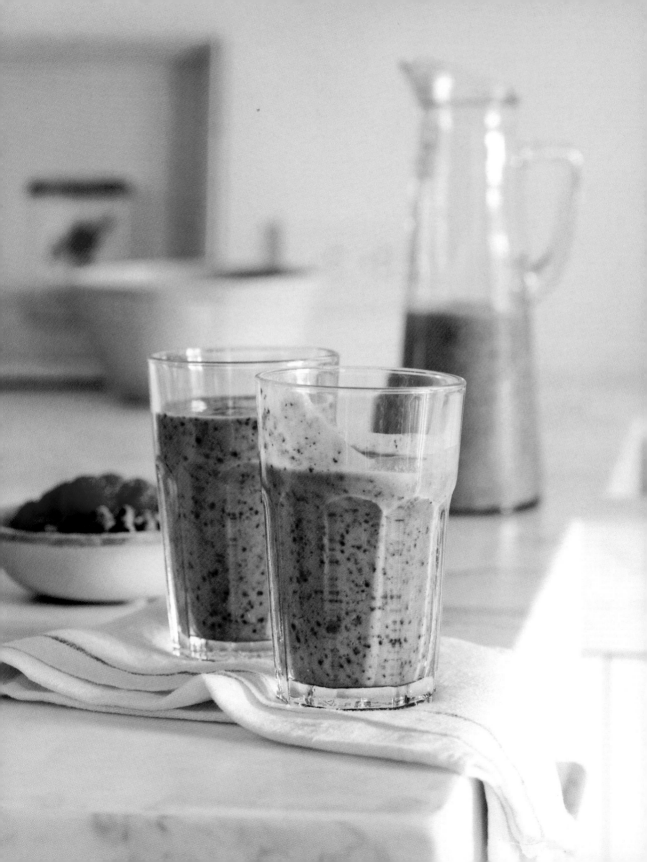

SUPER POWER SMOOTHIE

Servings: 3 x 1 cup
Prep time: 5 minutes
Cooking time:
0 minutes

This smoothie is called "Super Power" for a reason! It's packed with protein, brain-boosting carbs and healthy fats – everything you need for your best day yet! If your morning is rushed, try making it the night before – just keep it covered in the fridge. You'll have a super power breakfast waiting for you all ready to go!

INGREDIENTS

1 cup / 240 ml raspberries, fresh or frozen
1 cup / 240 ml blueberries, fresh or frozen
1 very ripe banana, fresh or frozen
1 cup / 240 ml plain low-fat yogurt
½ cup / 120 ml freshly squeezed orange juice, including pulp
¼ cup / 60 ml unsweetened natural protein powder
2 Tbsp / 30 ml oat bran
2 Tbsp / 30 ml flaxseed, cracked
1 Tbsp / 15 ml natural nut butter

METHOD

1. Add all ingredients to a blender and process on medium speed until smooth, scraping down the sides to ensure that all ingredients get incorporated. Pour into glasses and serve.

NUTRITIONAL VALUE
PER SERVING:

Calories: 278 |
Calories from Fat: 73 |
Protein: 17 g | Carbs: 39 g |
Total Fat: 8 g |
Saturated Fat: 1 g |
Trans Fat: 0 g | Fiber: 8 g |
Sodium: 155 mg |
Cholesterol: 5 mg

Servings:
4 x 2½ waffles
Prep time: 20 minutes
Cooking time:
30-40 minutes

SAVORY VEGETABLE WAFFLES

These waffles are delicious eaten as is – no toppings necessary! You can also use these waffles instead of bread to make an open-faced sandwich with your favorite toppings such as hummus, natural turkey lunch meat, greens, avocado, tomato, sprouts and more!

INGREDIENTS

1 cup / 240 ml plain, low-fat kefir

1 cup / 240 ml low-fat milk

½ cup / 120 ml old-fashioned rolled oats

1 Tbsp / 15 ml chia seeds

½ cup / 120 ml whole oat flour

½ cup / 120 ml whole wheat flour

½ cup / 120 ml whole grain corn flour

¼ cup / 60 ml whole grain cornmeal

2 tsp / 10 ml baking powder

½ tsp / 2.5 ml baking soda

½ tsp / 2.5 ml sea salt

1 egg

2 egg whites

3 Tbsp / 45 ml organic raw
turbinado sugar

1 cup / 240 ml grated zucchini
(about 1 baby zucchini)

½ cup / 120 ml grated carrot
(about 1 medium carrot)

½ cup / 120 ml marinated artichoke
hearts, drained and finely chopped

¼ cup / 60 ml julienne-cut sun-dried
tomatoes in extra virgin olive oil
with Italian herbs (do not drain)

2 Tbsp / 30 ml chopped chives

Eat-Clean Cooking Spray (see page 348)

METHOD

1. Preheat a waffle iron, placing it on a baking sheet to catch any batter that spills out. In a medium bowl, mix together kefir, milk, oats and chia seeds. In a large bowl, mix together oat, wheat and corn flours, cornmeal, baking powder, baking soda and salt. Mix egg, egg whites and turbinado sugar into kefir mixture, and then add all vegetables. Pour vegetable mixture into dry ingredients and mix until just combined. The batter will be lumpy. Do not over mix.

2. Spray the inside of waffle iron with Eat-Clean Cooking Spray, if necessary, and spread ½ cup / 120 ml to ⅔ cup / 160 ml batter over surface, stopping about half an inch from edge. Close and cook until golden brown and crispy, about 3 to 4 minutes. Use a fork or knife to lift waffle out of iron and transfer to a baking sheet. Repeat with remaining batter.

NUTRITIONAL VALUE
PER SERVING
(2½ WAFFLES):
Calories: 445 |
Calories from Fat: 98 |
Protein: 19 g | Carbs: 70 g |
Total Fat: 11 g |
Saturated Fat: 3 g |
Trans Fat: 0 g | Fiber: 11 g |
Sodium: 593 mg |
Cholesterol: 58 mg

TIP *Waffles can be kept warm in a 200°F / 95°C oven until ready to eat. Leftover waffles can be refrigerated for up to five days, or frozen for up to one month. Heat in a 350°F / 175°C oven, toaster oven or toaster. Microwaving not recommended.*

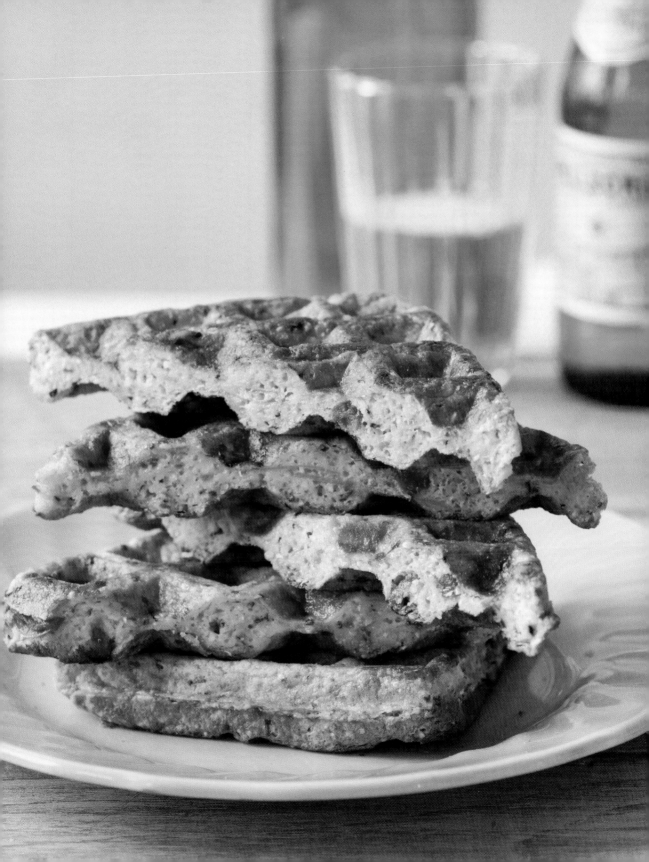

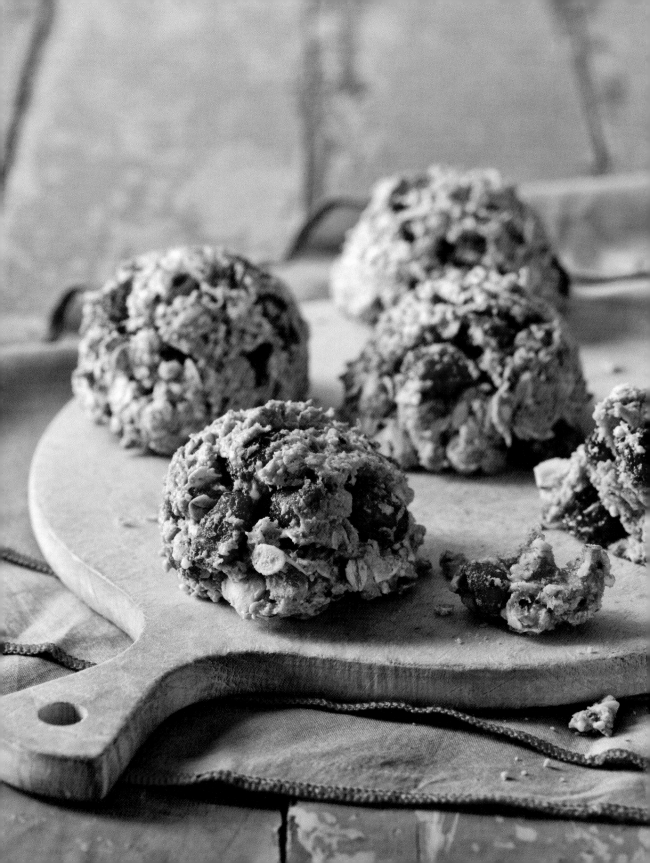

Servings: 15
Prep time: 10 minutes
Cooking time:
15-18 minutes

CHERRY PROTEIN POP 'EMS

Consider these delicious morsels an appetizer-style breakfast that will satisfy your sweet tooth – you'll never reach for a donut hole again! Pop a few into a plastic zipper bag and you've got a tasty meal-on-the-run that will fuel you all morning long.

INGREDIENTS

1 cup / 240 ml old-fashioned rolled oats
2 Tbsp / 30 ml wheat germ
1 Tbsp / 15 ml millet
1 Tbsp / 15 ml chia seeds
½ cup / 120 ml dried unsweetened bing cherries
¼ cup / 60 ml natural protein powder
¼ cup / 60 ml unsalted cashew pieces
¼ cup / 60 ml honey
¼ cup / 60 ml natural cashew butter
1 tsp / 5 ml real vanilla
1 egg white
Eat-Clean Cooking Spray (see page 348)

METHOD

1. Preheat the oven to 325°F / 160°C. In a large bowl, mix together oats, wheat germ, millet, chia seeds, cherries, protein powder and cashew pieces. In a separate small bowl, stir or whisk together honey, cashew butter, vanilla and egg white. Combine wet and dry ingredients and mix together well.

2. Using a spoon, scoop out golf-ball sized domes and place on a baking sheet misted with Eat-Clean Cooking Spray. Bake for 15 to 18 minutes until golden brown and crunchy. Remove and let cool before storing in an airtight container. Eat within one week, or freeze for up to three months.

NUTRITIONAL VALUE
PER SERVING:
Calories: 103 |
Calories from Fat: 27 |
Protein: 5 g | Carbs: 14 g |
Total Fat: 3 g |
Saturated Fat: 1 g |
Trans Fat: 0 g | Fiber: 2 g |
Sodium: 25 mg |
Cholesterol: 0 mg

Servings: 2 x 2 tacos
Prep time: 10 minutes
Cooking time:
2 minutes

CHILI AND SCRAMBLED EGG BREAKFAST TACOS

Did you know that the main difference between a taco and a burrito is the size of the wrapper? (Burritos use bigger shells.) A hit with kids and adults alike, breakfast tacos are typically made with eggs, vegetables and meat. Adding Clean chili really makes these tacos sizzle!

INGREDIENTS

1 egg
5 egg whites
⅛ tsp / 0.625 ml sea salt
Pinch freshly ground black pepper
4 whole grain sprouted corn or wheat tortillas, 5 to 6 inches in diameter
1 cup / 240 ml Clean chili, heated
¼ cup / 60 ml plain low-fat yogurt
4 heaping tsp / 20 ml finely chopped red onion
Eat-Clean Cooking Spray (see page 348)
Mexican hot sauce, to garnish

METHOD

1. Heat a large nonstick skillet over medium heat and coat with Eat-Clean Cooking Spray, if necessary. Add egg, egg whites, salt and pepper, and mix using a rubber spatula. Cook until whites are set, about 2 minutes.

2. Place tortillas on plates and divide eggs evenly among them. Top each egg mound with ¼ cup / 60 ml chili, 1 Tbsp / 15 ml yogurt, and 1 heaping tsp / 5 ml red onion. Sprinkle with hot sauce, if desired, and serve.

NUTRITIONAL VALUE
PER SERVING:
Calories: 516 |
Calories from Fat: 132 |
Protein: 33 g | Carbs: 61 g |
Total Fat: 16 g |
Saturated Fat: 3 g |
Trans Fat: 0 g | Fiber: 13 g |
Sodium: 711 mg |
Cholesterol: 123 mg

NOTE *For a great Clean chili recipe, see the Friday Night Chili on page 290 of The Eat-Clean Diet for Family & Kids.*

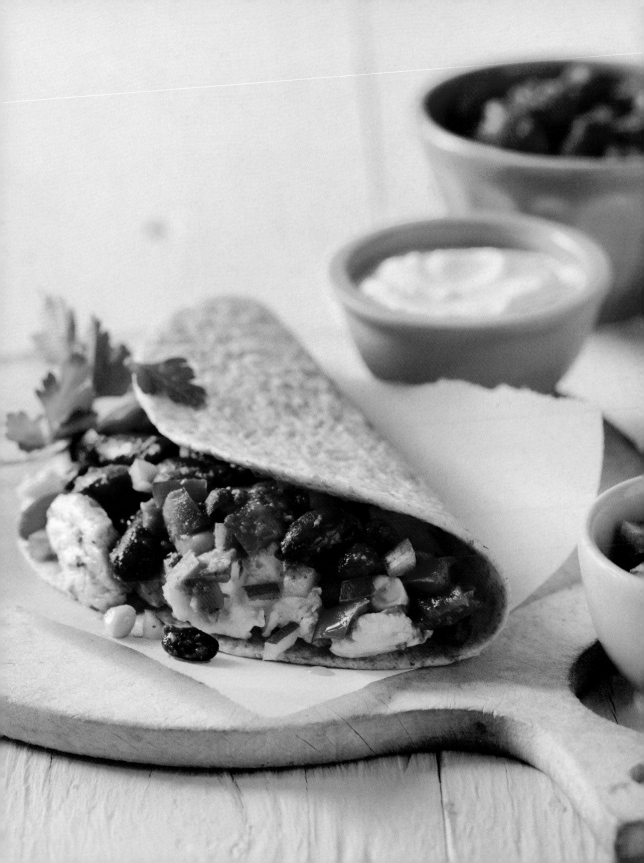

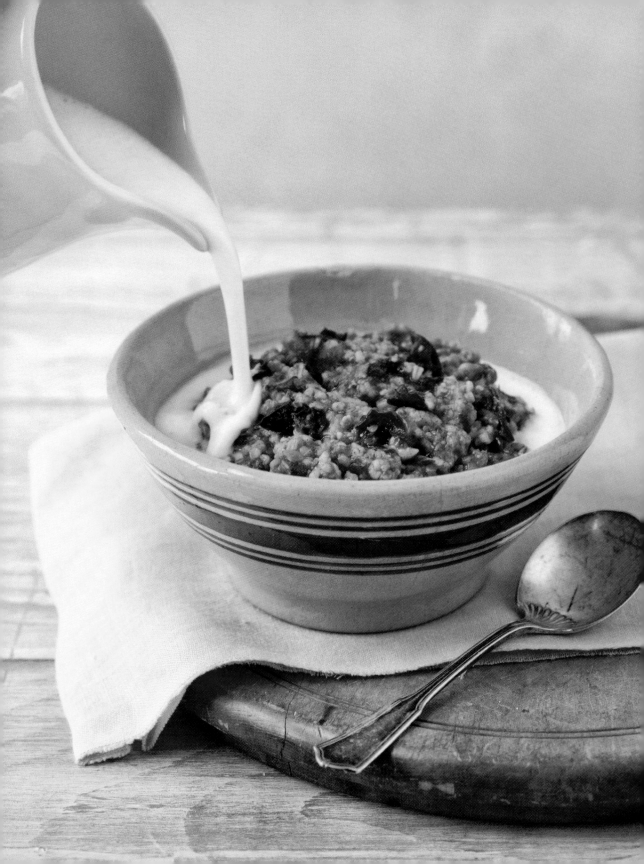

Servings: 4 x 1 cup
Prep time: 5 minutes
Cooking time:
13-15 minutes

OAT PORRIDGE
with Holiday Spices

It's no secret that I love oats. I also love the holiday season! There is something about cuddling up indoors with loved ones that makes me feel so cozy inside. I make this dish throughout the year and it always reminds me of those special celebrations.

INGREDIENTS

1 cup / 240 ml steel-cut oats
2 Tbsp / 30 ml oat bran
2 Tbsp / 30 ml chia seeds
1 Tbsp / 15 ml cracked flaxseed
8 dates, roughly chopped
8 dried plums (prunes), roughly chopped
¼ tsp / 1.25 ml ground cinnamon
⅛ tsp / 0.625 ml ground cloves
⅛ tsp / 0.625 ml ground ginger
Pinch sea salt

METHOD

1. Place all ingredients in a medium saucepan with 3 cups of water. Bring to a boil, then reduce heat to simmer gently, stirring occasionally. Cook 10 minutes for a chewier texture and 12 minutes for softer texture. Remove from heat, cover, and let sit for 3 minutes. Serve hot with low-fat kefir, low-fat milk or milk replacement, such as soy, rice or almond milk.

NUTRITIONAL VALUE
PER SERVING (1 CUP):
Calories: 286 |
Calories from Fat: 52 |
Protein: 6 g | Carbs: 53 g |
Total Fat: 6 g |
Saturated Fat: 1 g |
Trans Fat: 0 g | Fiber: 11 g |
Sodium: 61 mg |
Cholesterol: 0 mg

Servings: 3 x 1 cup
Prep time: 5 minutes
Cooking time:
0 minutes

STRAWBERRY PEACH KEFIR SMOOTHIE
with Chia Seeds

Chia seeds are one of nature's little wonders. They are an excellent source of fiber, protein and essential fatty acids. They also gel up when you add them to liquid, which makes them an excellent thickening agent for smoothies and puddings.

INGREDIENTS

1 peach, pitted and sliced, or 1 cup / 240 ml frozen peach slices
1 cup / 240 ml strawberries, fresh or frozen
1 cup / 240 ml plain low-fat kefir
2 Tbsp / 30 ml unsweetened natural protein powder
1 Tbsp / 15 ml chia seeds
1 Tbsp / 15 ml organic raw blue agave nectar
½ tsp / 2.5 ml real vanilla

METHOD

1. Add all ingredients to blender and blend until smooth. Pour into glasses and enjoy.

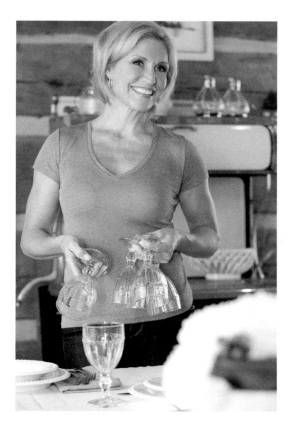

NUTRITIONAL VALUE
PER SERVING:
Calories: 148 |
Calories from Fat: 23 |
Protein: 12 g | Carbs: 21 g |
Total Fat: 3 g |
Saturated Fat: 1 g |
Trans Fat: 0 g | Fiber: 5 g |
Sodium: 105 mg |
Cholesterol: 3 mg

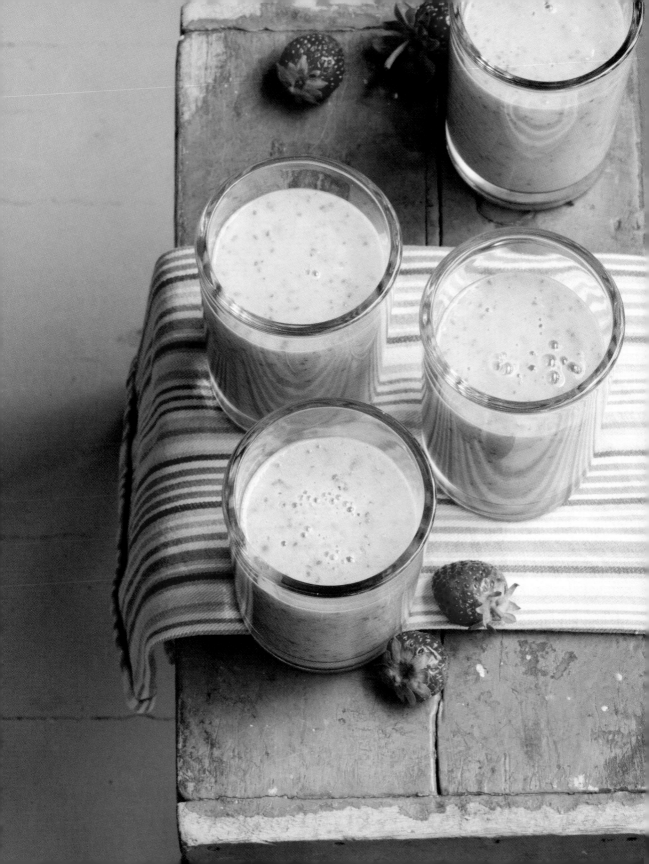

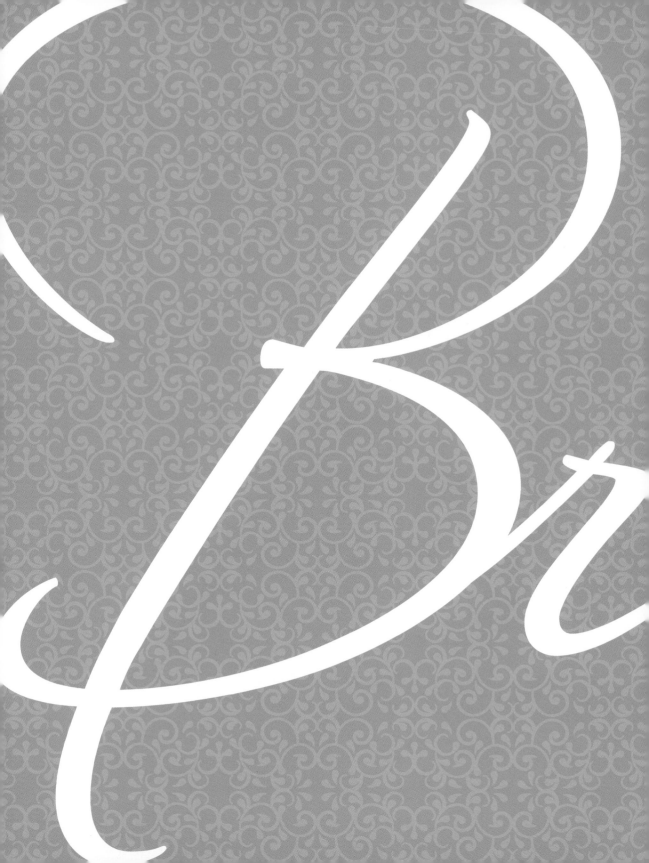

2

Brunch

40 CITRUS SALAD *with Mint*

43 MULTIGRAIN WAFFLES *with Raspberry Sauce*

44 EGGS SARDOU *with Warm Orange Vinaigrette*

47 WHITE PEACH AND BLACK CHERRY BELLISSIMO

48 SUMMER VEGETABLE PLATTER
with Baby Heirloom Tomatoes and Scallion Pistou

51 SUPER MOIST BANANA WALNUT BREAD

52 SMOKED SALMON ASPARAGUS BUNDLES

57 CHEDDAR JALAPEÑO CORN MUFFINS

58 TURKEY APPLE BREAKFAST SAUSAGE

61 OATMEAL "SCUFFINS"
with Currants and Dates

62 ROASTED PORK TENDERLOIN
with Sweet Sage Glaze

65 PRAWN AND HERBED YOGURT CHEESE CANAPÉS

66 CRUSTLESS BROCCOLI QUICHE
with Caramelized Onions and Blue Cheese

69 MEXICAN MOCHA CALIENTE

70 SEAFOOD PLATTER
of Crab, Prawns and Oysters on the Half Shell with Clean Cocktail Sauce and Cucumber Mignonette

73 POTATOES O'BRIEN

74 *Cheese Please*

Servings: 4 x 2 cups
Prep time: 20 minutes
Cooking time:
0 minutes

CITRUS SALAD
with Mint

Any dish that includes pineapple makes me think of vacation – lying on the beach, soaking up the sun... ah... I wish I were there right now! This fruit salad is sweet and juicy, and brings me back to the tropics any time of year.

INGREDIENTS

2 grapefruit, peeled and segmented, cut into 1-inch pieces
2 oranges, peeled and segmented, cut into 1-inch pieces
½ fresh pineapple, peeled and cored, cut into 1-inch pieces
4 cups / 960 ml watermelon, rind removed and cut into 1-inch cubes
1 Tbsp / 15 ml fresh key lime or lime juice
1 Tbsp / 15 ml finely chopped fresh mint

METHOD

1. Combine all ingredients in a large bowl and gently toss to combine. Can be served immediately, or chilled for a few hours and then served.

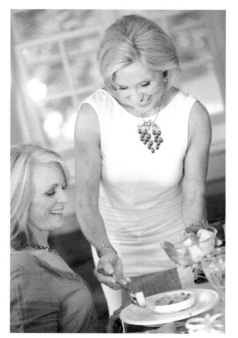

NUTRITIONAL VALUE
PER SERVING:
Calories: 184 |
Calories from Fat: 5 |
Protein: 4 g | Carbs: 47 g |
Total Fat: 0.1 g |
Saturated Fat: 0 g |
Trans Fat: 0 g | Fiber: 6 g |
Sodium: 4 mg |
Cholesterol: 0 mg

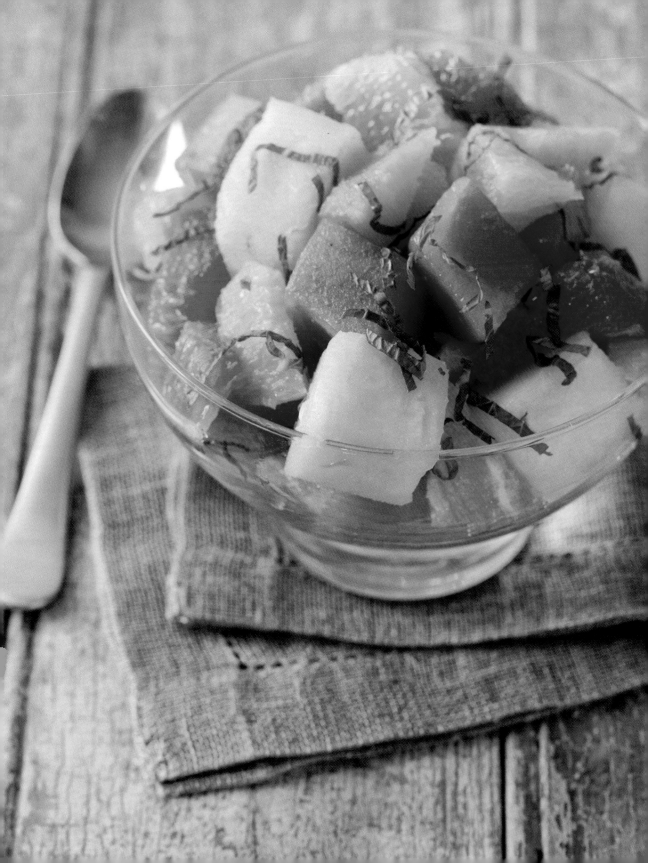

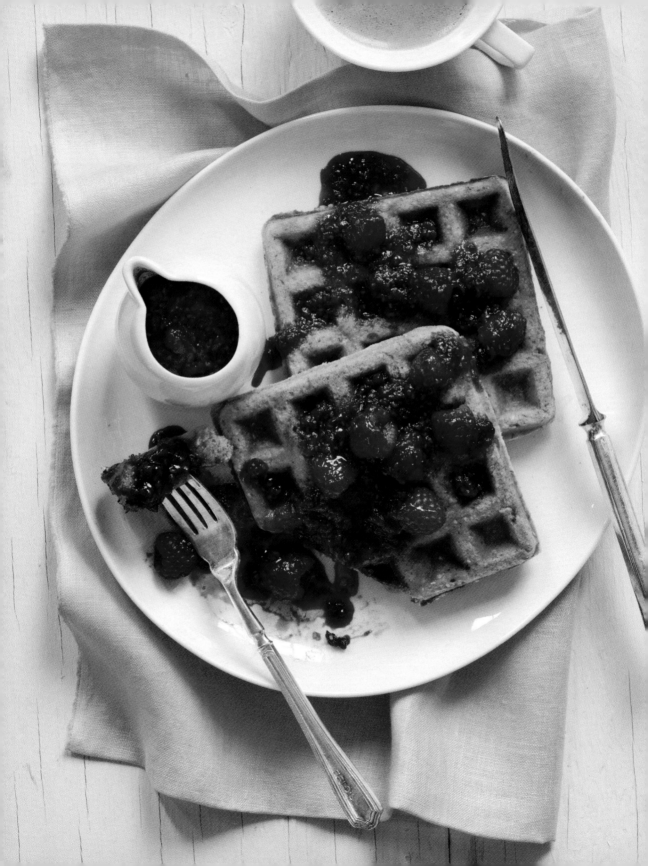

Servings:
4 x 2½ waffles
Prep time: 20 minutes
Cooking time:
12-14 minutes

MULTIGRAIN WAFFLES
with Raspberry Sauce

I love making waffles for family brunch when all my girls are home on the weekend. If you have trouble finding it in the supermarket, whole grain corn flour is usually called cornmeal. Don't confuse this product with cornstarch, which is known as "cornflour" across the pond in the UK.

INGREDIENTS

2 cups / 480 ml low-fat buttermilk
½ cup / 120 ml old-fashioned rolled oats
1 cup / 240 ml whole wheat flour
½ cup / 120 ml whole grain stone ground corn flour
¼ cup / 60 ml whole grain stone ground cornmeal
2 tsp / 10 ml baking powder
½ tsp / 2.5 ml baking soda
¼ tsp / 1.25 ml sea salt
1 egg
2 egg whites
¼ cup / 60 ml raw organic turbinado sugar
2 Tbsp / 30 ml safflower oil
1 tsp / 5 ml real vanilla
Eat-Clean Cooking Spray (see page 348)
Raspberry Sauce (see recipe on page 350)

METHOD

1. Preheat a waffle iron and place a baking sheet underneath to catch any batter drips. Mix buttermilk and oats in a medium bowl and set aside.

2. In a large bowl, whisk together wheat flour, corn flour, cornmeal, baking powder, baking soda and salt. Stir egg, egg whites, sugar, safflower oil and vanilla into reserved oat and buttermilk mixture, and pour into dry ingredients. Using a rubber spatula, mix until just moistened (the batter will be a little lumpy). Do not over mix.

3. Coat the waffle iron with Eat-Clean Cooking Spray. Spoon batter into center and spread out to almost completely cover the surface, stopping about a quarter inch from the edge (you will need about 2/3 cup / 160 ml batter for a 4 x 8-inch waffle iron). Cook until waffles are crisp and lightly browned, 3 to 4 minutes. Repeat with remaining batter. If waffles are not going to be eaten right away, place on a baking sheet in a single layer and keep warm in a 200°F / 90°C oven. Divide waffles among plates, and serve with warm Raspberry Sauce (see recipe on page 350).

NUTRITIONAL VALUE
PER SERVING
(2 ½ WAFFLES):
Calories: 426 |
Calories from Fat: 118 |
Protein: 15 g | Carbs: 65 g |
Total Fat: 14 g |
Saturated Fat: 2 g |
Trans Fat: 0 g | Fiber: 6 g |
Sodium: 452 mg |
Cholesterol: 58 mg

Servings:
4 eggs Sardou
Prep time:
15-20 minutes
Cooking time:
10-15 minutes

EGGS SARDOU
with Warm Orange Vinaigrette

Eggs Sardou is a Louisiana Creole cuisine dish consisting of poached eggs, artichokes, spinach and Hollandaise sauce. It is named after Victorien Sardou, a French dramatist from the 1800s, who was a guest in New Orleans when the dish was invented. I've cut the fat (substantially!) by subbing a Warm Orange Vinaigrette for the sauce.

INGREDIENTS
EGGS SARDOU

Eat-Clean Cooking Spray (see page 348)
8 egg whites
1 tsp / 5 ml extra virgin olive oil
8 oz / 226 g frozen artichoke
   hearts, thawed and drained
1 clove garlic, minced
3 cups / 720 ml baby spinach
¼ tsp / 1.25 ml sea salt
⅛ tsp / 0.625 ml freshly ground black pepper
2 whole wheat English muffins,
   split and toasted

WARM ORANGE VINAIGRETTE

1 tsp / 5 ml extra virgin olive oil
1 tsp / 5 ml minced shallot
¼ cup / 60 ml freshly squeezed orange juice
¼ cup / 60 ml low-sodium
   vegetable or chicken broth
2 Tbsp / 30 ml Champagne or
   white wine vinegar
1 tsp / 5 ml Dijon mustard
½ tsp / 2.5 ml fresh lemon juice
⅛ tsp / 0.625 ml sea salt
Pinch freshly ground black pepper
Pinch cayenne pepper

METHOD FOR EGGS SARDOU

1. Spray four cups of an egg poacher with Eat-Clean Cooking Spray and poach egg whites, two per cup, until opaque and cooked through, about 6 minutes.

2. In the meantime, heat olive oil in a large skillet over medium-high heat. Add artichoke hearts and sauté until heated through and golden brown, about 3 minutes. Fold in garlic and spinach, season with salt and pepper, and cook for 1 to 2 minutes until spinach is slightly wilted.

3. Divide English muffin halves among four plates and top each with a ¼ cup / 60 ml of artichoke and spinach mixture. Slide a knife around edge of poached egg whites to loosen them from cups and invert them on top of artichoke and spinach mixture. Spoon 1 Tbsp / 15 ml Warm Orange Vinaigrette over top of each Sardou and serve immediately.

METHOD FOR WARM ORANGE VINAIGRETTE

NUTRITIONAL VALUE
PER SERVING:
Calories: 154 |
Calories from Fat: 27 |
Protein: 14 g | Carbs: 21 g |
Total Fat: 3 g |
Saturated Fat: 0.4 g |
Trans Fat: 0 g | Fiber: 5 g |
Sodium: 531 mg |
Cholesterol: 0 mg

1. Heat olive oil in a small saucepan over medium-high heat. Add shallots and sauté until translucent, 1 minute. Add orange juice, broth and vinegar, and bring to a boil. Reduce heat and simmer until mixture reduces by half, about 3 minutes. Whisk in Dijon mustard and lemon juice, and season with salt, pepper and cayenne. Set aside, covered to keep warm.

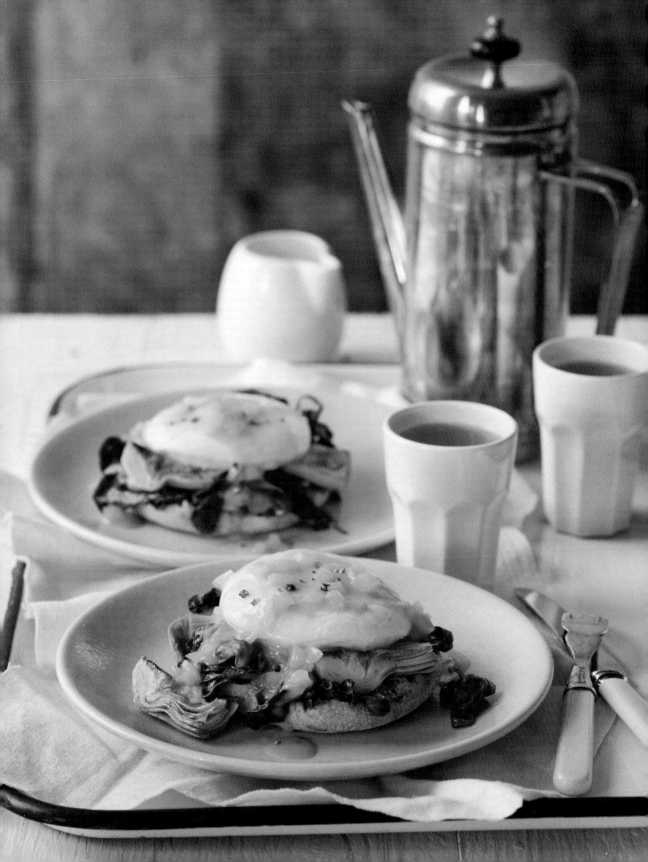

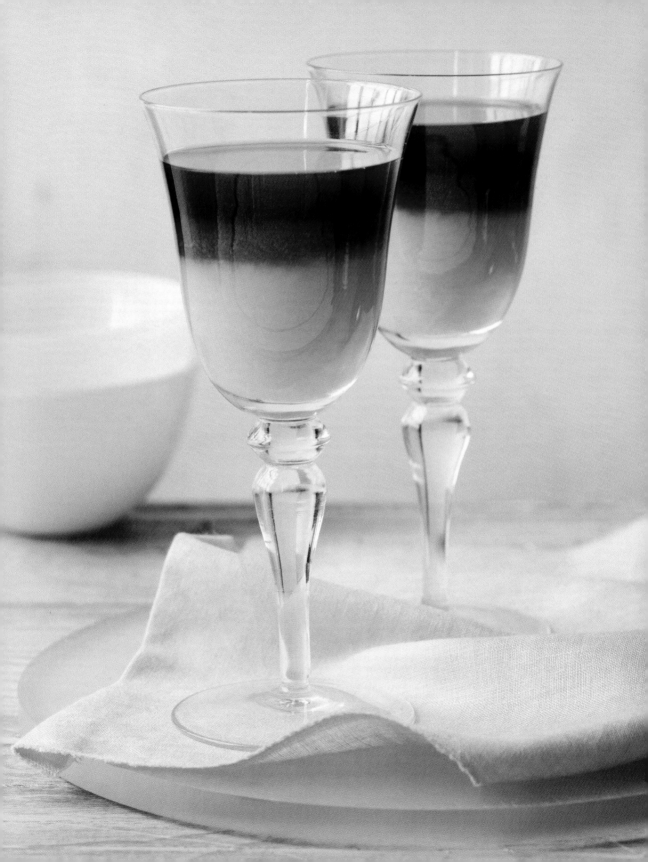

WHITE PEACH AND
BLACK CHERRY BELLISSIMO

Bellissimo is the Italian word for "lovely," and that's just what this colorful, fresh drink is. Kombucha, a fermented tea often used for medicinal purposes, can usually be found in the organic section of your grocery store or specialty health-food stores.

INGREDIENTS

2 ripe white peaches, peeled and pitted
1 cup / 240 ml natural unsweetened black cherry juice
1 cup / 240 ml organic unsweetened kombucha
1 cup / 240 ml sparkling mineral water

METHOD

1. In a blender, purée peaches until very smooth. In a small pitcher or four-cup measuring cup, combine cherry juice, kombucha and mineral water.

2. Set out four champagne flutes. Divide peach purée among flutes, about ¼ cup / 60 ml in each. Slowly pour ¾ cup / 180 ml of cherry juice mixture into each flute. Serve immediately without mixing two layers. Guests may choose to mix Bellissimo before drinking it.

NUTRITIONAL VALUE
PER SERVING:
Calories: 97 |
Calories from Fat: 2 |
Protein: 2 g | Carbs: 21 g |
Total Fat: 0 g |
Saturated Fat: 0 g |
Trans Fat: 0 g | Fiber: 7 g |
Sodium: 15 mg |
Cholesterol: 0 mg

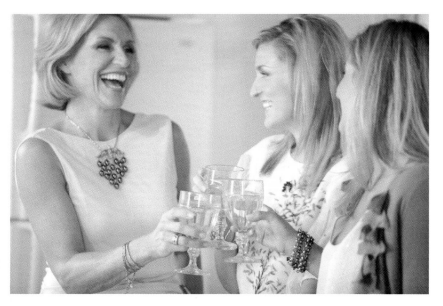

Servings: 6
Prep time: 10 minutes
Cooking time:
4-5 minutes

SUMMER VEGETABLE PLATTER
with Baby Heirloom Tomatoes and Scallion Pistou

There is nothing healthier, or more refreshing, than a platter of freshly grilled vegetables – they are a natural detox. You can serve this dish for brunch, or lunch, or dinner... you get the picture!

Note: Scallion Pistou must be made ahead of time.

INGREDIENTS

2 baby zucchini, sliced diagonally into ¼-inch pieces
2 yellow summer squash, sliced diagonally into ¼-inch pieces
1 cup / 240 ml baby heirloom cherry and pear tomatoes, stemmed
¼ cup / 60 ml Scallion Pistou (see recipe on page 352)
1 tsp / 5 ml sea salt
½ tsp / 2.5 ml freshly ground black pepper
Eat-Clean Cooking Spray (see page 348)

METHOD

1. Heat a grill or grill pan to medium-high heat.

2. Spread out zucchini and squash slices on a baking sheet and spray with Eat-Clean Cooking Spray. Season with half of salt and pepper, and place on grill in a single layer, seasoned side down. Spray dry topside of zucchini and squash slices with more Eat-Clean Cooking Spray, and season with remaining salt and pepper. Cook 4 to 5 minutes, turning once, until marked by grill and softened.

3. Remove and fan out on a large platter. Top with tomatoes and spoon Scallion Pistou over top. Can be served hot, at room temperature or chilled.

NUTRITIONAL VALUE
PER SERVING:
Calories: 30 |
Calories from Fat: 15 |
Protein: 1 g | Carbs: 3 g |
Total Fat: 2 g |
Saturated Fat: 0 g |
Trans Fat: 0 g | Fiber: 1 g |
Sodium: 315 mg |
Cholesterol: 0 mg

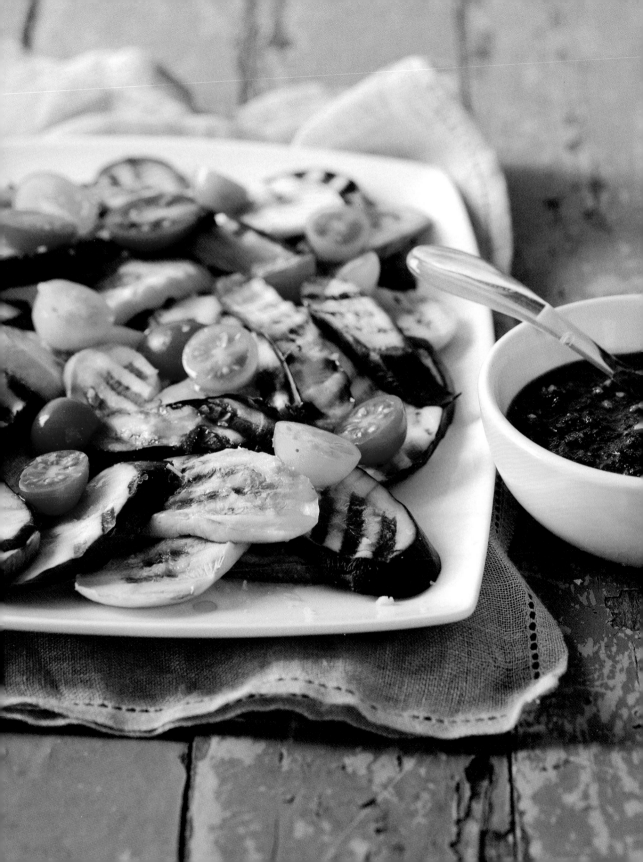

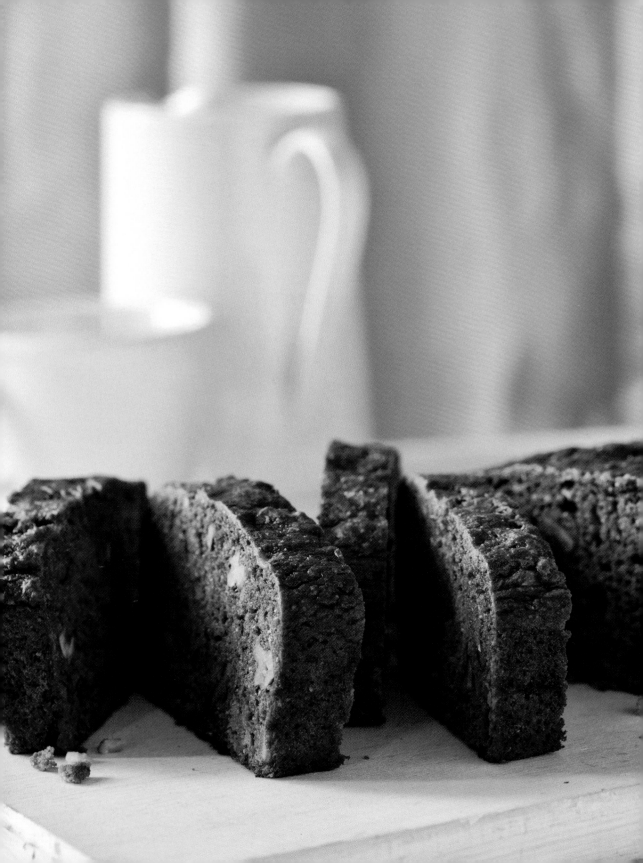

Servings: 9
Prep time: 15 minutes
Cooking time:
55-60 minutes

SUPER MOIST
BANANA WALNUT BREAD

Whenever I spot browning bananas on the kitchen counter I know there is banana bread in my future! Serve alongside fresh Yogurt Cheese (see recipe on page 348) with berries, or heat and spread with natural nut butter... heavenly!

INGREDIENTS

¼ cup / 60 ml + ½ tsp / 2.5 ml organic raw coconut butter, divided
1 ⅓ cup / 320 ml whole wheat pastry flour
2 Tbsp / 30 ml ground flaxseed
½ tsp / 2.5 ml sea salt
½ tsp / 2.5 ml baking soda
¼ tsp / 1.25 ml baking powder
¼ cup / 60 ml organic raw turbinado sugar
2 Tbsp / 30 ml unsulfured blackstrap molasses
½ cup / 120 ml low-fat milk or soymilk
3 large very ripe bananas, mashed
⅓ cup / 80 ml chopped unsalted walnuts

METHOD

1. Place oven rack in lower third of oven and preheat to 350°F / 175°C. Grease a 5 x 9-inch loaf pan with ½ tsp / 2.5 ml coconut butter.

2. In a medium bowl, whisk together flour, flaxseed, salt, baking soda and baking powder. In bowl of an electric mixer, combine remaining coconut butter with sugar and molasses on medium-high speed until thoroughly mixed. Add flour mixture and mix on medium speed until mixture resembles coarse grains of wet sand. Stop mixer and use a rubber spatula to scrape sides and bottom of the bowl, and then mix for a few more seconds to ensure that all ingredients get thoroughly combined. Add milk and mix on low speed until just combined. Remove bowl from mixing stand, and fold in bananas and walnuts until just combined.

3. Scrape batter into greased baking pan and place in oven to bake until a toothpick inserted into center comes out clean, 55 to 60 minutes. Remove and let cool slightly before unmolding from pan. Serve warm or let finish cooling on a rack. Can be stored for two days at room temperature with a tea towel draped over top, and then in refrigerator for an additional three days, if there is any left!

NUTRITIONAL VALUE
PER SERVING:
Calories: 222 |
Calories from Fat: 70 |
Protein: 4 g | Carbs: 35 g |
Total Fat: 8 g |
Saturated Fat: 4 g |
Trans Fat: 0 g | Fiber: 6 g |
Sodium: 187 mg |
Cholesterol: 0 mg

Servings: 8
Prep time: 10 minutes
Cooking time:
10 minutes

SMOKED SALMON ASPARAGUS BUNDLES

You'll love this simple recipe for its flavor and color! Smoked salmon lox is cold-smoked, which means that the fish remains uncooked. It's thinly sliced with a rich taste and silky texture. Don't confuse this with regular smoked salmon, which is smoked over wood, packaged and sealed to protect the moisture and flavor.

INGREDIENTS

1 bunch baby asparagus (about 24 asparagus)
½ tsp / 2.5 ml extra virgin olive oil
½ tsp / 2.5 ml finely chopped fresh tarragon
Pinch sea salt
Pinch freshly ground black pepper
3 oz all-natural wild smoked salmon lox
Lemon wedges, to garnish

METHOD

1. Preheat oven to 425°F / 220°C. Trim stalks of asparagus about one to two inches, to remove dry ends. Discard trimmings. Place asparagus on a baking sheet and toss with olive oil, tarragon, salt and pepper until asparagus is evenly coated. Spread out in a single layer and roast until lightly browned, about 10 minutes. Remove and let cool slightly.

2. Separate smoked salmon lox into pieces, laying them out on a clean work surface. You will need at least eight strips of lox (one for each bundle of three asparagus). Place three asparagus across a strip of lox and wrap the lox around the bundle. Transfer to a serving platter. Repeat with remaining lox and asparagus. Place lemon wedges around platter for guests to squeeze over top. Serve immediately.

NUTRITIONAL VALUE
PER SERVING:
Calories: 32 |
Calories from Fat: 10 |
Protein: 4 g | Carbs: 2 g |
Total Fat: 1 g |
Saturated Fat: 0 g |
Trans Fat: 0 g | Fiber: 1 g |
Sodium: 103 mg |
Cholesterol: 11 mg

NOTE *This dish can be made the night before and stored, tightly covered, in the refrigerator.*

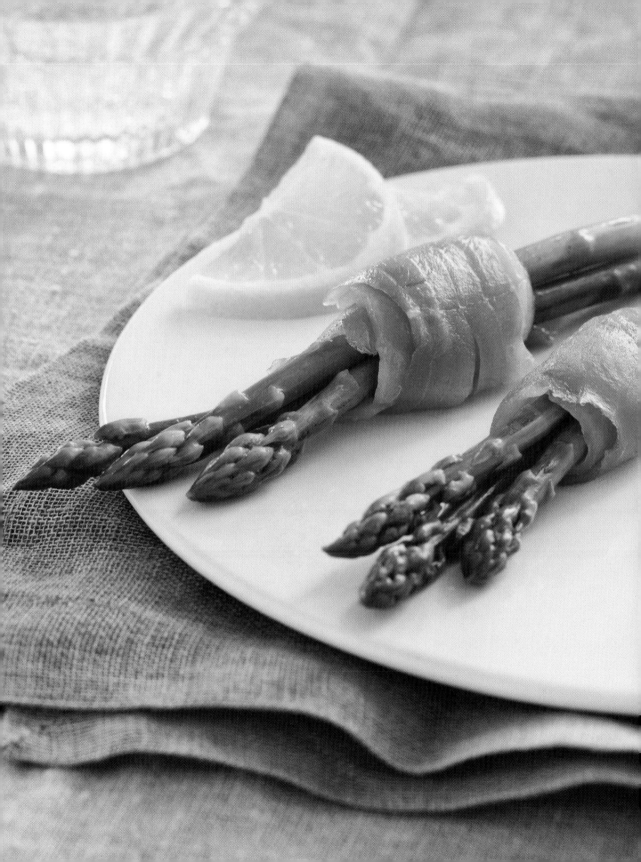

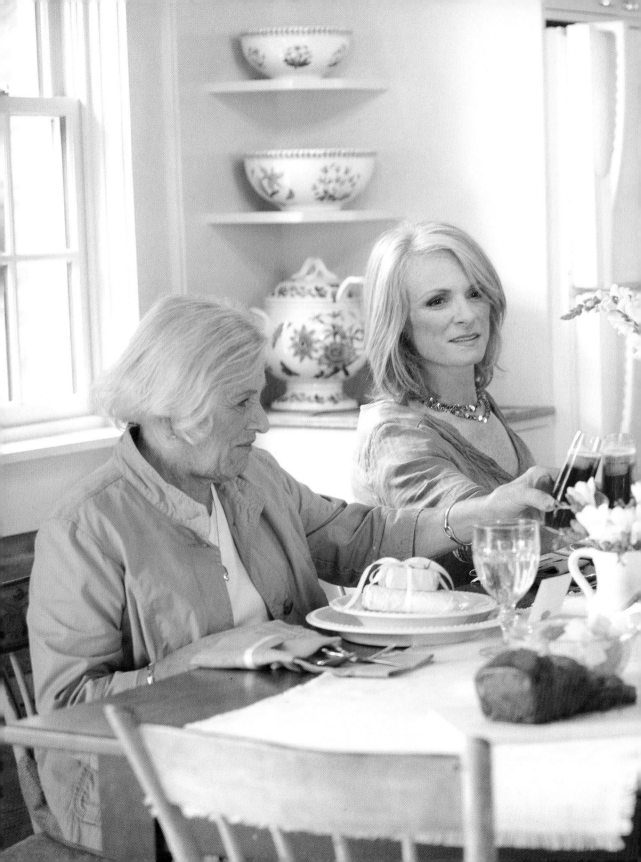

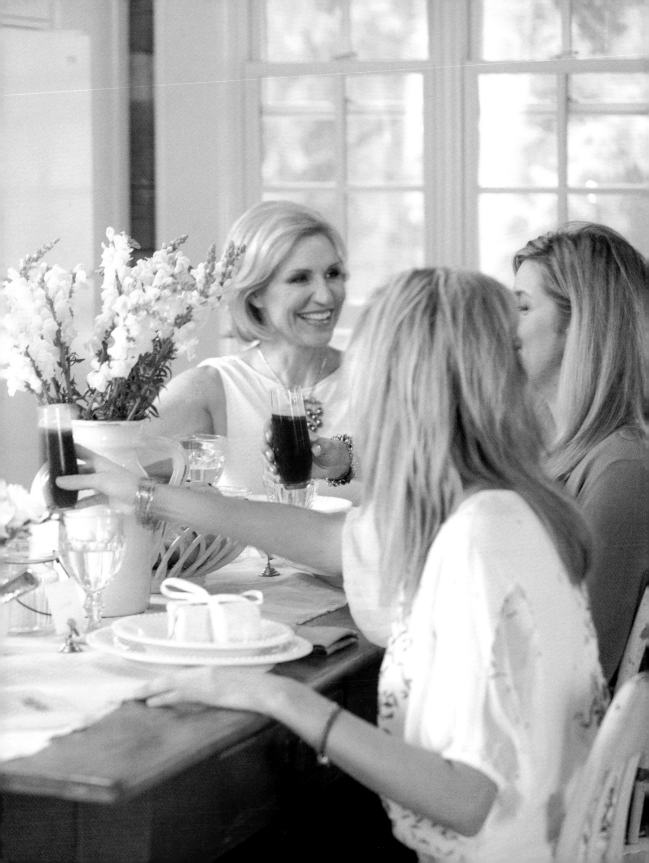

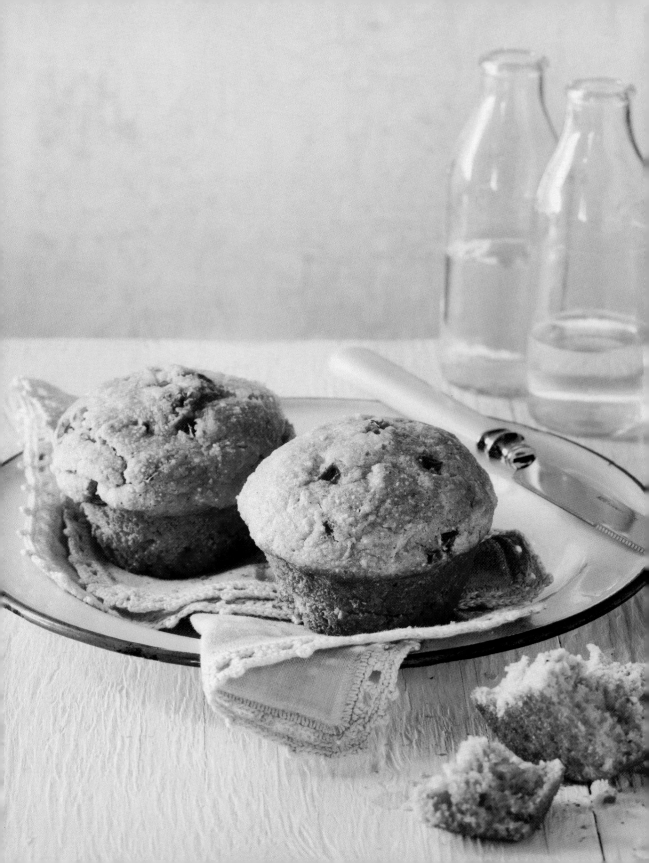

Servings: 8
Prep time: 15 minutes
Cooking time:
22 minutes

CHEDDAR JALAPEÑO CORN MUFFINS

These muffins are a sweet and spicy treat, perfect as a side to scrambled eggs or a frittata. Using sharp cheddar allows you to use less cheese without sacrificing taste. Delicious!

INGREDIENTS

Eat-Clean Cooking Spray (see page 348)
1 jalapeño, seeds and ribs removed, finely diced
1 cup / 240 ml whole grain stone ground cornmeal
½ cup / 120 ml whole grain stone ground corn flour
½ cup / 120 ml whole wheat pastry flour
¼ cup / 60 ml organic raw turbinado sugar
1 Tbsp / 15 ml + 1 tsp / 5 ml baking powder
½ tsp / 2.5 ml sea salt
1 egg
1 cup / 240 ml plain, low-fat kefir
3 Tbsp / 45 ml skim milk
¼ cup / 60 ml safflower oil
1 cup / 240 ml grated reduced-fat sharp cheddar

METHOD

1. Preheat the oven to 425°F / 220°C. Spray an eight-cup muffin tin with Eat-Clean Cooking Spray. Heat a small skillet over medium heat and spray with Eat-Clean Cooking Spray. Add jalapeño and cook until soft but not brown, 3 minutes. Remove skillet from heat and set aside.

2. In the large bowl of a mixer, add cornmeal, corn flour, pastry flour, sugar, baking powder and sea salt, and mix on low speed until thoroughly combined. Add egg, kefir, milk and oil, and mix on medium speed until just combined, 1 minute. Add reserved cooked jalapeño pepper and cheese, and fold into batter.

3. Pour batter evenly into muffin cups and bake in oven until golden brown and a toothpick comes out clean when inserted into the center, about 18 minutes. Let cool slightly before removing. If muffins don't easily unmold, slide a small sharp knife around edges to loosen muffin from tin and ease it out gently. Eat warm, or transfer to a rack to finish cooling.

NUTRITIONAL VALUE
PER SERVING:
Calories: 278 |
Calories from Fat: 93 |
Protein: 9 g | Carbs: 38 g |
Total Fat: 11 g |
Saturated Fat: 2 g |
Trans Fat: 0 g | Fiber: 3 g |
Sodium: 244 mg |
Cholesterol: 31 mg

TURKEY APPLE BREAKFAST SAUSAGE

These sausage patties are extremely versatile. Try one over a simple bed of greens or pop one on a whole grain bun and top with your favorite condiments. I find sauerkraut to be the perfect accoutrement.

INGREDIENTS

1 tsp / 5 ml extra virgin olive oil
½ granny smith apple, cored and diced
½ yellow onion, diced
1 large clove garlic, minced
1 lb / 454 g extra-lean ground turkey
1 Tbsp / 15 ml 100% pure maple syrup
1 Tbsp / 15 ml chopped fresh sage
1 tsp / 5 ml chopped fresh marjoram or oregano
1 tsp / 5 ml chopped fresh thyme
½ tsp / 2.5 ml chopped fresh rosemary
¼ tsp / 1.25 ml sweet paprika
¼ tsp / 1.25 ml ground nutmeg
1 tsp / 5 ml sea salt
¼ tsp / 1.25 ml freshly ground black pepper
Eat-Clean Cooking Spray (see page 348)

METHOD

1. Heat oil in a large skillet over medium-high heat. Add apple and onion, and sauté until soft and starting to brown, 3 to 5 minutes. Add garlic and cook for 1 minute longer. Remove from heat and set aside to cool slightly.

2. In a large bowl, add ground turkey and rest of ingredients, up to and including black pepper. Add reserved cooked apple and onion mixture that has been cooling. Using clean hands, mix together all ingredients until well combined. Score mixture into four equal parts and form into four large patties.

3. Preheat oven to 350°F / 175°C. Heat a large nonstick skillet over medium-low heat and coat with Eat-Clean Cooking Spray. Add patties in a single layer and cook until browned on both sides, about 5 minutes. Transfer to a baking sheet and finish cooking in oven, about 5 to 7 minutes. This will allow sausage patties to cook through without burning on the outside. Serve hot.

NUTRITIONAL VALUE
PER SERVING:
Calories: 166 |
Calories from Fat: 24 |
Protein: 26 g | Carbs: 12 g |
Total Fat: 3 g |
Saturated Fat: 1 g |
Trans Fat: 0 g | Fiber: 1 g |
Sodium: 541 mg |
Cholesterol: 56 mg

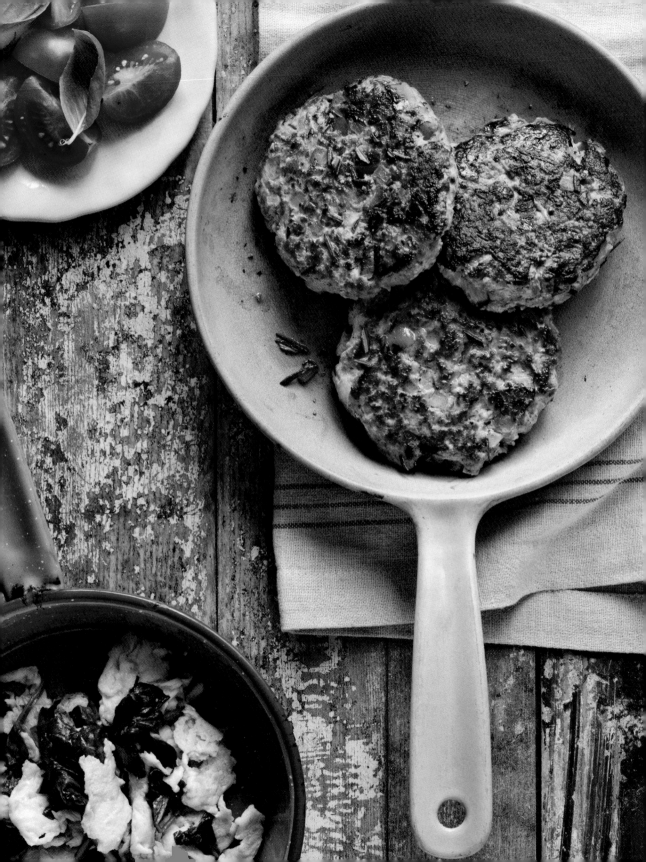

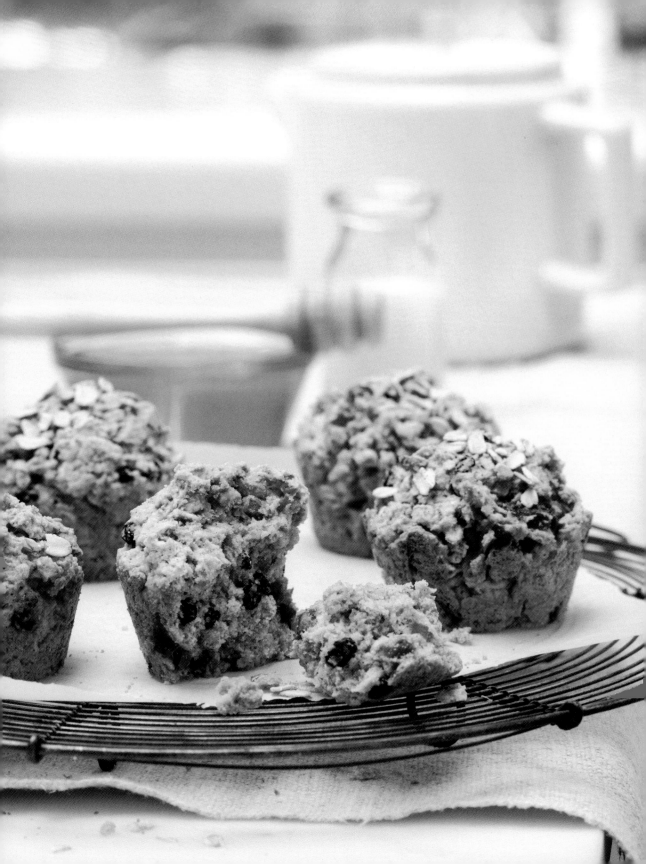

Servings: 8
Prep time: 15 minutes
Cooking time:
20-22 minutes

OATMEAL "SCUFFINS"
with Currants and Dates

A "scuffin" is the perfect blend between a muffin and scone. It's not light and fluffy like a muffin, but not flaky like a scone either. The result is a heartier muffin with the texture of a biscuit.

INGREDIENTS

1½ cups / 360 ml whole grain oat flour
1½ cups / 360 ml old-fashioned rolled oats
3 Tbsp / 45 ml raw organic turbinado sugar
1 Tbsp / 15 ml baking powder
¼ tsp / 1.25 ml ground cinnamon
½ tsp / 2.5 ml sea salt
8 dates, finely chopped (about ¼ cup / 60 ml)
¼ cup / 60 ml unsweetened dried currants
2 egg whites
3 Tbsp / 45 ml raw organic coconut butter, melted
¼ cup / 60 ml unsweetened applesauce
⅓ cup / 80 ml low-fat milk
Eat-Clean Cooking Spray (see page 348)

METHOD

1. Preheat oven to 400°F / 200°C. In a large bowl, thoroughly whisk together oat flour, oats, turbinado sugar, baking powder, cinnamon and salt. Stir in chopped dates and currants.

2. In a small bowl, whisk together egg whites, coconut butter, applesauce and milk. Add to dry ingredients and, using a rubber spatula or wooden spoon, stir until just combined. Spray muffin tins with Eat-Clean Cooking Spray. Divide batter among eight muffin cups. Bake until golden brown and a toothpick inserted in center comes out clean, 20 to 22 minutes. Remove and let cool for 5 minutes.

NUTRITIONAL VALUE
PER SERVING:
Calories: 262 |
Calories from Fat: 64 |
Protein: 8 g | Carbs: 43 g |
Total Fat: 7 g |
Saturated Fat: 4 g |
Trans Fat: 0 g | Fiber: 5 g |
Sodium: 148 mg |
Cholesterol: 0 mg

TIP *To remove your scuffins from the muffin tin, bang the bottom on the counter a few times to loosen, then remove to a wire rack to finish cooling or eat warm (the best way to eat scuffins!).*

Servings: 4
Prep time: 10 minutes
Cooking time:
15-20 minutes
Marinating Time:
2 hours to overnight

ROASTED PORK TENDERLOIN
with Sweet Sage Glaze

Serving this dish at your next brunch (or dinner) party will surely bring a level of decadence to the mid-morning affair. Since pork tenderloin is small and lean, it is prone to overcooking. An instant-read thermometer is a must when cooking tenderloin.

INGREDIENTS

2 Tbsp / 30 ml cider vinegar
1 Tbsp / 15 ml extra virgin olive oil
1 Tbsp / 15 ml unsulfured molasses
1 Tbsp / 15 ml unrefined sugar
2 cloves garlic, minced
1 tsp / 5 ml finely chopped fresh sage
1 tsp / 5 ml finely chopped fresh thyme
1 tsp / 5 ml alderwood smoked salt or other natural smoked salt
¼ tsp / 1.25 ml freshly ground black pepper
1 lb / 454 g pork tenderloin, trimmed of excess fat

METHOD

1. In a small bowl, whisk together all ingredients except pork and pour into a large plastic zipper bag. Add pork loin, press out air and seal tightly. Distribute glaze around tenderloin until thoroughly coated. Place bagged tenderloin in a small container to catch any drips and place in the refrigerator to marinate between 2 hours and overnight.

2. After marinating, remove tenderloin from fridge and bring to room temperature. Preheat the oven to 425°F / 220°C. Remove tenderloin from zipper bag and allow marinade to drip off into bag. Place tenderloin on a baking sheet or in a baking pan lined with aluminum foil, for easier cleanup. Reserve marinade and set aside. Roast tenderloin in oven until well browned and cooked to desired doneness, 15 to 17 minutes for medium rare, 17 to 20 minutes for medium. Remove from heat and let rest for 10 minutes to allow juices to be reabsorbed and temperature to reach 160°F / 71°C.

3. While tenderloin rests, pour reserved marinade into a small saucepan and place on stove over medium-high heat. Bring to a gentle boil and cook for 1 minute until slightly thickened, swirling the pan. Immediately remove from heat and set aside. (The marinade is completely safe to eat once boiled.) To serve, thinly slice the tenderloin at an angle across the grain. Pour cooked marinade over top and serve.

NUTRITIONAL VALUE
PER SERVING:
Calories: 217 |
Calories from Fat: 85 |
Protein: 23 g | Carbs: 8 g |
Total Fat: 10 g |
Saturated Fat: 3 g |
Trans Fat: 0 g | Fiber: <1 g |
Sodium: 526 mg |
Cholesterol: 75 mg

TIP *Using a thermometer is the most accurate way to determine when pork or any other meat is done cooking.*

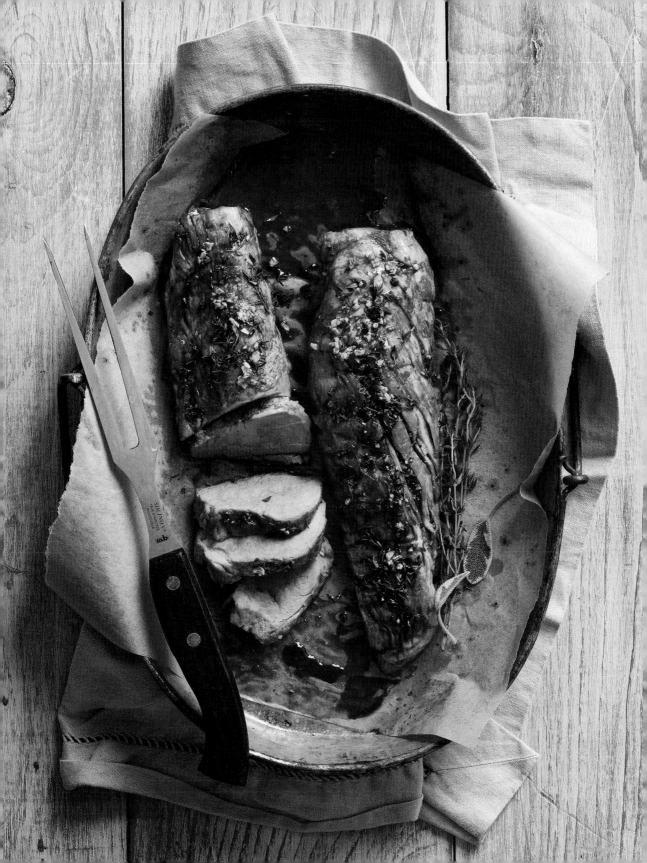

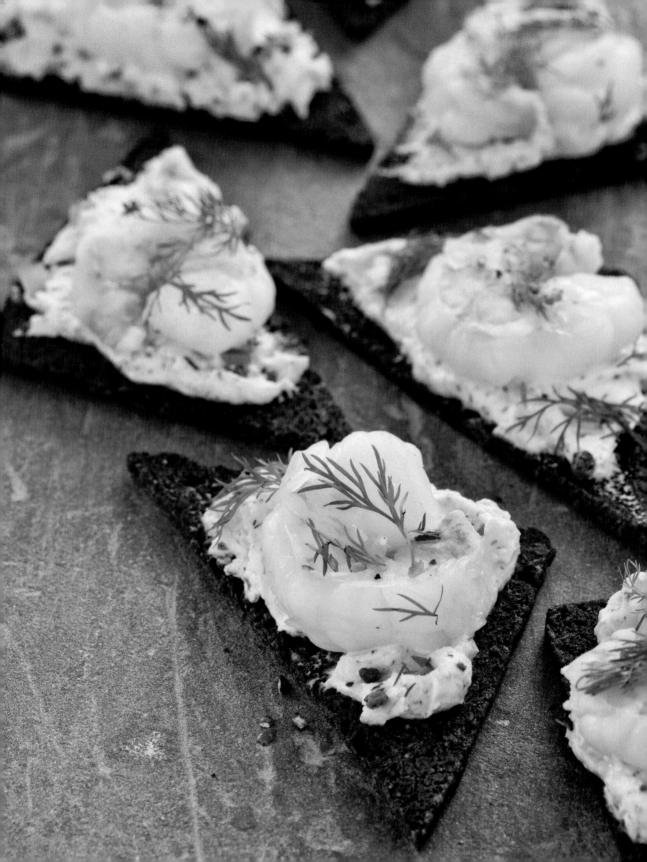

PRAWN AND HERBED YOGURT CHEESE CANAPÉS

Servings:
4 x 2 canapés
Prep time: 10 minutes
Cooking time:
15-20 minutes

I like to serve up these little gems when I'm trying to impress my brunch guests. They are so simple to make (only four ingredients) and yet they taste gourmet! Be smart and whip up a batch of Yogurt Cheese at the beginning of each week – you can use it in a multitude of recipes (many in this book!) and you'll never have to wait to make something while it strains.

INGREDIENTS
4 pieces whole grain dark rye bread (3½ inches square), thinly sliced
4 large prawns (12/15 per pound), peeled, deveined and cooked
8 heaping tsp / 50 ml Herbed Yogurt Cheese (see recipe on page 351)
Fresh dill, to garnish

METHOD

1. Preheat the oven to 350°F / 175°C. Cut bread slices in half diagonally to make triangles and place on a baking sheet. Bake until toasted and slightly crispy, but still a little soft and flexible, 15 to 20 minutes. Remove and set aside to cool.

2. Carefully remove tail shells to keep prawn meat intact. Cut prawns in half lengthwise, following butterfly cut on topside of prawns that was made to remove the vein. (You now have two identical prawn halves.)

3. Place toasted rye triangles on a serving platter, and top each with a heaping teaspoon of Herbed Yogurt Cheese. Place prawn halves on top, cut side down. Garnish each with a small piece of dill. Serve immediately.

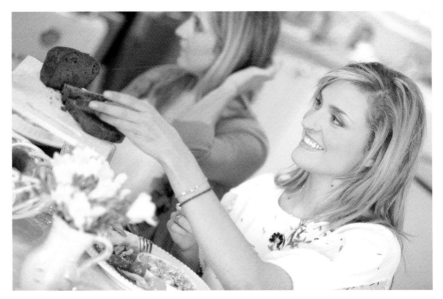

NUTRITIONAL VALUE
PER SERVING:
Calories: 64 |
Calories from Fat: 3 |
Protein: 3 g | Carbs: 13 g |
Total Fat: 0.3 g |
Saturated Fat: 0 g | Trans
Fat: 0 g | Fiber: 1 g |
Sodium: 128 mg |
Cholesterol: 11 mg

Servings: 8
Prep time: 10 minutes
Cooking time:
50-55 minutes

CRUSTLESS BROCCOLI QUICHE
with Caramelized Onions and Blue Cheese

This crustless quiche is healthy, simple and filling. To cut down the prep and cooking time on the morning of your brunch, prepare the filling ingredients the night before and spread them on the bottom of your quiche dish. The next morning, whisk the eggs with the milk and seasonings, then pour into the quiche dish and bake.

INGREDIENTS

Eat-Clean Cooking Spray (see page 348)
1 tsp / 5 ml extra virgin olive oil
1 onion, halved and thinly sliced
¼ tsp / 1.25 ml dried Herbes de Provence
Pinch sea salt
Pinch freshly ground black pepper
1 cup / 240 ml broccoli florets

1 egg
2 egg whites
1 cup / 240 ml low-fat milk
⅛ tsp / 0.625 ml freshly grated nutmeg
2 Tbsp / 30 ml Danish or
   French blue cheese
Freshly ground black pepper, to taste

METHOD

1. Position a rack in the upper third of oven and preheat to 400°F / 200°C. Coat a 9-inch glass or ceramic quiche dish with Eat-Clean Cooking Spray and place on a baking sheet to catch any spills.

2. Heat olive oil in a large skillet over medium-high heat. Add onion and Herbes de Provence, and season with a pinch of salt and pepper. Stir to combine and spread out in a single layer to cook, undisturbed, until starting to caramelize, about 3 minutes. Stir and reduce heat to medium low. Continue to cook onions, stirring occasionally, until they reduce in volume and are well caramelized, 20 to 25 minutes.

3. In the meantime, heat a small pot of boiling water over high heat and prepare an ice bath. Blanch broccoli florets in boiling water for 10 seconds, then drain and immediately submerge in ice bath to stop cooking process. Drain and chop florets into half- to one-inch pieces.

4. Whisk together egg, egg whites, milk and nutmeg, and season with a pinch of salt and pepper. Spread caramelized onions, broccoli and blue cheese in bottom of prepared quiche dish. Pour egg mixture over top and push under any ingredients not covered by egg to prevent burning. Bake uncovered until set and golden brown around edges and a knife inserted in the center comes out clean, about 25 minutes. Let quiche rest at room temperature for 10 minutes to settle, then cut into eight slices and serve.

NUTRITIONAL VALUE
PER SERVING:
Calories: 61 |
Calories from Fat: 28 |
Protein: 4 g | Carbs: 35 g |
Total Fat: 3 g |
Saturated Fat: 1 g | Trans
Fat: 0 g | Fiber: 1 g |
Sodium: 118 mg |
Cholesterol: 30 mg

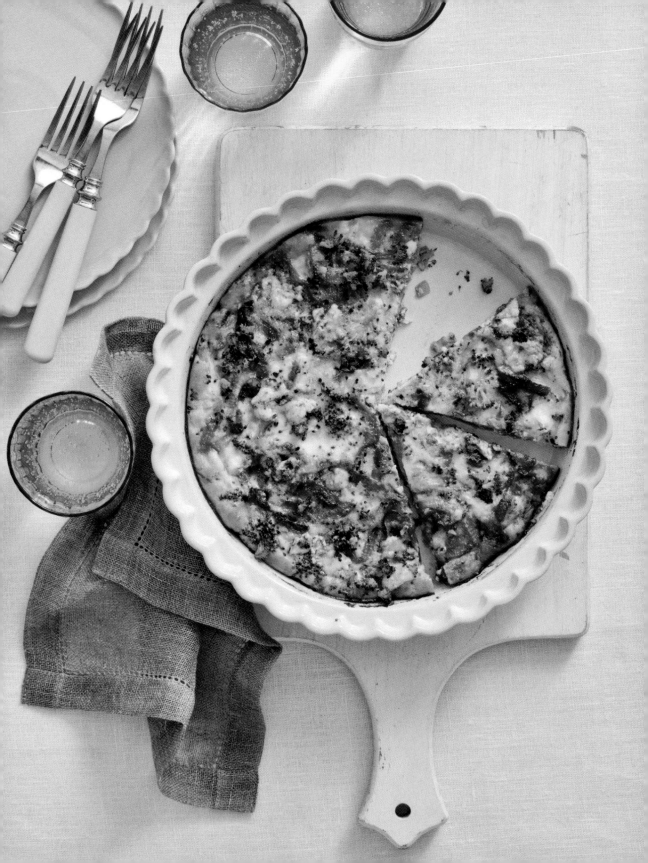

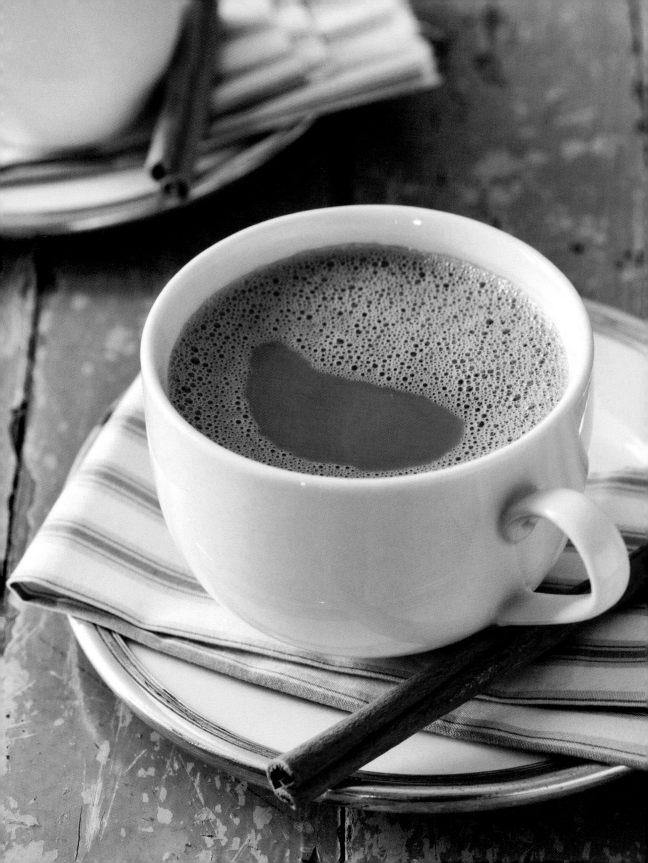

MEXICAN MOCHA CALIENTE

The Aztec people, native to central Mexico in the 14th, 15th and 16th centuries, were the first to serve chocolate as a drink. They mixed it with hot chili pepper to give it a kick. This version contains cayenne pepper, known to stimulate your metabolism and reduce LDL (bad) cholesterol. See, chocolate can be good for you!

INGREDIENTS

¼ cup / 60 ml cocoa powder
⅛ tsp / 0.625 ml ground cinnamon
Pinch cayenne pepper
1 cup / 240 ml low-fat milk
1 cup / 240 ml freshly brewed strong coffee or espresso (can be decaf)
2 Tbsp / 30 ml honey or agave nectar
Cinnamon sticks, to garnish

METHOD

1. In a heavy-bottomed small saucepan, whisk together cocoa powder, cinnamon, cayenne pepper and milk until thoroughly combined. Set burner to medium-high heat, and add coffee and honey. Heat, whisking frequently, until hot and frothy. Do not let mixture boil. Immediately remove from heat and pour into mugs. Serve garnished with whole cinnamon sticks.

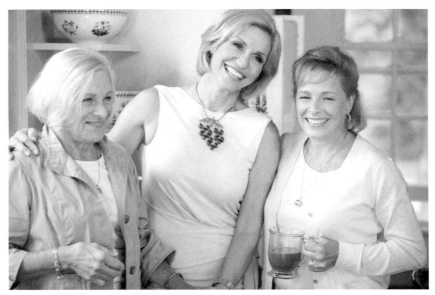

NUTRITIONAL VALUE
PER SERVING:
Calories: 152 |
Calories from Fat: 25 |
Protein: 7 g | Carbs: 30 g |
Total Fat: 4 g |
Saturated Fat: 1 g |
Trans Fat: 0 g | Fiber: 4 g |
Sodium: 91 mg |
Cholesterol: 5 mg

SEAFOOD PLATTER
of Crab, Prawns and Oysters on the Half Shell with Clean Cocktail Sauce and Cucumber Mignonette

Wow your brunch guests with this introduction-to-shellfish dish that is just as much about presentation as is it about taste. Serve alongside fresh whole grain breads, fruits and raw vegetables.

INGREDIENTS

Crushed or shaved ice, for serving
1 to 2 lbs / 454 to 908 g Dungeness crab, steamed, cleaned and chilled
12 raw oysters, cleaned and chilled
1 lb / 454 g cooked prawns, deveined, tails on, chilled
Lemon wedges, for serving
Clean Cocktail Sauce (see recipe on page 351)
Cucumber Mignonette (see recipe on page 354)

METHOD

1. Fill a large, shallow serving bowl or platter with shaved or crushed ice. Separate crab legs from crab body. Cut body of meat into quarters. Place crab in center of ice, placing two legs with claws on top.

2. To shuck oysters, hold oyster firmly in a kitchen towel, deep shell down, with hinge facing out. Using an oyster-shucking knife, which has a strong pointed blade but is not sharp, insert point of knife into hinge between two shells, pointing tip of knife away from hinge. Turn knife to pry open oyster, and slide blade under oyster to cut muscle attaching it to bottom shell. Run knife between two shells to completely open oyster shell and remove top shell. Run knife under oyster to ensure that it's detached, but do not remove it from shell. Place oyster in its shell on ice on one side of platter. Repeat with remaining oysters, fanning them around edge of platter.

3. Fan out prawns on ice across from oysters. Place lemon wedges around platter to fill in any gaps and to squeeze over seafood. Serve immediately with Clean Cocktail Sauce for crab and prawns, and Cucumber Mignonette for Oysters.

NUTRITIONAL VALUE
PER SERVING:
Calories: 128 |
Calories from Fat: 16 |
Protein: 25 g | Carbs: 1 g |
Total Fat: 2 g |
Saturated Fat: 0 g |
Trans Fat: 0 g | Fiber: 0 g |
Sodium: 377 mg |
Cholesterol: 158 mg

NOTE *You will need one or two nutcrackers or small mallets to crack the crab's claws. Keep all seafood well chilled until ready to prepare and serve.*

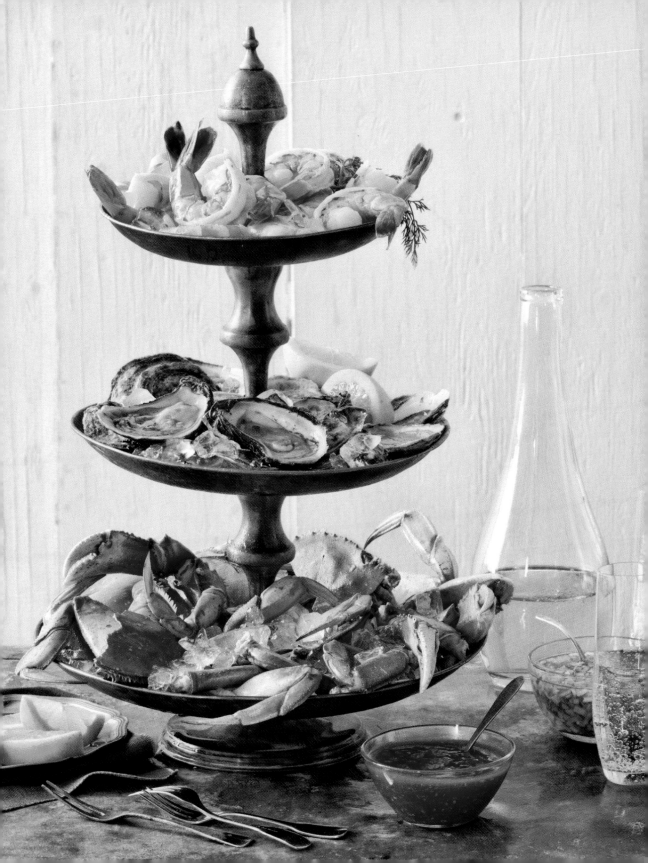

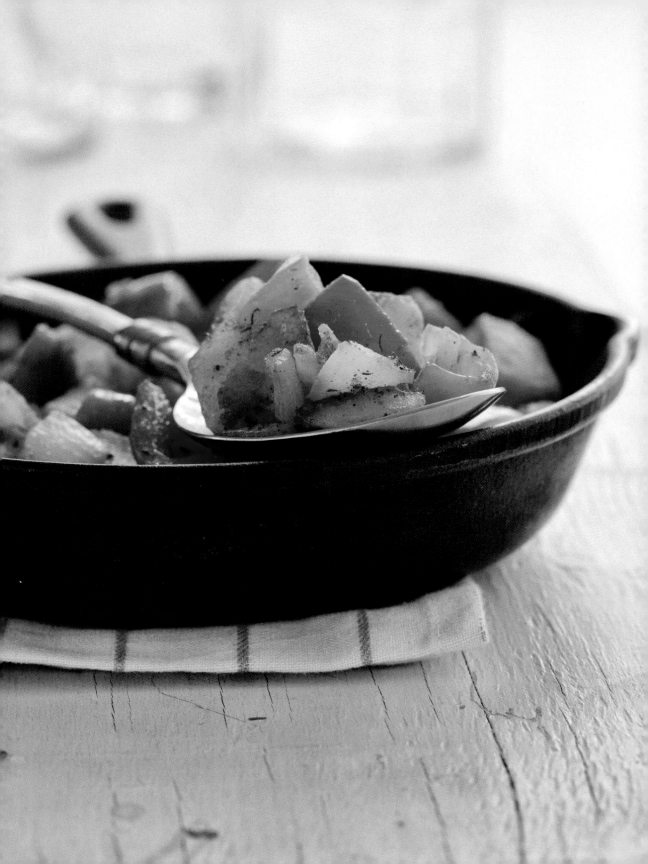

POTATOES O'BRIEN

Potatoes O'Brien is a dish that hails from Boston at the beginning of the 20th century. Simply put, it's potatoes and red and green bell peppers, fried and served hot. I like mine with a little hot sauce for an extra spicy kick.

INGREDIENTS

4 Yukon gold potatoes, cut into 1-inch cubes
1 tsp / 5 ml sea salt, divided
2 Tbsp / 30 ml extra virgin olive oil
1 yellow onion, chopped
½ each red and green pepper, seeded and chopped
1 clove garlic, minced
1 tsp / 5 ml chopped fresh thyme
¼ tsp / 1.25 ml freshly ground black pepper
Tobasco or other hot sauce, to taste

METHOD

1. Add potatoes to a medium pot filled with cold water; season with ½ tsp / 2.5 ml salt and bring to a boil over high heat. Reduce heat to simmer until potatoes are cooked through, but still hold their shape, about 12 minutes. Drain in a colander and set aside.

2. Heat olive oil in a very large skillet over medium-high heat and add drained potatoes, spreading them out evenly in pan. Let cook without stirring for a few minutes until well browned on the bottom. Stir and allow potatoes to cook for a few more minutes, undisturbed, until well browned. (Potatoes will need to cook for a total of 7 to 10 minutes to be well browned.)

3. Add onion and peppers and toss to combine, so vegetables contact bottom of pan. Cook until onion is translucent and peppers are soft and starting to brown, 3 to 5 minutes. Stir in garlic and thyme, and cook for 1 minute longer. Season with remaining ½ tsp / 2.5 ml salt and pepper. Serve immediately with hot sauce, if desired.

NUTRITIONAL VALUE
PER SERVING:
Calories: 122 |
Calories from Fat: 40 |
Protein: 3 g | Carbs: 21 g |
Total Fat: 5 g |
Saturated Fat: 1 g |
Trans Fat: 0 g | Fiber: 3 g |
Sodium: 320 mg |
Cholesterol: 0 mg

Cheese Please

One of the foods I am most commonly questioned about is cheese. Is cheese part of Eating Clean? Why do some of your recipes contain cheese? Why don't you talk more about cheese? Can I really eat cheese and lose weight? You know by now that Eating Clean is not about depriving yourself of the foods you love; instead, it's about making better food choices and eating foods that are as close to nature as possible. Cheese does contain healthful nutrients including protein, calcium and phosphorus; however, it's also a major source of saturated fat. Saturated fats raise LDL (bad) cholesterol and total blood cholesterol, as well as clogging your arteries.

My official position on cheese is that it is a treat food. Most cheese is at least 30 percent or higher in fat content and I'm not talking about healthy fats here. If you are trying to lose weight, cheese is something you want to eat sparingly and by that I mean not every day and perhaps not even every week.

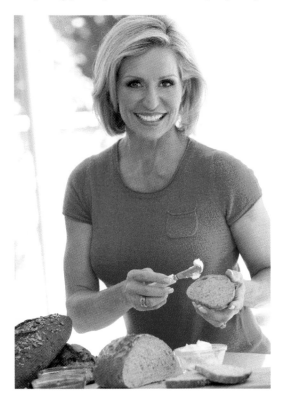

Think of it this way: If you have a lot of weight to lose, you need to be stricter with your food choices until you have met your goals. The cheese isn't going anywhere. It will still be available to you three months, six months or even a year from now. If you have already met your weight-loss goals, you can be a little less strict with yourself – although this isn't permission to get crazy with the Cheez Whiz. I do eat cheese myself but I eat it rarely and sparingly.

A portion of cheese is one ounce, or a little smaller than your thumb. That is not very much! When I do indulge in cheese, I stick to hard, older cheeses, which have less fat and a higher flavor value. If you decide to include cheese in your diet, eat a very good one and not too much of it. If you do include cheeses such as cheddar or mozzarella in your diet, choose low-fat or nonfat varieties. And please know that cheese in a jar or in prewrapped slices does not qualify as "real" food.

Some of my favorite cheeses are:

*C*ottage cheese is a stereotypical dieter's food, and with reason, as long as you choose a low-fat or nonfat, plain variety. High in protein and somewhat bland in flavor, cottage cheese is a fresh cow's milk cheese that is made from cheese curd byproduct. You can eat cottage cheese on its own or bake it into dishes. Make sure to read the label before purchasing! Most cottage cheese contains additives.

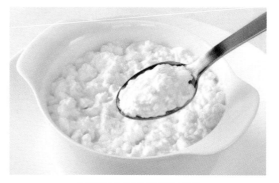

*R*icotta cheese is similar to cottage cheese but is made from whey product. It can be used interchangeably with cottage cheese, but is a thicker cheese and therefore preferred for cannoli, lasagna and other dishes that require a soft, mild cheese. Again, if you are using ricotta cheese in your recipes, choose a low-fat or nonfat variety.

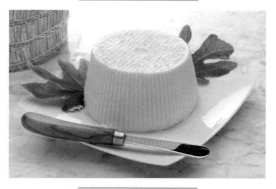

*P*armigiano-Reggiano (also known as Parmesan) is a very hard cheese with a distinct salty flavor. It's made with pure cow's milk and very few additives. Grate your own fresh Parmesan instead of purchasing it pre-grated – the flavor will be much more intense and you'll use less. Asiago, Romano and Pecorino cheeses are all hard cheeses that can be used in the same way.

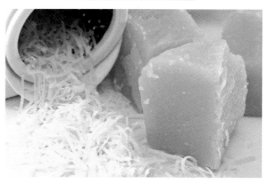

*G*oat cheese is a strong-tasting, tangy, easily spread cheese made from goat's milk. If I am craving something creamy, I often opt for goat cheese because the protein content is high and it's lower in fat than other cheeses. If you have an intolerance to lactose, products made from goat's milk are a good choice for you, as goat's milk is more similar to human milk than cow's milk.

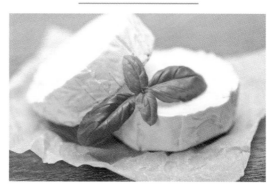

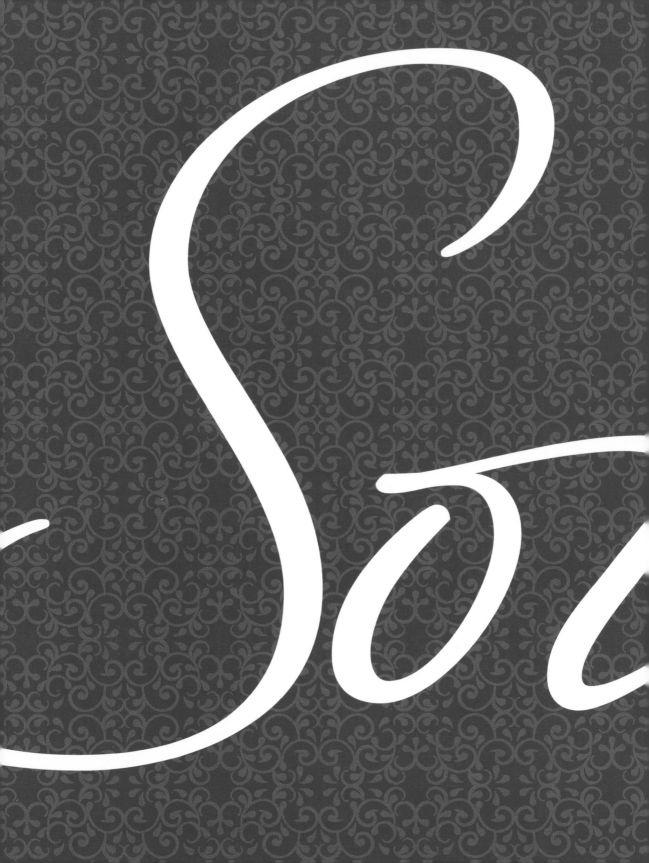

3

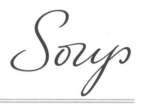

78   SMOOTH AND HEARTY BORSCHT-STYLE BEET SOUP

81   CREAMY ARTICHOKE SOUP

82   FRENCH ONION SOUP
with Parmesan Croutons

85   GREEN LENTIL AND VEGETABLE SOUP

86   JAPANESE VEGETABLE AND TOFU SOUP
(Kenchinjiru)

89   MEXICALI CABBAGE PATCH SOUP

90   EGG DROP SOUP

93   TOMATO FENNEL SOUP
with Lima Beans

94   GAZPACHO

97   PURÉE OF PARSNIP, CELERIAC AND APPLE SOUP
with Crispy Sage

Servings: 6 x 1 cup
Prep time: 10 minutes
Cooking time:
31-36 minutes

SMOOTH AND HEARTY BORSCHT-STYLE BEET SOUP

Borscht is a beet soup that is popular in Eastern and Central European countries. This version is borscht-style because it begins with beets, but ends as a smooth and creamy version of the classic. Try it with whole grain crackers or toast for dipping.

INGREDIENTS

1 Tbsp / 15 ml **extra virgin olive oil**
2 **red beets**, peeled and diced into ½-inch cubes (about 2 cups / 480 ml)
2 **carrots**, peeled and diced into ½-inch cubes
½ large **yellow onion**, or 1 **medium onion**, diced
1 tsp / 5 ml **sea salt**
¾ tsp / 3.75 ml freshly ground **black pepper**
1 clove **garlic**, chopped
½ cup / 120 ml **red lentils**, rinsed and drained
4 cups / 960 ml low-sodium **vegetable broth**
1 **bay leaf**
Juice of ½ **lemon**
½ cup / 120 ml plain, low-fat **yogurt**, drained, plus more to garnish
Fresh **dill**, to garnish

METHOD

1. Heat oil in a large heavy-bottomed soup pot over medium-high heat. Add beets, carrots, onions, salt and pepper, and sauté for 5 minutes, stirring occasionally. Add garlic and cook for 1 minute longer. Add lentils, vegetable broth and bay leaf. Bring soup to a boil, then cover and reduce heat to simmer until ingredients are cooked through and soft, 25 to 30 minutes.

2. Remove bay leaf and ladle soup into a blender. Add lemon juice and yogurt. Purée soup until velvety smooth, taking care because hot liquids can expand when blended. Ladle into bowls and serve garnished with a dollop of yogurt and a few pieces of chopped dill.

NUTRITIONAL VALUE
PER SERVING:
Calories: 93 |
Calories from Fat: 24 |
Protein: 3 g | Carbs: 13 g |
Total Fat: 3 g |
Saturated Fat: 0.5 g |
Trans Fat: 0 g | Fiber: 4 g |
Sodium: 409 mg |
Cholesterol: 1 mg

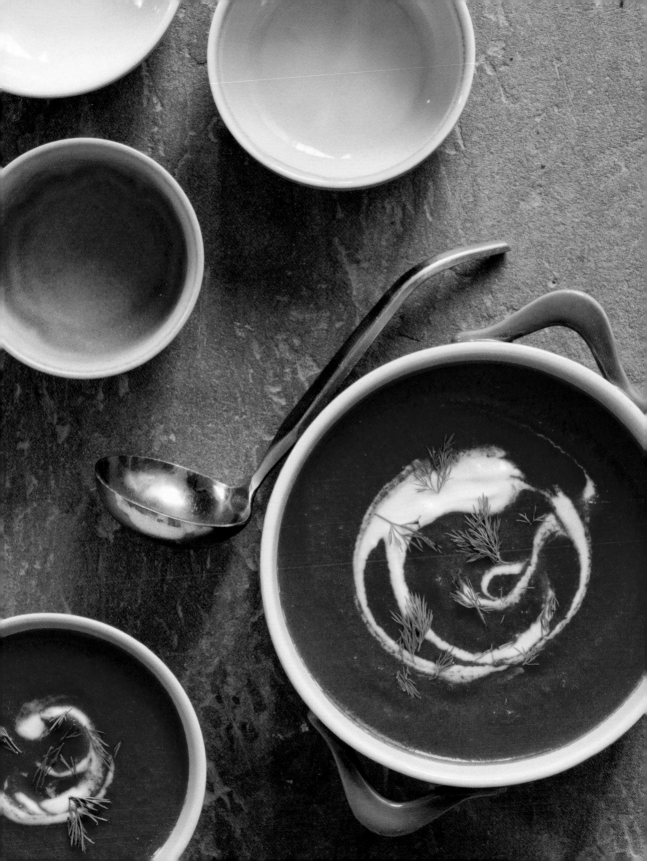

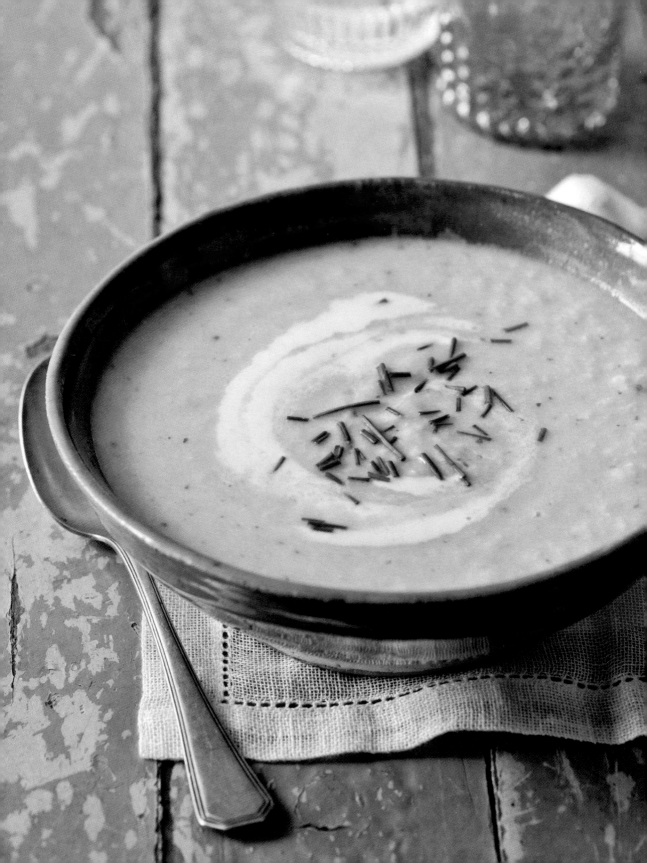

CREAMY ARTICHOKE SOUP

Servings: 4 x 1 cup
Prep time: 10 minutes
Cooking time: 25 minutes

This soup is the ultimate comfort food. The creaminess comes from the goat's milk, an easily digestible alternative to cow's milk that can be consumed by those with an intolerance to lactose. Goat's milk also contains 20 percent less cholesterol, but if you can't find it, go ahead and use cow's milk instead.

INGREDIENTS

1 Tbsp / 15 ml **extra virgin olive oil**
2 **leeks**, white and light green parts only, chopped and rinsed well
2 cloves **garlic**, chopped
1 x 8-oz package frozen **artichoke hearts**, slightly thawed
1 tsp / 5 ml chopped fresh **thyme**
1 tsp / 5 ml **sea salt**
¼ tsp / 1.25 ml freshly ground **black pepper**
1 **russet potato**, peeled and cut into 1-inch cubes
2 cups / 480 ml low-sodium **chicken broth**
½ cup / 120 ml low-fat **goat's milk**
Juice of ½ **lemon**
2 tsp / 10 ml chopped **chives**, to garnish

METHOD

1. Heat olive oil in a heavy-bottomed pot over medium heat. Add leeks, garlic, artichoke hearts, thyme, sea salt and black pepper. Cook, stirring occasionally, until leeks are soft but garlic is not yet brown, about 5 minutes. Add potatoes and chicken broth. Bring to a boil, cover and reduce heat to simmer for 20 minutes until all ingredients are soft and flavors are combined.

2. Remove from heat and blend until smooth using a hand-held immersion blender. (You can also use a stand blender and work in batches.) Add goat's milk and lemon juice; blend again to combine. Taste, and make any final adjustments to seasoning with salt, pepper and/or lemon juice. Ladle into four bowls and sprinkle each with ½ tsp / 2.5 ml chopped chives.

NUTRITIONAL VALUE PER SERVING:
Calories: 150 |
Calories from Fat: 41 |
Protein: 6 g | Carbs: 23 g |
Total Fat: 4 g |
Saturated Fat: 1 g |
Trans Fat: 0 g | Fiber: 4 g |
Sodium: 571 mg |
Cholesterol: 1 mg

TIP *Be careful when blending hot liquids using a stand blender because hot liquids can expand. Always leave one corner of the blender lid lifted and cover with a towel.*

Servings: 4 x 1 cup
Prep time: 10 minutes
Cooking time:
75-85 minutes

FRENCH ONION SOUP
with Parmesan Croutons

There is a myth that states French onion soup was created by King Louis XIV or XV in a hunting lodge after finding the pantry bare, except for onions, champagne and stale bread. I'm not sure if this is true or not, but I do know that this soup has been around for a long time and for good reason – it's comforting and delicious.

INGREDIENTS

1 Tbsp / 15 ml **extra virgin olive oil**
3 large **yellow onions**, thinly sliced
½ tsp / 2.5 ml **sea salt**
¼ tsp / 1.25 ml freshly ground **black pepper**
1 clove **garlic**, peeled and slightly smashed
3 sprigs fresh **thyme**
1 **bay leaf**
¼ tsp / 1.25 ml whole **black peppercorns**
1 tsp / 5 ml **Cognac, brandy** or **dry sherry**
1 tsp / 5 ml **white wine vinegar**
1 tsp / 5 ml **sherry vinegar**
4 cups / 960 ml low-sodium **beef broth**
Dash **Worcestershire**
8 **Parmesan croutons** (see recipe on page 353)

METHOD

1. Heat olive oil in a large heavy-bottomed soup pot or Dutch oven over medium heat. Add onions, salt and pepper, and sweat onions until they reduce in volume, stirring occasionally, about 10 minutes. Reduce heat to medium low and continue to cook onions slowly until they are well browned, using a wooden spoon to stir and scrape bottom of the pot regularly, 45 to 55 minutes. (This is a slow process to caramelize onions, so don't try to rush browning them over high heat.)

2. While onions are browning, cut a 3 x 3-inch square of double layered cheesecloth. Place garlic clove, thyme sprigs, bay leaf and black peppercorns on cheesecloth, gather corners and tie it closed with butcher twine or food-safe string. Set aside.

3. When onions are evenly browned and have reduced down greatly, add Cognac and both vinegars. Scrape bottom of pot to loosen brown crusty bits, and allow liquid to infuse its flavor into onions and cook out the alcohol, about 30 seconds. Add beef broth, a dash of Worcestershire and cheesecloth sachet. Bring soup to a boil, partially cover, reduce heat and simmer for 30 minutes. Remove cheesecloth sachet and discard. Ladle soup into four bowls and top each with two Parmesan croutons.

NUTRITIONAL VALUE
PER SERVING:
Calories: 152 |
Calories from Fat: 49 |
Protein: 8 g | Carbs: 17 g |
Total Fat: 6 g |
Saturated Fat: 1 g |
Trans Fat: 0 g | Fiber: 3 g |
Sodium: 404 mg |
Cholesterol: 1 mg

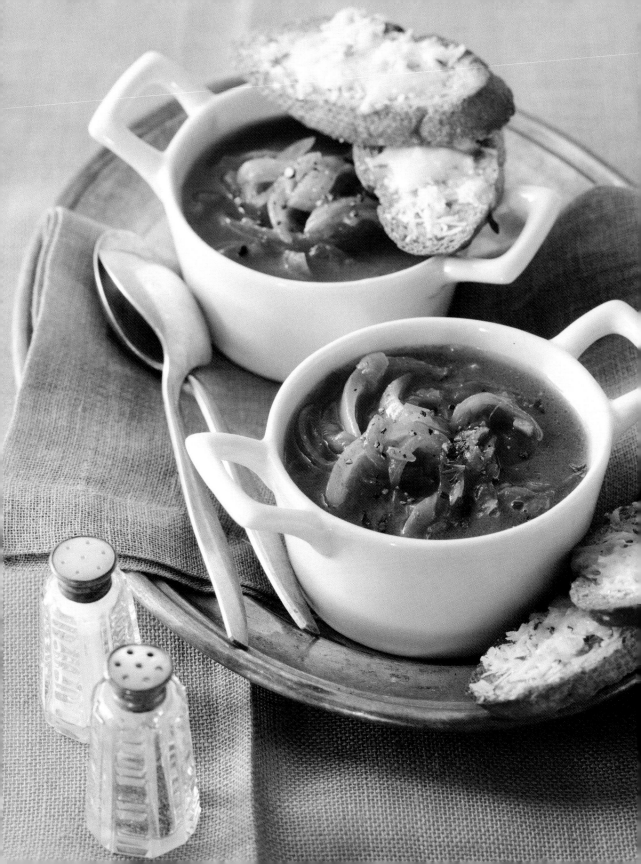

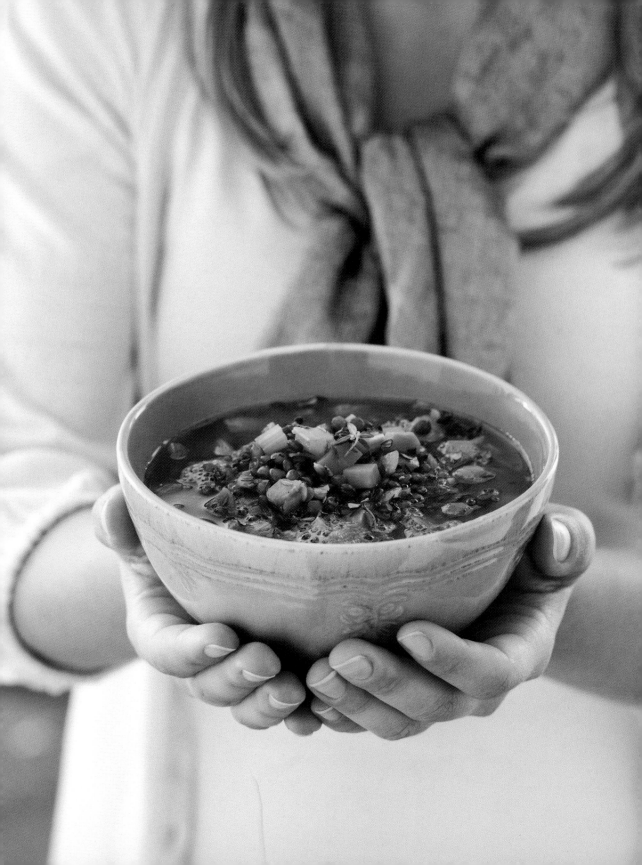

Servings: 4 x 1 cup
Prep time: 10 minutes
Cooking time:
51 minutes

GREEN LENTIL AND VEGETABLE SOUP

I often add lentils to my soups and salad for added bulk and protein – they can turn any dish into something satisfying. French green lentils, also called "lentilles du Puy," are peppery tasting and delicate – they take longer to cook than other lentils, but hold their shape well. (They won't turn to mush!)

INGREDIENTS

1 Tbsp / 15 ml **extra virgin olive oil**
½ large **yellow onion**, diced
1 large **carrot**, peeled and diced
2 ribs **celery**, diced
1 tsp / 5 ml **sea salt**
¼ tsp / 1.25 ml freshly ground **black pepper**
2 cloves **garlic**, chopped
1 tsp / 5 ml chopped fresh **thyme**
1 tsp / 5 ml chopped fresh **rosemary**
½ cup / 120 ml **French green lentils** (lentilles du Puy)
2 cups / 480 ml low-sodium **vegetable broth**
2 cups / 480 ml **water**
1 **bay leaf**

METHOD

1. Heat olive oil in a medium soup pot over medium-high heat. Add onion, carrot, celery, salt and pepper. Sauté until vegetables are soft and starting to turn golden brown, about 5 minutes. Add garlic, thyme and rosemary, and cook for 1 minute longer.

2. Add lentils, vegetable broth, water and bay leaf. Bring soup to a simmer, cover and cook until the lentils are tender, 45 minutes. Remove bay leaf and ladle into four bowls.

NUTRITIONAL VALUE
PER SERVING:
Calories: 149 |
Calories from Fat: 36 |
Protein: 6 g | Carbs: 23 g |
Total Fat: 4 g |
Saturated Fat: 0.5 g |
Trans Fat: 0 g | Fiber: 6 g |
Sodium: 541 mg |
Cholesterol: 0 mg

Servings: 4 x 1¼ cups
Prep time: 20 minutes
Cooking time: 6-8 minutes

JAPANESE VEGETABLE AND TOFU SOUP

(Kenchinjiru)

Kenchinjiru is a Japanese clear soup made with tofu and sautéed vegetables. Popular ingredients include mushrooms and potatoes. This soup is as hearty and filling as you want it to be, depending on the ingredients you choose to include.

Note: Dashi must be made ahead of time.

INGREDIENTS

4 cups / 960 ml **Dashi** (see recipe on page 353)
1 **carrot**, peeled and cut into thin quarter-rounds
4 inches **daikon radish**, peeled and cut into thin quarter-rounds
1 cup / 240 ml finely shredded **green cabbage**
1 **portobello mushroom**, stem removed, gills scraped out, halved and thinly sliced
1 medium **Yukon gold potato**, peeled and diced into ½-inch cubes
1 tsp / 5 ml **wakame** (edible dried seaweed)
1 tsp / 5 ml **sesame oil**
2 tsp / 10 ml low-sodium **soy sauce** or **tamari**
¾ tsp / 3.75 ml **sea salt**
4 oz / 125 g firm **tofu**, diced into ½-inch cubes

METHOD

1. In a medium soup pot, bring to a simmer Dashi, carrot, daikon, cabbage, portobello mushroom and potato. Cook until vegetables are tender and potato still holds its shape, 5 to 7 minutes. Turn heat off and stir in wakame, sesame oil, soy sauce and salt. Add tofu and let sit for 1 minute to heat. Ladle into four bowls and serve.

NUTRITIONAL VALUE PER SERVING:
Calories: 112 | Calories from Fat: 31 | Protein: 9 g | Carbs: 13 g | Total Fat: 3 g | Saturated Fat: 0.3 g | Trans Fat: 0 g | Fiber: 4 g | Sodium: 556 mg | Cholesterol: 0 mg

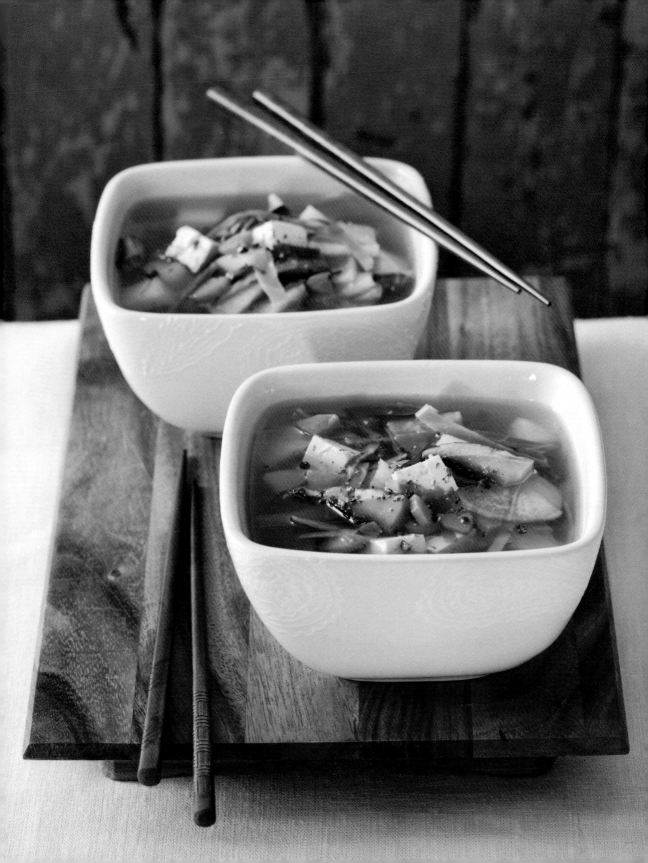

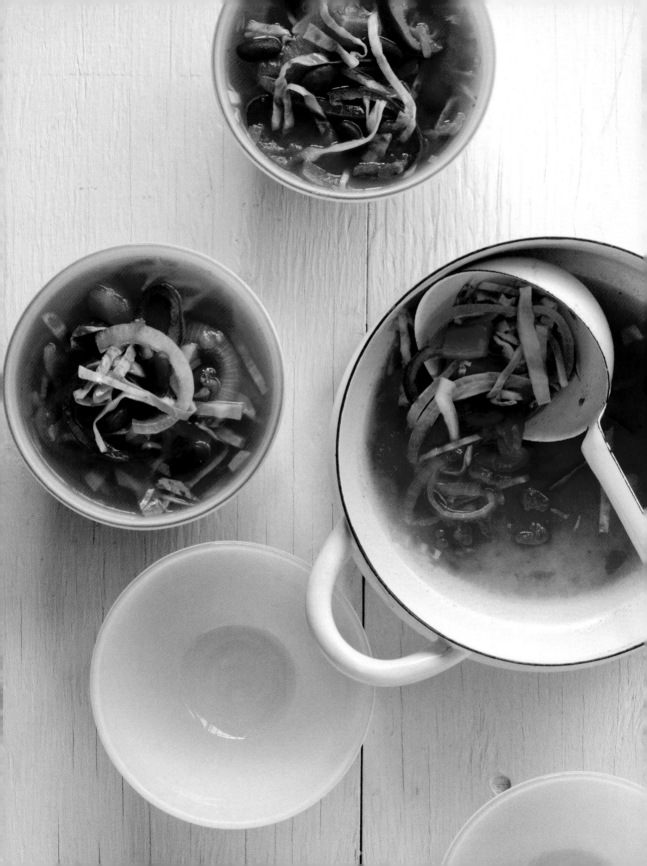

Servings: 4 x 1 cup
Prep time: 10 minutes
Cooking time:
25-32 minutes

MEXICALI CABBAGE PATCH SOUP

I know, I know. You read the words "cabbage soup" and are immediately put off. Trust me when I say, this is not your traditional tasteless "diet" cabbage soup. Bursting with Mexican flavor, this soup will have you screaming "olé!"

INGREDIENTS

1 Tbsp / 15 ml **extra virgin olive oil**
1 **yellow onion**, halved and thinly sliced
1 **poblano pepper**, halved, seeded and thinly sliced
½ head **green cabbage**, cored and thinly sliced
2 cloves **garlic**, chopped
1 tsp / 5 ml **sea salt**
¾ tsp / 3.75 ml freshly ground **black pepper**
1 **chipotle pepper** in adobo sauce, chopped
2 tsp / 10 ml **chili powder**
1 tsp / 5 ml ground **cumin**
¼ tsp / 1.25 ml dried **Mexican oregano**
1 **bay leaf**
1½ cups / 360 ml cooked **kidney beans**
2 cups / 480 ml diced **tomatoes**
4 cups / 960 ml low-sodium **vegetable broth**
1 cup / 240 ml **water**

METHOD

1. Heat olive oil in a large heavy-bottomed soup pot over medium-high heat. Add onion and poblano pepper, and sauté until onion is translucent, 3 to 5 minutes. Add cabbage, garlic, salt and pepper, and cook until cabbage is wilted, about 2 minutes. Add rest of ingredients and bring soup to a boil.

2. Cover pot and reduce heat to simmer until all ingredients are tender and cooked through, and flavors have combined, 20 to 25 minutes. Taste, and make any final adjustments to seasoning with salt and pepper. Remove bay leaf and ladle into bowls.

NUTRITIONAL VALUE
PER SERVING:
Calories: 103 |
Calories from Fat: 18 |
Protein: 4 g | Carbs: 17 g |
Total Fat: 2 g |
Saturated Fat: 0 g |
Trans Fat: 0 g |
Fiber: 5 g | Sodium: 289 mg |
Cholesterol: 0 mg

Servings: 4 x 1 cup
Prep time: 5 minutes
Cooking time:
3-5 minutes

EGG DROP SOUP

Egg drop soup is just what the name suggests: a soup of beaten eggs dropped into boiled stock. It originated in China, but is now popular all over the world. A successful soup is created by slowly dripping a thin stream of egg into the hot liquid, making thin strands or flakes of cooked egg that float in the soup.

Note: Dashi must be made ahead of time.

INGREDIENTS

4 cups / 960 ml **Dashi** (see recipe on page 353)
3 **egg whites** + 1 whole **egg**, beaten well
1 tsp / 5 ml **wakame** (dried edible seaweed)
1 tsp / 5 ml **sake rice wine**
1 tsp / 5 ml low-sodium **tamari**
¾ tsp / 3.75 ml **sea salt**
1 **scallion**, finely chopped

METHOD

1. In a medium saucepan, bring Dashi to a very gentle simmer. Using a fork, slowly stir beaten eggs into broth, 1 Tbsp / 15 ml at a time to create "ribbons." Add wakame, sake, tamari, sea salt and scallion, and stir to combine. Serve immediately.

NUTRITIONAL VALUE
PER SERVING:
Calories: 48 |
Calories from Fat: 13 |
Protein: 7 g | Carbs: 3 g |
Total Fat: 2 g |
Saturated Fat: 0.5 g |
Trans Fat: 0 g | Fiber: 1 g |
Sodium: 527 mg |
Cholesterol: 61 mg

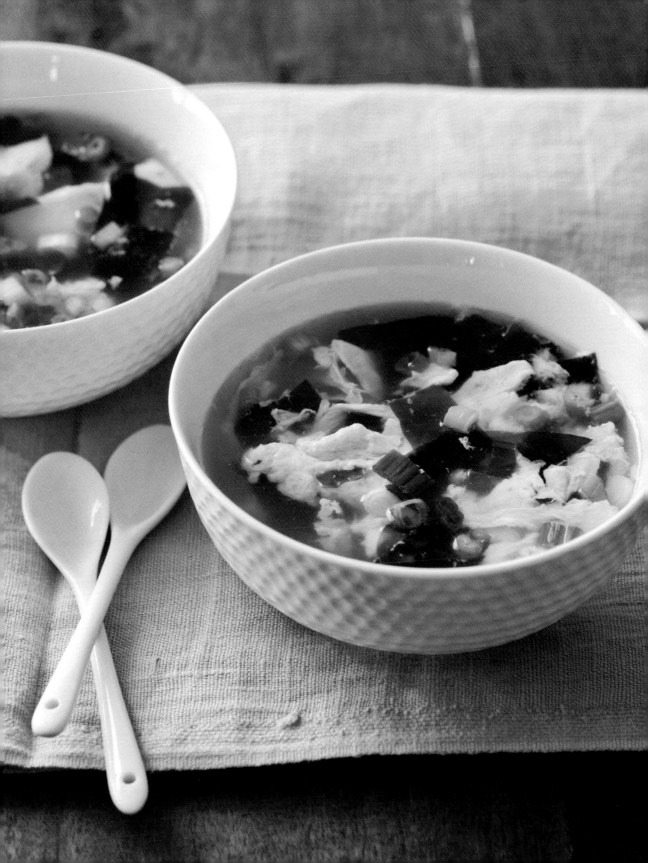

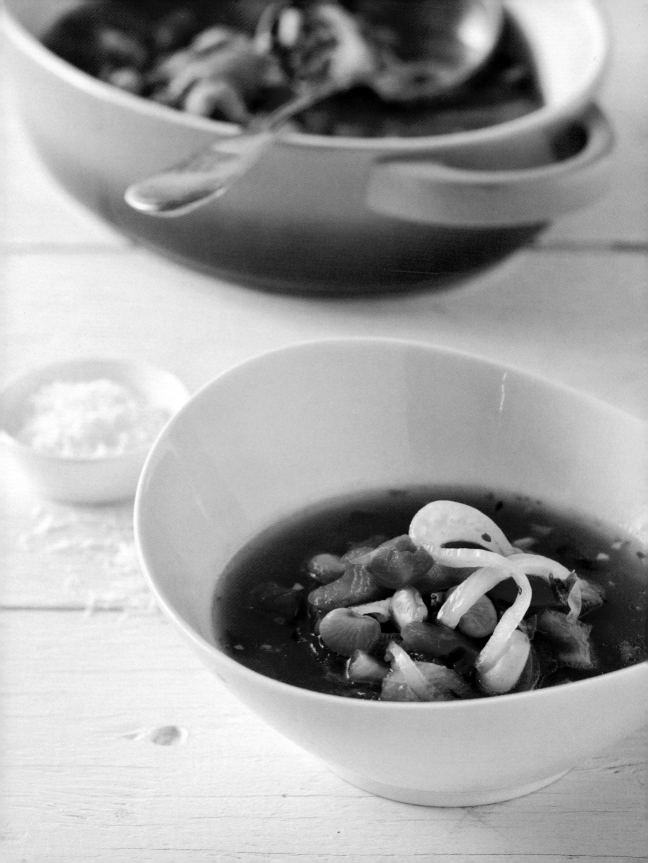

Servings: 8 x 1 cup
Prep time: 10 minutes
Cooking time:
26 minutes

TOMATO FENNEL SOUP
with Lima Beans

This harvest soup is sure to boost your spirit and your immune system. Lima beans, with their rich buttery smoothness, add protein to this dish to make it a complete meal – perfect for an easy reheated lunch or quick dinner.

INGREDIENTS

1 Tbsp / 15 ml **extra virgin olive oil**
1 medium **yellow onion**, halved and thinly sliced
1 **bulb fennel**, halved and thinly sliced
2 stalks **celery** with leaves, thinly sliced on the diagonal
⅛ tsp / 0.675 ml crushed **red pepper flakes**
1 tsp / 5 ml **sea salt**
¼ tsp / 1.25 ml freshly ground **black pepper**
2 cloves **garlic**, chopped
1 Tbsp / 15 ml chopped fresh **thyme**
2 cups diced **roma tomatoes**
3 cups / 720 ml low-sodium **vegetable broth**
1 cup / 240 ml frozen **baby lima beans**
1 rind **Parmigiano Reggiano cheese** (see note)

METHOD

1. Heat olive oil in a large pot over medium heat. Add onion, fennel, celery, red pepper flakes, salt and pepper, and cook, stirring occasionally, until soft but not brown, about 5 minutes. Add garlic and thyme, and cook for 1 more minute.

2. Add diced tomatoes, broth, lima beans and Parmigiano Reggiano rind. Increase heat to bring to a boil. Cover, reduce heat and simmer, stirring occasionally, until ingredients are cooked through and flavors combine, about 20 minutes. As it cooks, the Parmigiano rind infuses the soup with a delicious creamy, salty, nutty flavor, just like the cheese (but you don't have to actually add any cheese to the soup!).

NUTRITIONAL VALUE
PER SERVING:
Calories: 78 |
Calories from Fat: 18 |
Protein: 3 g | Carbs: 12 g |
Total Fat: 2 g |
Saturated Fat: 0 g |
Trans Fat: 0 g | Fiber: 4 g |
Sodium: 447 mg |
Cholesterol: 0 mg

NOTE *You must use a rind from real Italian Parmigiano Reggiano cheese. If you don't want to buy the wedge of Parmigiano Reggiano, you can usually get the rind at no cost from a cheese shop or cheese department of finer grocery stores.*

Servings: 4 x 1½ cups
Prep time: 20 minutes
Cooking time:
0 minutes

GAZPACHO

Often described as liquid salad, gazpacho is a Spanish, raw vegetable, tomato-based soup. Delightfully fresh and healthy, this soup is usually consumed in summertime – it's refreshingly cool and acidic.

INGREDIENTS

4 ripe **tomatoes**
1 **English cucumber**, peeled and seeded
1 **green pepper**, ribs and seeds removed
1 **red pepper**, ribs and seeds removed
1 cup / 240 ml all-natural low-sodium sugar-free **vegetable juice**
¼ cup / 60 ml **sherry vinegar** or **red wine vinegar**
2 Tbsp / 30 ml **extra virgin olive oil**
2 cloves **garlic**, minced
1 tsp / 5 ml **sea salt**
½ tsp / 2.5 ml freshly ground **black pepper**

METHOD

1. Dice tomatoes, cucumber and green and red peppers into ¼-inch pieces and place in a large bowl. Add rest of ingredients and stir to combine.

2. Scoop out half of gazpacho and place in a food processor or blender and pulse-blend until mostly smooth. Pour blended gazpacho back into bowl and stir to combine. (Alternatively, you can blend entire batch of gazpacho if you prefer a smoother soup.) Taste, and make any adjustments to seasoning with salt and pepper. Chill for at least 2 hours to marry the flavors before serving.

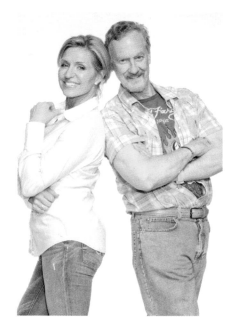

NUTRITIONAL VALUE
PER SERVING:
Calories: 124 |
Calories from Fat: 64 |
Protein: 2 g | Carbs: 13 g |
Total Fat: 7 g |
Saturated Fat: 1 g |
Trans Fat: 0 g | Fiber: 3 g |
Sodium: 521 mg |
Cholesterol: 0 mg

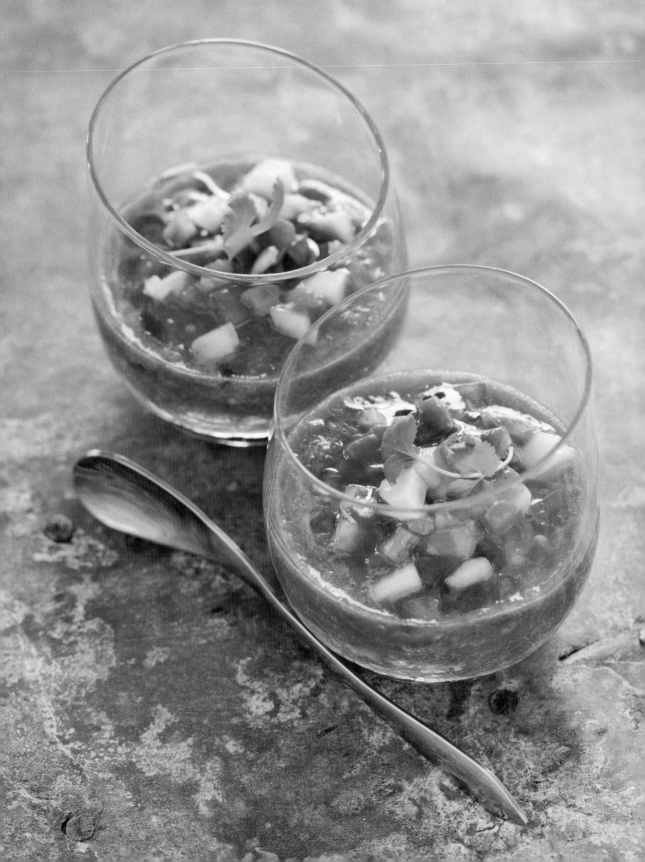

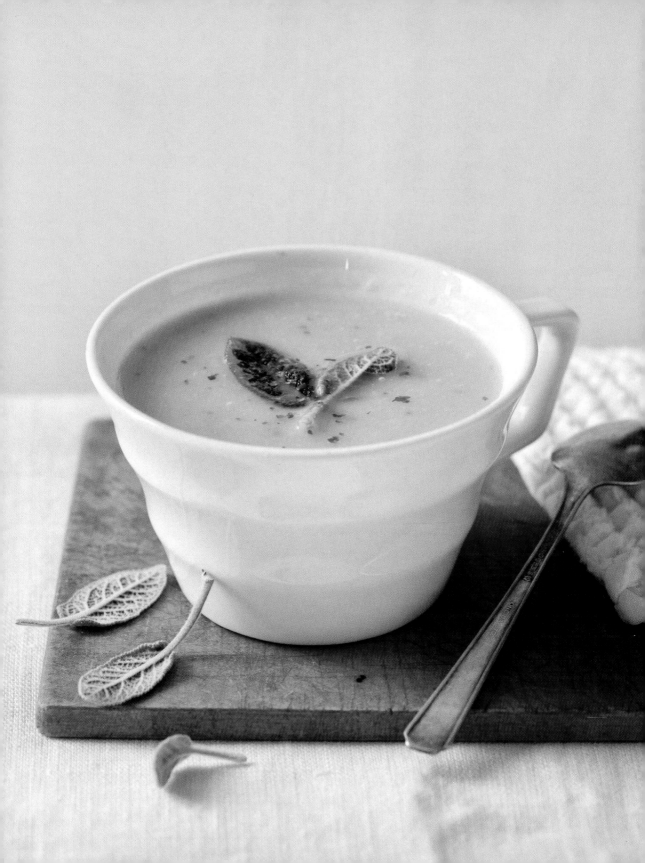

Servings: 6 x 1 cup
Prep time: 15 minutes
Cooking time:
30-36 minutes

PURÉE OF PARSNIP, CELERIAC AND APPLE SOUP
with Crispy Sage

This soup is a terrific introduction to the fall season. The nutty smoothness of parsnip pairs well with the tart sweetness of apple for a taste that is comforting, nourishing and good for the soul.

INGREDIENTS

1 Tbsp / 15 ml extra virgin olive oil
1 large leek, cleaned well and chopped (about 2 cups / 480 ml)
2 cloves garlic, chopped
2 parsnips, peeled and chopped
1 medium celeriac (also known as celery root), chopped
1 apple, peeled and chopped
1 heaping tsp / 6 ml each chopped fresh sage and chopped fresh thyme
3 cups / 720 ml low-sodium chicken or vegetable broth
1 tsp / 5 ml sea salt
½ tsp / 2.5 ml freshly ground black pepper
½ cup / 120 ml low-fat milk, or unsweetened soy, rice or almond milk
1 tsp / 5 ml fresh lemon juice
1 to 2 Tbsp / 15 to 30 ml unsalted butter or extra virgin olive oil
6 fresh sage leaves

METHOD

1. Heat olive oil in a medium soup pot over medium heat. Add leek and cook until soft but not brown, 4 to 5 minutes. Add garlic and cook for 1 minute longer. Add parsnips, celeriac, apple, sage, thyme, broth, salt and pepper. Stir to combine and bring soup to a boil. Reduce heat and partially cover to simmer until all vegetables are very soft, 25 to 30 minutes.

2. Transfer soup to a blender or use a hand-held immersion blender to purée soup until very smooth. Add milk and lemon juice, and blend again to combine. Taste, and make any final adjustments to seasoning with salt, pepper and lemon juice.

3. In a very small low-sided saucepan or skillet, melt 1 to 2 Tbsp / 15 to 30 ml butter (enough to completely cover the bottom of your pan once melted) over medium heat and add sage leaves. Swirl pan to coat leaves in butter. Allow sage to sizzle gently making sure butter does not burn. As soon as butter starts to brown, immediately remove it from heat. (If using olive oil, it won't brown as butter does, so cook sage leaves until they're crispy and then remove from heat.)

4. To serve, ladle soup into bowls, top each with a crispy sage leaf and use a spoon to drizzle browned butter over top. Serve immediately.

NUTRITIONAL VALUE
PER SERVING:
Calories: 115 |
Calories from Fat: 42 |
Protein: 2 g | Carbs: 16 g |
Total Fat: 5 g |
Saturated Fat: 1 g |
Trans Fat: 0 g |
Fiber: 3 g |
Sodium: 581 mg |
Cholesterol: 0 mg

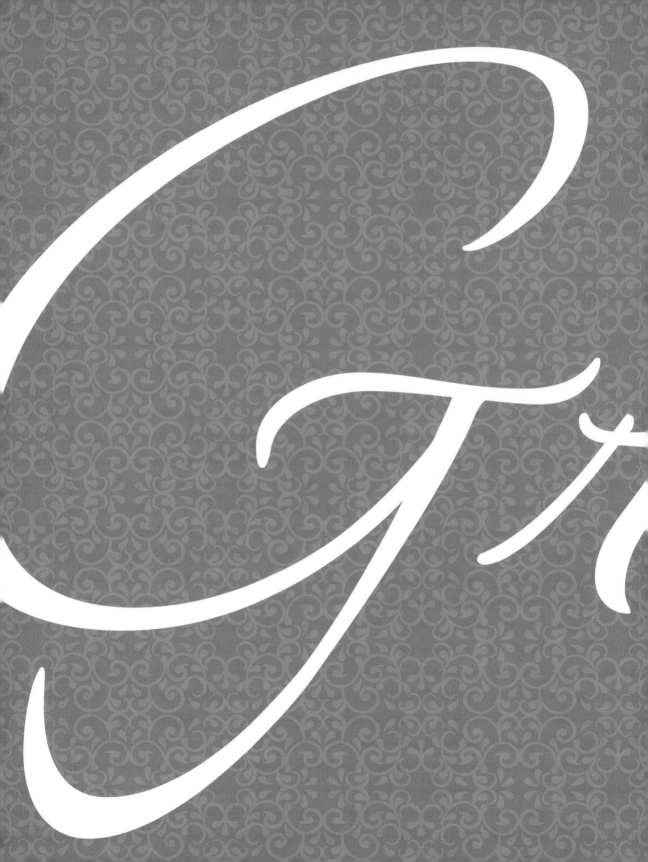

4

Grains & Legumes

100   ISRAELI COUSCOUS SALAD

103   OAT GROAT RISOTTO
with Mushrooms

104   FRESH FAVA BEANS
with Lemon Anchovy Vinaigrette

107   GREEK BROWN RICE DOLMAS

108   TABOULI
with Quinoa

111   SPANISH RICE

112   THREE BEAN SALAD
with Grilled Corn and Peppers

115   QUINOA
with Sausage and Peppers

ISRAELI COUSCOUS SALAD

Servings: 4 x ½ cup
Prep time: 20 minutes
Cooking time:
25-30 minutes

Israeli couscous or "ptitim" was invented in Israel in the 1950s as a substitute for rice, which was scarce at the time. This couscous is made by roasting hard wheat flour in an oven. In Israel, ptitim is mainly a food for children. In North America, it's considered a gourmet delicacy used by top chefs!

INGREDIENTS

1 sweet potato, peeled and
   diced into ½-inch cubes
Eat-Clean Cooking Spray (see page 348)
Pinch + ¼ tsp / 1.25 ml sea salt
Pinch + ⅛ tsp / 0.625 ml freshly
   ground black pepper
1 tsp / 5 ml + 1 Tbsp / 15 ml extra
   virgin olive oil, divided
1⅓ cup / 320 ml Israeli couscous
1¾ cups / 420 ml boiling water
1 bay leaf

Zest of ½ orange
⅓ cup / 80 ml freshly squeezed
   orange juice
¼ cup / 60 ml red wine vinegar
½ cup / 120 ml pitted dried cherries
¼ cup / 60 ml dried currants
¼ cup / 60 ml roasted, shelled
   pistachios, chopped
¼ cup / 60 ml finely chopped scallions
1 Tbsp / 15 ml chopped flat leaf parsley

METHOD

1. Preheat oven to 375°F / 190°C. Place diced sweet potato on a baking sheet and spray liberally with Eat-Clean Cooking Spray; season with a pinch of salt and pepper. Toss to combine and spread out in a single layer. Roast in oven for 10 to 12 minutes until soft and lightly browned. Remove and set aside.

2. Heat 1 tsp / 5 ml olive oil in a heavy-bottomed medium saucepan over medium-high heat. Add Israeli couscous, stir to coat with oil and then toast, stirring, for 3 minutes. Slowly pour in boiling water and add bay leaf. Cover, reduce heat to very low and simmer for 12 minutes or until the water is absorbed and the couscous is cooked through but still holds its shape. Uncover, fluff gently with a wooden spoon, cover and set aside.

3. While couscous is cooking, in a small saucepan place orange zest, orange juice, vinegar, cherries and currants and bring to a boil over medium-high heat. Remove from heat and let sit until cherries and currants are plumped up, about 3 minutes. Drain, reserving the liquid.

4. Scrape couscous into a large bowl and add the roasted sweet potatoes, drained cherries and currants. Add the pistachios, scallions, remaining salt and pepper, and parsley. Add 2 Tbsp / 30 ml reserved orange and vinegar mixture and remaining 1 Tbsp / 15 ml olive oil. Toss to combine. If salad is not moist enough, add another 1 Tbsp / 15 ml of reserved orange and vinegar mixture. Can be served at room temperature or chilled.

NUTRITIONAL VALUE
PER SERVING:
Calories: 189 |
Calories from Fat: 40 |
Protein: 5 g | Carbs: 29 g |
Total Fat: 5 g |
Saturated Fat: 1 g |
Trans Fat: 0 g | Fiber: 2 g |
Sodium: 83 mg |
Cholesterol: 0 mg

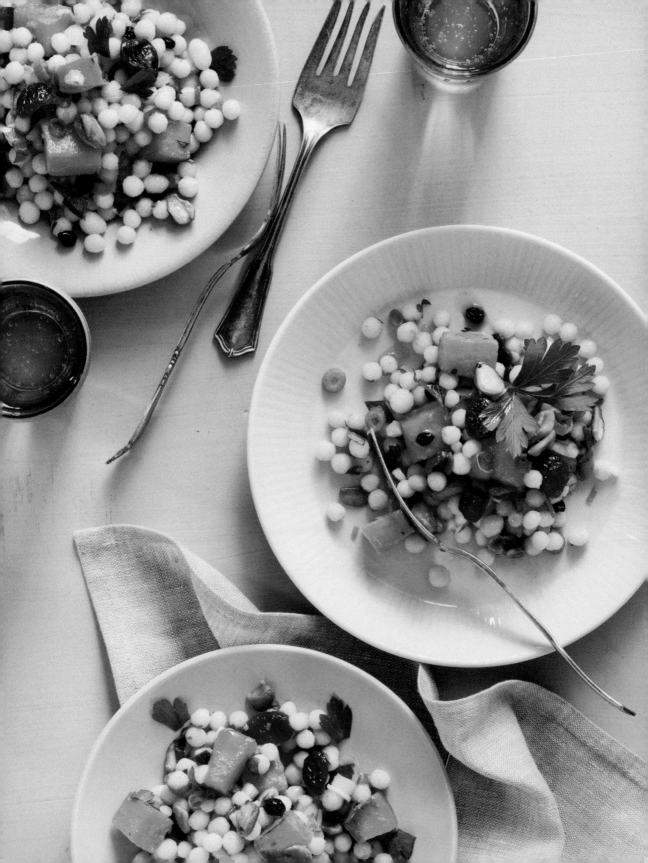

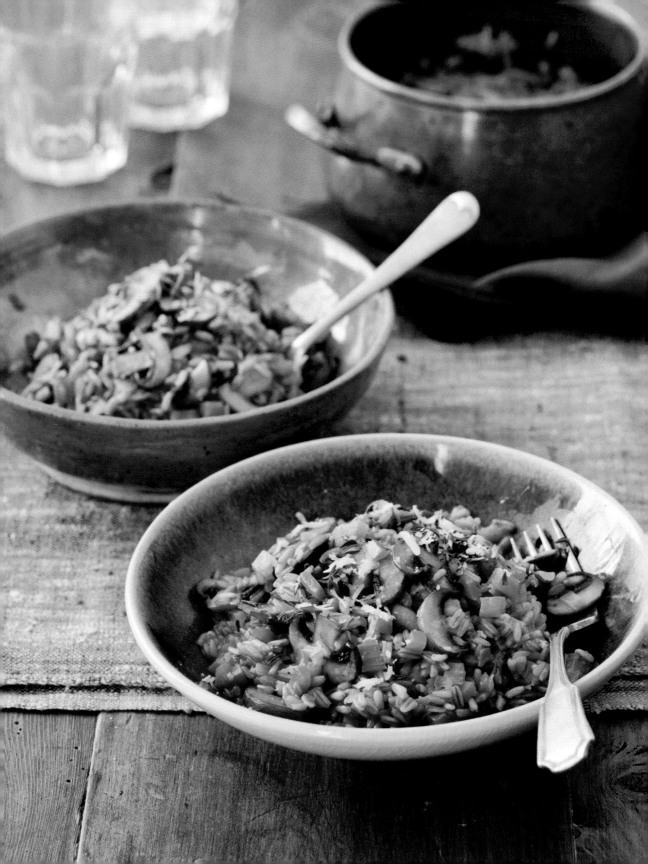

Servings: 5 x 1 cup
Prep time: 15 minutes
Cooking time:
50-55 minutes

OAT GROAT RISOTTO
with Mushrooms

I love trying different types of grains. Oat groats are whole oats that have been minimally processed, which means they are highly nutritious and perfect for a wide variety of Clean dishes. You can find oat groats in bulk food stores and the cereal section of some grocery stores.

INGREDIENTS

1 Tbsp / 15 ml plus 1 tsp / 5 ml extra virgin olive oil, divided
2 cups / 480 ml cremini mushrooms, thinly sliced
1 medium onion, diced into ½-inch pieces
1 medium carrot, diced into ½-inch pieces
1 rib celery, diced into ½-inch pieces
1½ cups / 360 ml whole oat groats
1 tsp / 5 ml fresh thyme
3 cups / 720 ml low-sodium mushroom or vegetable broth
½ cup / 120 ml dry white wine
1 tsp / 5 ml sea salt
¼ tsp / 1.25 ml freshly ground black pepper

METHOD

1. Heat 1 Tbsp / 15 ml olive oil in a large skillet over medium heat. Add mushrooms in a single layer and sauté until browned, about 3 minutes. Remove to a small bowl and set aside.

2. Return skillet to stove over medium heat and add remaining 1 tsp / 5 ml olive oil. Add onion, carrot and celery, and cook until soft but not brown, about 3 minutes. Add oat groats and thyme, and stir into vegetables, toasting oats for 3 minutes. Add mushrooms and any juices back into skillet. Add white wine and allow it to be absorbed by oats. Add broth, salt and pepper to oat groat mixture, and stir to combine.

3. Bring to a boil, then cover skillet and reduce heat to simmer until mixture is tender but still chewy, stirring occasionally, 40 to 45 minutes. When risotto is done, mixture will be "loose." If broth gets completely absorbed, add more broth to "loosen." Serve topped with freshly grated Parmesan, if desired.

NUTRITIONAL VALUE
PER SERVING:
Calories: 161 |
Calories from Fat: 43 |
Protein: 4 g | Carbs: 7 g |
Total Fat: 5 g |
Saturated Fat: 0.5 g |
Trans Fat: 0 g | Fiber: 3 g |
Sodium: 483 mg |
Cholesterol: 0 mg

Servings: 4 x ½ cup
Prep time: 20 minutes
Cooking time:
3 minutes

FRESH FAVA BEANS
with Lemon Anchovy Vinaigrette

Fava beans, also known as Windsor beans, broad beans, pigeon beans and horse beans, are actually a member of the pea family! They've been around for a long time – all the way back to ancient Greece and Rome – and their interesting flavor and creamy texture makes them a delightful addition to soups and grain salads. Here, however, they are the star.

INGREDIENTS

2 cups / 480 ml shucked fresh fava beans (2 lbs / 908 g fava bean pods)
1½ Tbsp / 22.5 ml fresh lemon juice
1 Tbsp / 15 ml extra virgin olive oil
1 small clove garlic, minced
⅛ tsp / 0.625 ml anchovy paste
¼ tsp / 1.25 ml sea salt
¼ tsp / 1.25 ml freshly ground black pepper
1 tsp / 5 ml finely chopped tarragon
2 Tbsp / 30 ml shaved curls of Pecorino Romano cheese (if desired)

METHOD

1. Fill a large bowl with ice water. Bring a pot of water to boil over high heat. Add fava beans to boiling water and cook until tender, about 3 minutes. Drain and place beans in ice water bath. Let cool then drain again. Press beans out of their membranes and add to a medium bowl.

2. In a small bowl, whisk together lemon juice, olive oil, garlic, anchovy paste, salt and pepper. Pour over fava beans and add tarragon. Gently toss to combine all ingredients. Divide mixture among four plates and serve. If desired, shave curls of Pecorino Romano overtop.

NUTRITIONAL VALUE
PER SERVING:
Calories: 134 |
Calories from Fat: 36 |
Protein: 10 g | Carbs: 18 g |
Total Fat: 4 g |
Saturated Fat: 0.5 g |
Trans Fat: 0 g | Fiber: 5 g |
Sodium: 188 mg |
Cholesterol: 0 mg

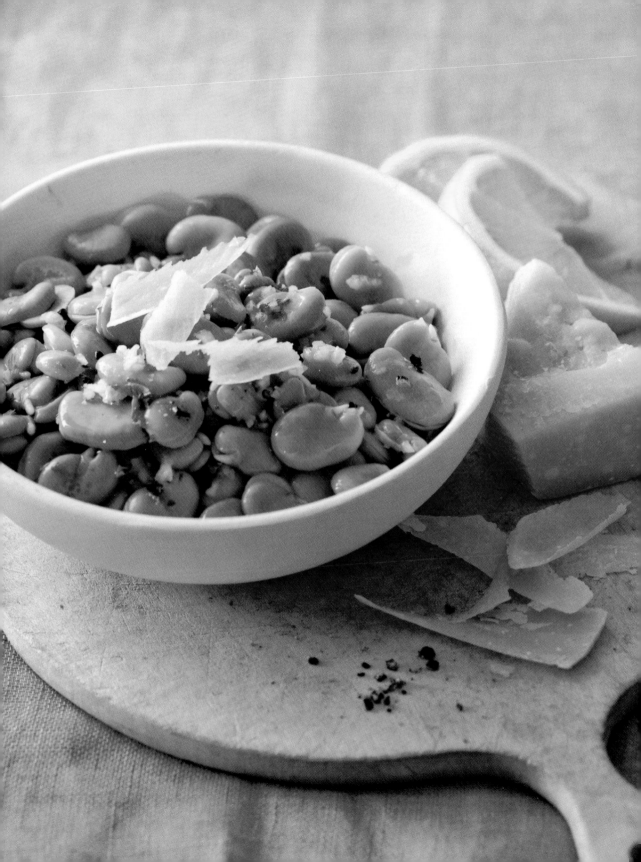

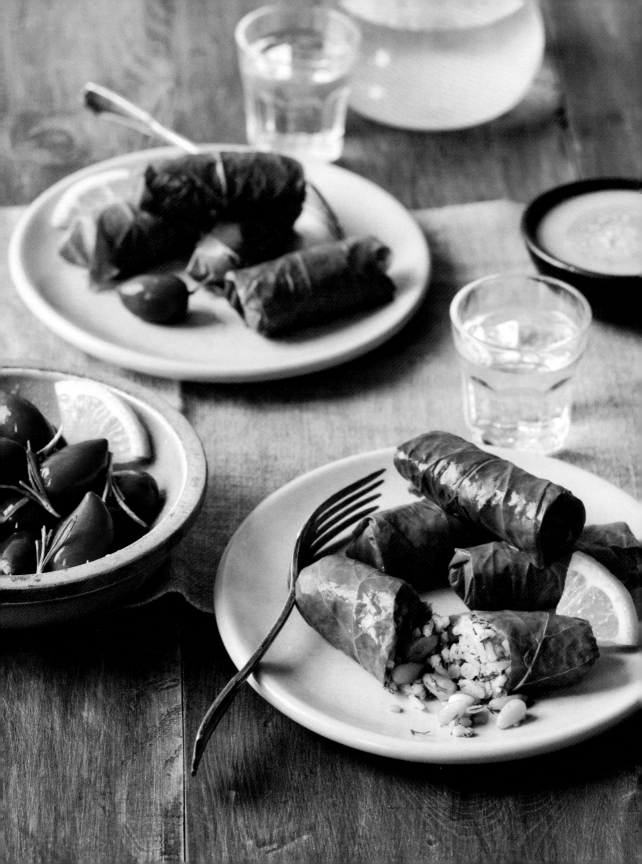

Servings: 8 x 6 dolmas
Prep time: 45 minutes
Cooking time:
65-70 minutes

GREEK BROWN RICE DOLMAS

Popular in Mediterranean cuisine, dolmas are stuffed grape leaves, usually containing a mixture of lamb and rice. This vegetarian version is packed with onions, nuts, seasonings and fresh herbs.

INGREDIENTS

2 Tbsp / 30 ml extra virgin olive oil, divided
½ large red onion, finely chopped
4 green onions, finely chopped
2 cups / 480 ml cooked brown rice
3 Tbsp / 45 ml chopped fresh mint
3 Tbsp / 45 ml chopped fresh dill
Zest of 1 lemon
Juice of 2 lemons, divided
¼ cup / 60 ml lightly toasted pine nuts
½ tsp / 2.5 ml sea salt
¼ tsp / 1.25 ml freshly ground black pepper
50 grape leaves, drained
¼ cup / 60 ml low-sodium vegetable broth

METHOD

1. Preheat oven to 350°F / 175°C.

2. Heat 1 Tbsp / 30 ml olive oil in a large skillet over medium heat. Add red and green onion, and cook until soft but not brown, 5 to 7 minutes. Remove from heat and add rice, mint, dill, lemon zest, juice of one lemon, pine nuts, salt and pepper. Stir to combine.

3. Rinse grape leaves in warm water and drain again. Separate leaves and lay them out on a clean working surface with stems toward you and veins facing up. Place 1 Tbsp / 15 ml of rice mixture in center of leaf and fold stem side over filling. Bring sides of leaf toward center and roll up tightly, like a cigar. Place dolma seam side down in a large baking dish. Repeat until all filling is used.

4. Add broth, remaining olive oil and lemon juice to baking dish, and then add enough water to almost cover dolmas. Cover tightly and place in oven to cook for one hour. Let dolmas cool to room temperature in cooking liquid. Transfer to a large platter and serve with Tahini Sauce for dipping (see recipe on page 354).

NUTRITIONAL VALUE
PER SERVING:
Calories: 140 |
Calories from Fat: 61 |
Protein: 3 g | Carbs: 18 g |
Total Fat: 7 g |
Saturated Fat: 0.5 g |
Trans Fat: 0 g | Fiber: 3 g |
Sodium: 126 mg |
Cholesterol: 0 mg

Servings: 6 x 1¼ cups
Prep time: 20 minutes
Cooking time:
10-12 minutes
Resting time:
5 minutes

TABOULI
with Quinoa

Tabouli, often spelled tabbouleh, is a grain salad made with bulgur, parsley, mint, tomato, onion, lemon juice and olive oil. I've swapped the bulgur (a good-for-you grain) for protein-packed quinoa to make this dish a healthy side or a complete Clean meal on its own. Fun fact: According to the Guinness Book of World Records, *the largest recorded dish of tabouli weighed 7,842 pounds!*

INGREDIENTS
¼ cup / 60 ml quinoa
½ cup / 120 ml water
1 bunch green onions, thinly sliced
1 English cucumber, seeded and chopped
1 cup / 240 ml chopped tomatoes
2 cups / 480 ml chopped curly parsley
½ cup / 120 ml chopped fresh mint
1 clove garlic, minced
¼ cup / 60 ml fresh lemon juice
2 Tbsp / 30 ml extra virgin olive oil
1 tsp / 5 ml sea salt
⅛ tsp / 0.625 ml freshly ground black pepper

METHOD

1. Combine quinoa and water in a small saucepan and bring to a boil. Reduce heat and cover to simmer for 10 to 12 minutes until almost all water is absorbed. Remove from heat, fluff, cover and let stand for 5 minutes to finish absorbing water and plump up.

2. In a large bowl, add green onions, cucumber, tomatoes, parsley and mint. Add cooked quinoa. In a small bowl, whisk together garlic, lemon juice, olive oil, salt and pepper, and pour over tabouli in large bowl. Toss to combine. Tabouli can be served immediately but is also delicious the next day.

NUTRITIONAL VALUE
PER SERVING:
Calories: 59 |
Calories from Fat: 43 |
Protein: 2 g | Carbs: 9 g |
Total Fat: 7 g |
Saturated Fat: 1 g |
Trans Fat: 0 g | Fiber: 2 g |
Sodium: 327 mg |
Cholesterol: 0 mg

NOTE *Curly parsley holds its shape better in this dish than flat leaf parsley, and is traditionally used in tabouli.*

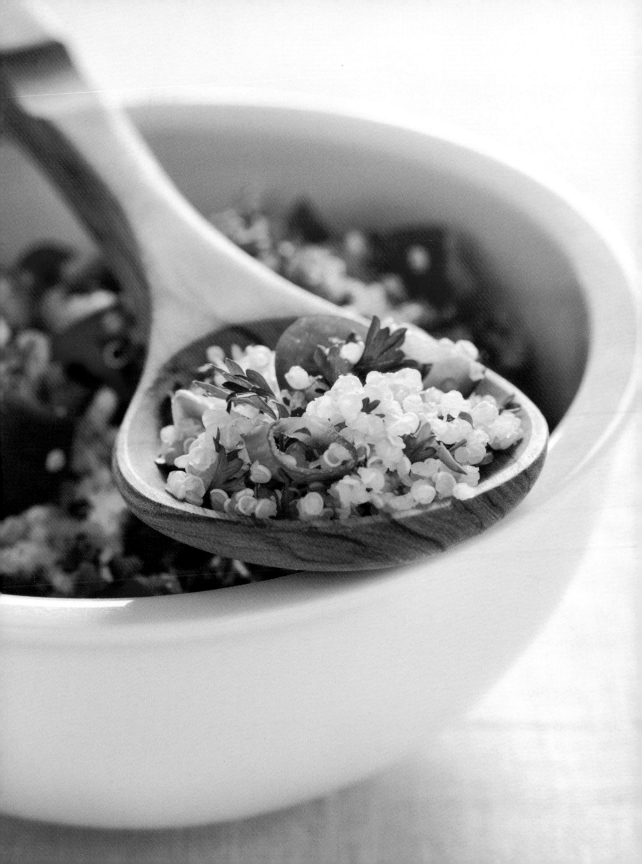

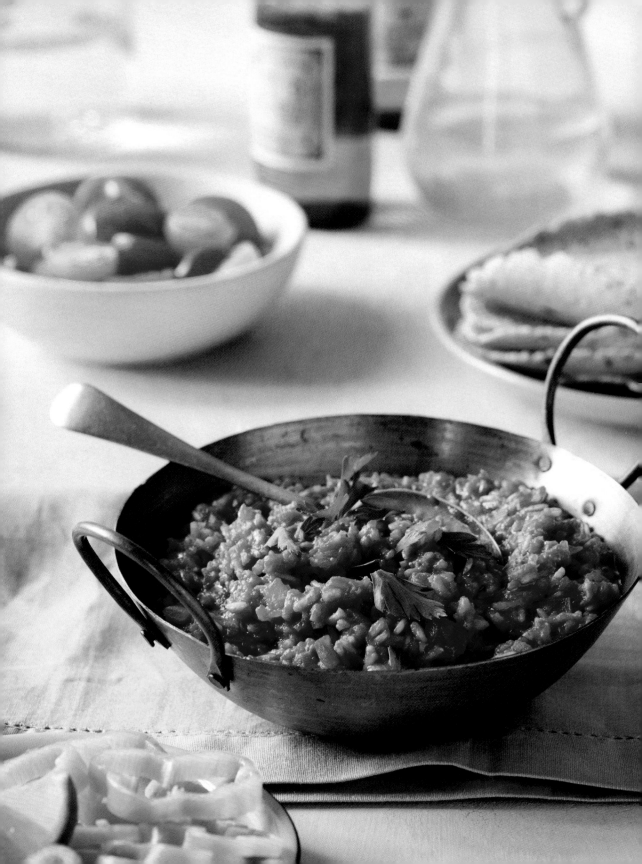

SPANISH RICE

Popular in the American southwest and unknown in Spain (despite its name!), Spanish rice is a side made with rice, spices and vegetables. It's typically made with white rice but I've Cleaned it up by using long-grain brown rice – an easy switch for added fiber and nutrients.

Servings: 7 x ½ cup
Prep time: 10 minutes
Cooking time:
55 minutes
Resting time:
5-10 minutes

INGREDIENTS

1 Tbsp / 15 ml extra virgin olive oil
½ large yellow onion, finely chopped
3 cloves garlic, minced
1 cup / 240 ml unrinsed long-grain brown rice
1 bay leaf
2 cups / 480 ml diced tomatoes (if using canned, make sure to purchase BPA-free cans)
⅓ cup / 80 ml low-sodium chicken broth
1 tsp / 5 ml sea salt
½ tsp / 2.5 ml freshly ground black pepper

METHOD

1. Heat olive oil in a medium heavy-bottomed saucepan over medium-high heat. Add onion and cook until translucent, stirring occasionally, about 3 minutes. Add garlic and cook for 30 seconds. Stir in rice and bay leaf and cook for 1 minute. Add tomatoes, chicken broth, salt and pepper. Bring to a boil, cover, then reduce to a gentle simmer and cook for 50 minutes.

2. Remove from heat and let sit for 5 to 10 minutes, covered, until all liquid is absorbed and rice is tender but not mushy. Uncover, fluff with a fork and serve.

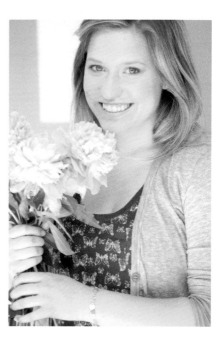

NUTRITIONAL VALUE
PER SERVING:
Calories: 65 |
Calories from Fat: 20 |
Protein: 2 g | Carbs: 10 g |
Total Fat: 2 g |
Saturated Fat: 0 g |
Trans Fat: 0 g | Fiber: 1 g |
Sodium: 301 mg |
Cholesterol: 0 mg

Servings: 6 x 1 cup
Prep time: 20 minutes
Cooking time:
5-7 minutes

THREE BEAN SALAD
with Grilled Corn and Peppers

Bean salads are remarkably easy to put together. Here I've used creamy pinto beans, rich black beans and kidney beans, which easily absorb the flavors of dressings, oils and herbs. This dish is sure to be a hit at your next summer BBQ.

INGREDIENTS

2 ears corn, husked
½ red pepper, seeds and ribs removed
½ green pepper, seeds and ribs removed
1 poblano pepper, seeds and ribs removed, halved
1 jalapeño pepper, seeds and ribs removed, halved
Eat-Clean Cooking Spray (see page 348)
1 cup / 240 ml each, cooked pinto, kidney and black beans
¼ cup / 60 ml red onion, diced into ¼-inch pieces
2 scallions, finely chopped
2 Tbsp / 30 ml extra virgin olive oil
2 Tbsp / 30 ml cider vinegar
Juice of 1 lime
1 tsp / 5 ml ground cumin
1 tsp / 5 ml chili powder
1½ tsp / 7.5 ml sea salt
½ tsp / 2.5 ml freshly ground black pepper

METHOD

1. Preheat a grill or grill pan to medium-high heat. Place corn and all pepper halves on a baking sheet and spray with Eat-Clean Cooking Spray. Place vegetables on grill and cook 5 to 7 minutes, turning peppers once and corn two or three times. Remove and let sit until cool enough to handle.

2. Cut kernels from corn and add to a large bowl. Cut peppers into half-inch pieces and add to bowl. Add beans, red onion and scallions. Add rest of ingredients and toss well to combine. Salad can be served immediately, though flavors will develop as the salad sits, so it will be even more flavorful the next day. Salad can be kept, covered, in the refrigerator for up to five days.

NUTRITIONAL VALUE
PER SERVING:
Calories: 224 |
Calories from Fat: 58 |
Protein: 9 g | Carbs: 34 g |
Total Fat: 7 g |
Saturated Fat: 1 g |
Trans Fat: 0 g | Fiber: 9 g |
Sodium: 483 mg |
Cholesterol: 0 mg

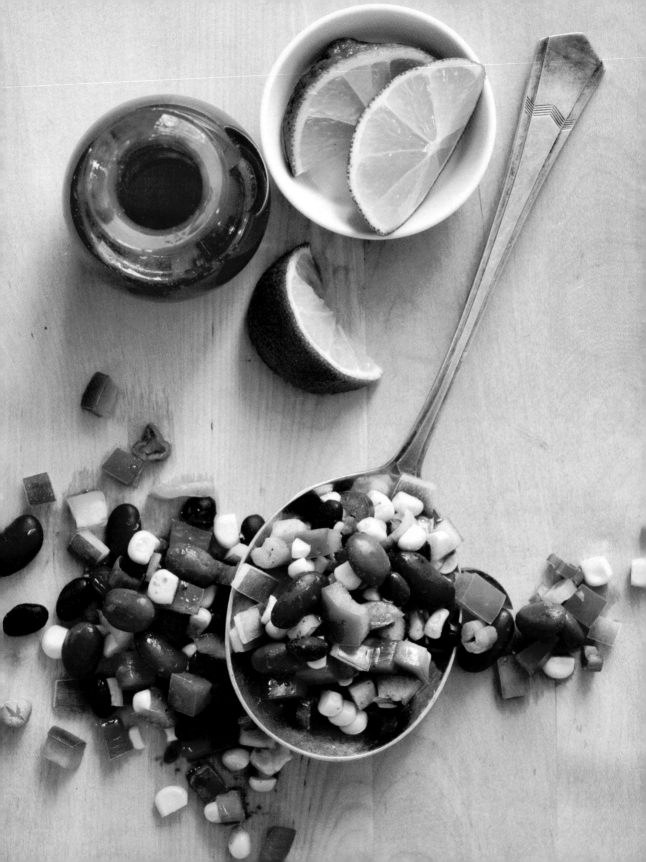

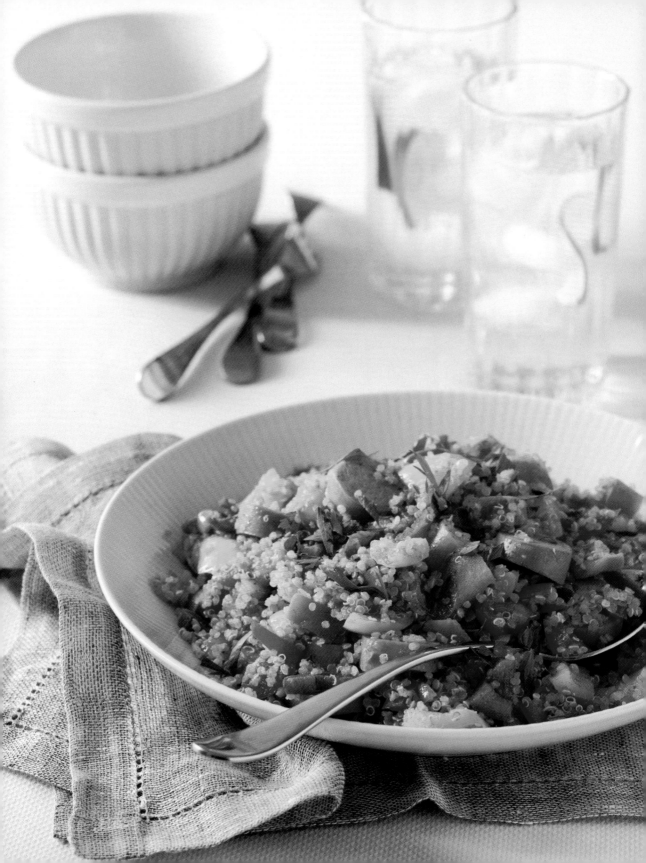

Servings: 4 x 1⅓ cups
Prep time: 20 minutes
Cooking time:
15-20 minutes

QUINOA
with Sausage and Peppers

I've said it before and I'll say it again: quinoa is a power food. It tastes like a grain but it's a complete protein; it's high in calcium and iron, and it's a good source of vitamins B and E. This dish is a protein powerhouse, guaranteed to fill you up and help you stay that way until your next meal.

INGREDIENTS

1 cup / 240 ml quinoa
Eat-Clean Cooking Spray (see page 348)
1 lb / 16 oz low-fat all-natural chicken
   or turkey sausages in casings
1 cup / 240 ml pale ale, amber ale,
   or other flavorful ale or beer (can
   substitute low-sodium chicken stock)
1 tsp / 5 ml extra virgin olive oil
1 jalapeño, halved and sliced
   (for a less spicy dish, remove
   seeds and membranes)
1 red chili pepper, halved and sliced
   (for a less spicy dish, remove
   the seeds and membranes)

½ green pepper, seeded and chopped
½ yellow or orange pepper,
   seeded and chopped
½ medium yellow onion, chopped
3 cloves garlic, chopped
1 tsp / 5 ml smoked paprika, divided
1 tsp / 5 ml chili powder, divided
½ tsp / 2.5 ml ground coriander
¼ tsp / 1.25 ml dried Italian seasoning
1 tsp / 5 ml sea salt
¼ tsp / 1.25 ml freshly ground
   black pepper
1 large tomato, diced

METHOD

1. In a medium saucepan, combine quinoa and 1½ cups / 360 ml water. Bring to a boil, cover and reduce heat to simmer until all water is absorbed and quinoa is plump, 10 to 15 minutes. Remove from heat, fluff with a fork, cover and set aside.

2. In the meantime, heat a large skillet over medium-high heat. Spray with Eat-Clean Cooking Spray and add sausages in a single layer. Cook until browned on both sides, turning at least once, about 4 to 5 minutes. Add ½ cup / 120 ml ale, cover, and reduce heat to simmer until sausages are cooked through and ale has almost completely evaporated, 5 to 10 minutes. Remove sausages to a cutting board and cut into half-inch pieces.

3. Return skillet to stove over medium-high heat and add olive oil. Add jalapeño, red chili, green and yellow peppers, and onion. Sauté, stirring occasionally, until soft and starting to brown, about 5 minutes. Add garlic, ½ tsp / 2.5 ml paprika, ½ tsp / 2.5 ml chili powder, coriander, Italian seasoning, salt and pepper. Stir to combine and cook for 2 minutes. Add tomato and remaining ½ cup / 120 ml ale, and using a sturdy spoon, scrape up any crusty bits from bottom of skillet. Simmer until ale is reduced by half.

4. Transfer quinoa to a large serving bowl and add remaining ½ tsp / 2.5 ml smoked paprika and ½ tsp / 2.5 ml chili powder. Add sliced sausages and pepper mixture, and toss to combine. Divide among plates and serve.

NUTRITIONAL VALUE
PER SERVING:
Calories: 187 |
Calories from Fat: 44 |
Protein: 17 g | Carbs: 14 g |
Total Fat: 5 g |
Saturated Fat: 1 g |
Trans Fat: 0 g | Fiber: 2 g |
Sodium: 1017 mg |
Cholesterol: 57 mg

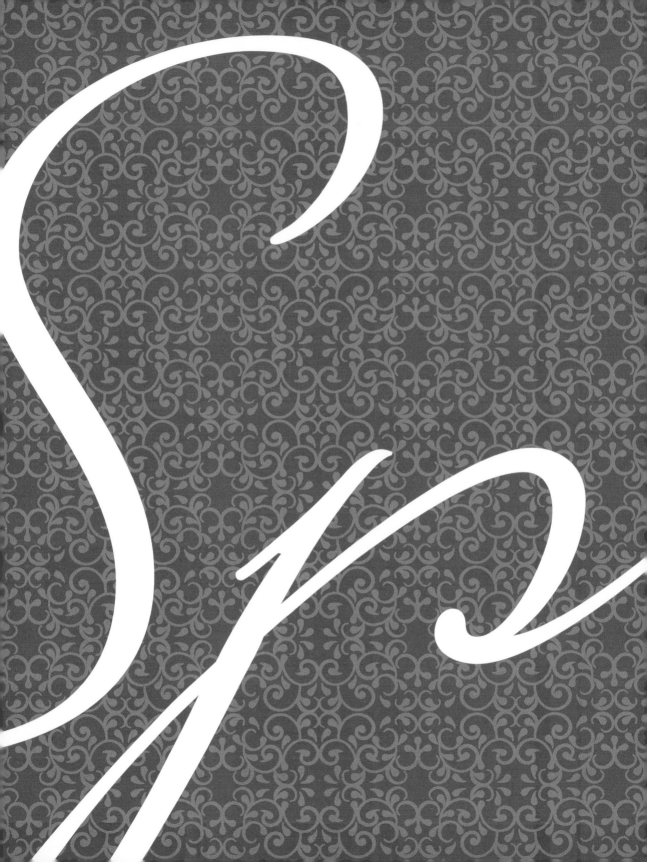

5

Sauces, Spreads & Salsas

118 SALSA ROJA

121 CREAMY GUACA-DE-GALLO

122 CLEAN MARINARA SAUCE

125 BABA GHANOUSH

126 BASIL LEMON PESTO

129 NO-COOK FRESH TOMATO SAUCE

130 CHICKEN LIVER PÂTÉ

133 SPICY CLEAN BBQ SAUCE

134 RAPINI PESTO

136 *Herbs*

SALSA ROJA

Servings: 6 x ½ cup
Prep time: 15 minutes
Cooking time:
6-7 minutes

The varieties of salsa are endless. Salsa roja, which means "red sauce" in Spanish, is used as a spicy condiment in Southwestern and Mexican cooking. It's delicious on tacos, burritos, fajitas, eggs, vegetables and grains, and adds a spicy, smoky zip to almost any dish.

INGREDIENTS

4 dried arbol chiles, stems removed
4 dried guajillo chiles, stems removed
2 dried pasilla chiles, stems removed
2 medium tomatoes, halved
½ yellow onion, peeled, cut into 4 wedges and layers separated
5 large cloves garlic, peeled
2 Tbsp / 30 ml fresh lime juice
2 Tbsp / 30 ml white vinegar
¼ tsp / 1.25 ml cayenne pepper
1 tsp / 5 ml sea salt

METHOD

1. Thoroughly heat a dry, non-oiled cast-iron skillet over medium heat. Add chiles to hot skillet and toast, stirring, until they are fragrant and dark in spots, 1 to 2 minutes. Remove to a heatproof bowl and cover with boiling water; let sit for 15 minutes while chiles rehydrate. Return skillet to burner and add tomatoes, cut side down. Cook until charred, about 1 minute, and then turn over and cook 1 minute longer. Transfer to a blender or food processor.

2. Add onion and garlic to skillet and allow to char and slightly soften, stirring occasionally, about 2 minutes. Transfer to blender with tomatoes. Drain chiles, reserving liquid. Add rehydrated chiles to blender. Add lime juice, vinegar, cayenne and salt. Blend until very smooth. Salsa should be spoonable. If too thick, add some of reserved chile liquid, a spoonful at a time, until desired consistency is achieved. Taste and adjust seasoning if necessary. Salsa will last in refrigerator, covered, for up to two weeks.

NUTRITIONAL VALUE
PER SERVING:
Calories: 34 |
Calories from Fat: 4 |
Protein: 1 g | Carbs: 7 g |
Total Fat: 0.4 g |
Saturated Fat: 0 g |
Trans Fat: 0 g | Fiber: 2 g |
Sodium: 267 mg |
Cholesterol: 0 mg

NOTE *If you desire a less spicy salsa, shake out most of the chiles' seeds and discard before starting this recipe.*

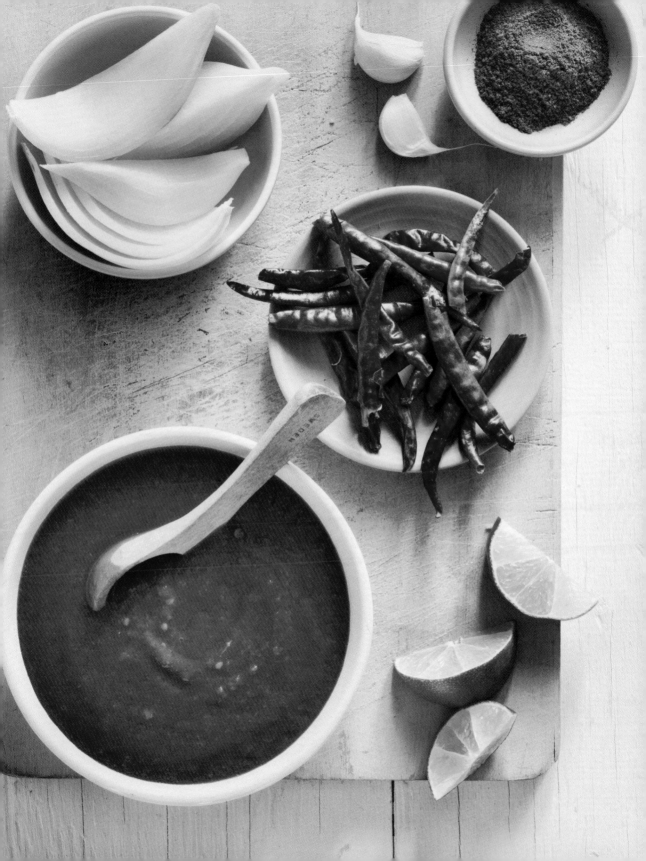

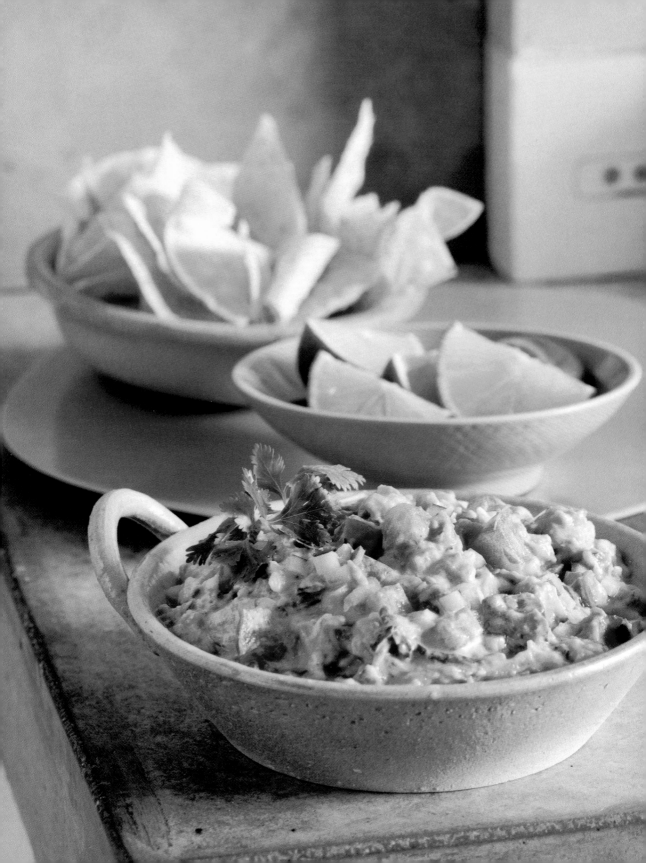

Servings: 12 x ¼ cup
Prep time: 20 minutes
Cooking time:
0 minutes

CREAMY GUACA-DE-GALLO

Guaca-de-Gallo is a cross between guacamole and pico de gallo, as the name suggests. It's spicy, fresh and perfect for your next party or no-guilt movie night.

INGREDIENTS

2 avocados, pitted
½ cup / 120 ml plain low-fat Greek yogurt or Yogurt Cheese (see recipe on page 348)
½ English cucumber, halved lengthwise, seeds removed
1 tomato, cored and diced (about 1 cup / 240 ml)
¼ cup / 60 ml diced red onion
1 jalapeño, seeds and membrane removed, diced
1 clove garlic, minced
¼ cup / 60 ml fresh lime juice
1 tsp / 5 ml sea salt
¼ tsp / 1.25 ml freshly ground black pepper

METHOD

1. Spoon avocado flesh out of skins and place in a medium bowl. Using a fork, mash avocados but keep slightly chunky. Add yogurt and mix in.

2. Grate cucumber and place in a colander. Using your hands, squeeze out liquid and allow it to drain away. (You can also use cheesecloth or a tea towel to squeeze liquid out.)

3. Add cucumber to avocado and yogurt mixture. Add tomato and rest of ingredients, and stir to thoroughly combine. Serve with baked pita chips or baked tortilla chips.

NUTRITIONAL VALUE
PER SERVING:
Calories: 68 |
Calories from Fat: 43 |
Protein: 2 g | Carbs: 5 g |
Total Fat: 5 g |
Saturated Fat: 1 g |
Trans Fat: 0 g | Fiber: 3 g |
Sodium: 138 mg |
Cholesterol: 0 mg

CLEAN MARINARA SAUCE

Servings: 6 x 1/2 cup
Prep time: 10 minutes
Cooking time:
35 minutes

There is nothing better than fresh marinara sauce – it's a very versatile ingredient. Once you realize how easy it is to make, you'll never go back to store-bought sauces again!

INGREDIENTS

1 Tbsp / 15 ml extra virgin olive oil
½ large yellow onion, diced
⅛ tsp / 0.625 ml red pepper flakes
1 large clove garlic, minced
1 Tbsp / 15 ml tomato paste
2 cups / 480 ml diced roma tomatoes (If using canned, make sure to use BPA-free cans.)
2 cups / 480 ml Clean bottled or homemade tomato sauce
1 Tbsp / 15 ml finely chopped fresh oregano leaves (or ½ tsp / 5 ml) dried
1 tsp / 5 ml sea salt
½ tsp / 2.5 ml freshly ground black pepper

METHOD

1. Heat olive oil in a medium saucepan with straight, shallow sides. Add onion and red pepper flakes, and sauté until onion is translucent, about 3 minutes. Add garlic and cook for 1 minute longer. Stir in tomato paste and allow it to cook for 1 minute. Add diced tomatoes, tomato sauce and oregano. Bring to a boil and reduce heat to simmer for 30 minutes, stirring occasionally.

2. Using a hand-held immersion blender, blend sauce until desired smoothness. (You can also use a stand blender, but you might have to work in batches, and be careful when blending because hot liquids can expand.) Season with salt and pepper. Sauce is ready to serve with pasta, grains, vegetables and more. Can be stored, covered, in refrigerator for up to one week, or in freezer for up to three months.

NUTRITIONAL VALUE
PER SERVING:
Calories: 67 |
Calories from Fat: 20 |
Protein: 1 g | Carbs: 11 g |
Total Fat: 2 g |
Saturated Fat: 0 g |
Trans Fat: 0 g | Fiber: 2 g |
Sodium: 307 mg |
Cholesterol: 0 mg

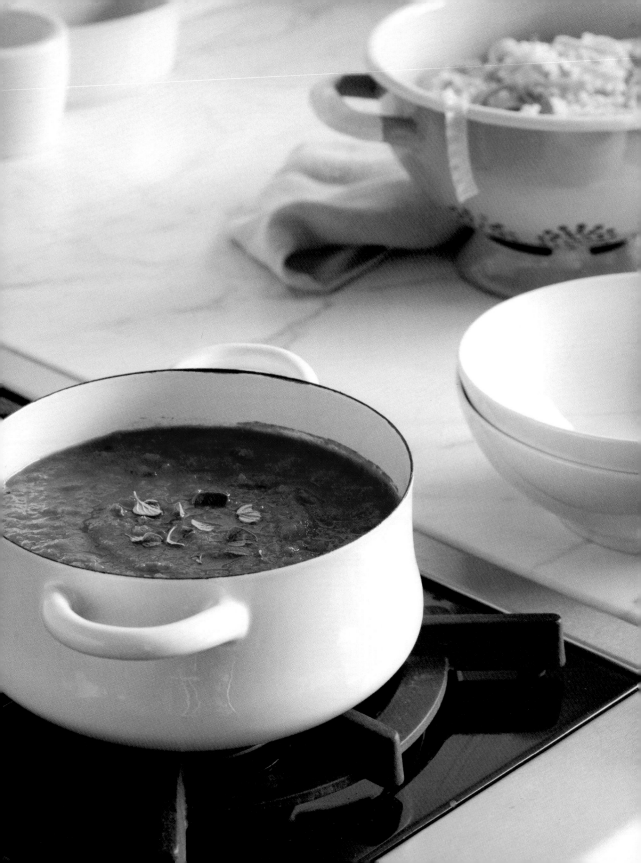

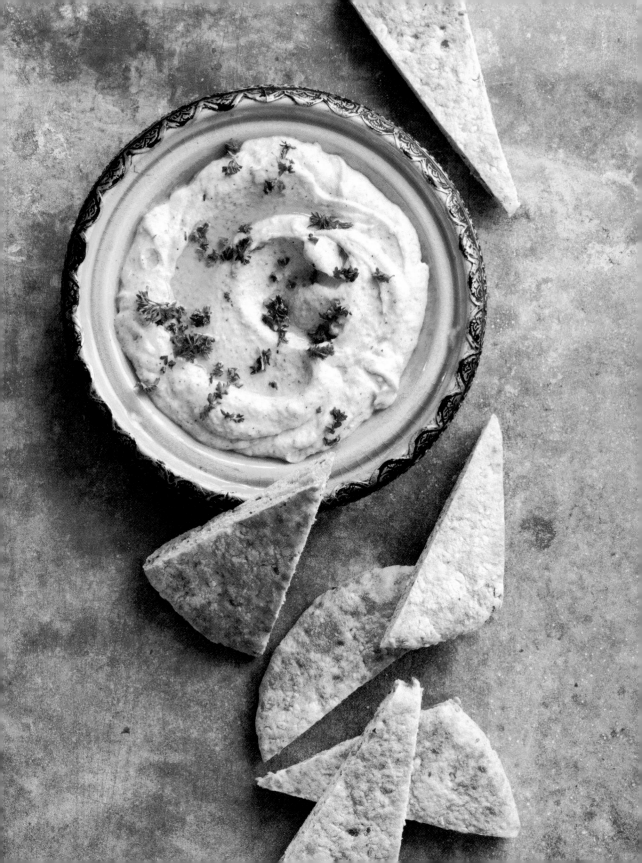

Servings: 12 x ¼ cup
Prep time: 5 minutes
Cooking time:
25-35 minutes

BABA GHANOUSH

Baba ghanoush is an eggplant-based dish that originated in the Middle East. In North America, it's used as a dip for pita and vegetables, but in Egypt it's a side dish. Grilling the eggplant before peeling the skin gives it a delightful, smoky flavor.

INGREDIENTS

1 large eggplant (1½ to 2 lbs / 681 to 908 g)
1 clove garlic, minced
¼ cup / 60 ml tahini
2 Tbsp / 30 ml fresh lemon juice
½ tsp / 2.5 ml ground cumin
¾ tsp / 3.75 ml sea salt
1 Tbsp / 15 ml extra virgin olive oil
1 Tbsp / 15 ml chopped fresh parsley

METHOD

1. Preheat the oven to 400°F / 200°C. Heat a grill or grill pan to medium-high heat. Using a fork, prick eggplant six to eight times. (This will keep the eggplant from exploding when it cooks.) Place eggplant on grill to char skin, turning two or three times, 10 to 15 minutes. When skin starts to easily peel away, it is charred well.

2. Using tongs, transfer eggplant to a baking sheet and finish cooking in the oven until very soft, 15 to 20 minutes. To test doneness, stick a bamboo skewer into center of widest part of eggplant and if it easily slides in without resistance, it is cooked through. Remove eggplant and let sit at room temperature until cool enough to handle. Peel away skin and discard.

3. Cut peeled eggplant into pieces to fit into a food processor or blender. Add garlic, tahini, lemon juice, cumin and salt, and blend until smooth. Scrape baba ghanoush into a shallow serving bowl and using a spoon, make a well in center. Drizzle olive oil over top and in center well. Sprinkle with fresh parsley. Serve with warm pita wedges or veggies, or use on a sprouted Ezekial tortilla to make a wrap.

NUTRITIONAL VALUE
PER SERVING:
Calories: 105 |
Calories from Fat: 72 |
Protein: 3 g | Carbs: 8 g |
Total Fat: 8 g |
Saturated Fat: 1 g |
Trans Fat: 0 g | Fiber: 4 g |
Sodium: 200 mg |
Cholesterol: 0 mg

Servings: 6 x 2 Tbsp
Prep time: 10 minutes
Cooking time:
0 minutes

BASIL LEMON PESTO

There is nothing quite so delicious as fresh pesto on whole wheat pasta. Best of all, it comes together quickly and doesn't require too many ingredients that aren't already in your cupboards. This light and lemony version also works well with chicken, fish and scallops.

INGREDIENTS

3 large cloves garlic
¼ cup / 60 ml pine nuts
3 cups / 720 ml fresh basil leaves, slightly packed
Juice and zest of ½ lemon
¾ tsp / 3.75 ml sea salt
⅛ tsp / 0.675 ml freshly ground black pepper
2 Tbsp / 30 ml extra virgin olive oil
¼ cup / 60 ml freshly grated Parmigiano Reggiano

METHOD

1. In a food processor, pulse garlic and pine nuts until chopped. Add basil, lemon juice and zest, salt and pepper. Pulse until chopped.

2. While processor is running, stream in olive oil until pesto is blended and fairly smooth. Stop processor and use a rubber spatula to scrape down sides. Add Parmigiano Reggiano and pulse blend until all ingredients are combined. Serve over pasta, as a sandwich spread, in wraps, on meats, or use your imagination! Can be refrigerated, covered, for up to one week.

NUTRITIONAL VALUE
PER SERVING:
Calories: 62 |
Calories from Fat: 41 |
Protein: 3 g | Carbs: 3 g |
Total Fat: 10 g |
Saturated Fat: 1 g |
Trans Fat: 0 g | Fiber: 1 g |
Sodium: 248 mg |
Cholesterol: 3 mg

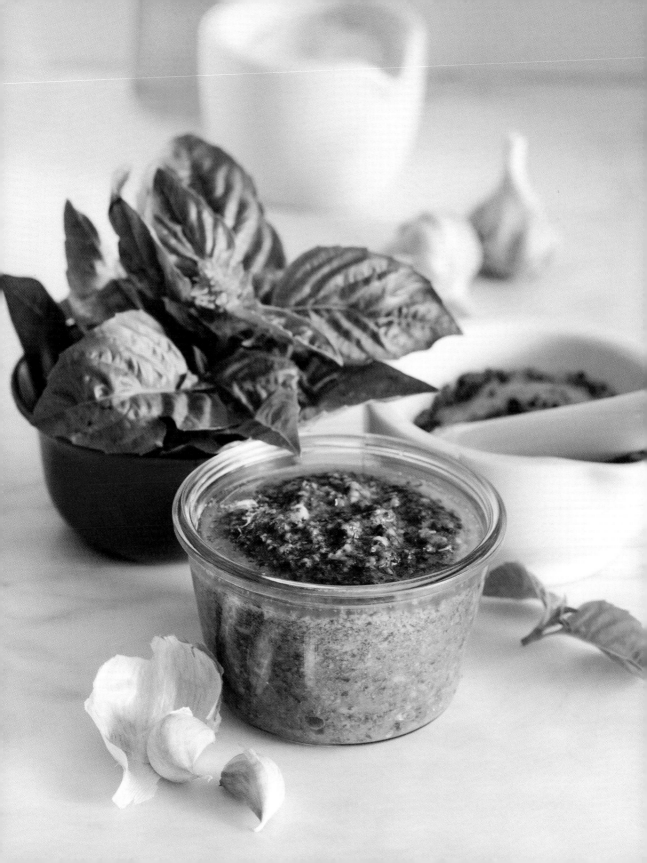

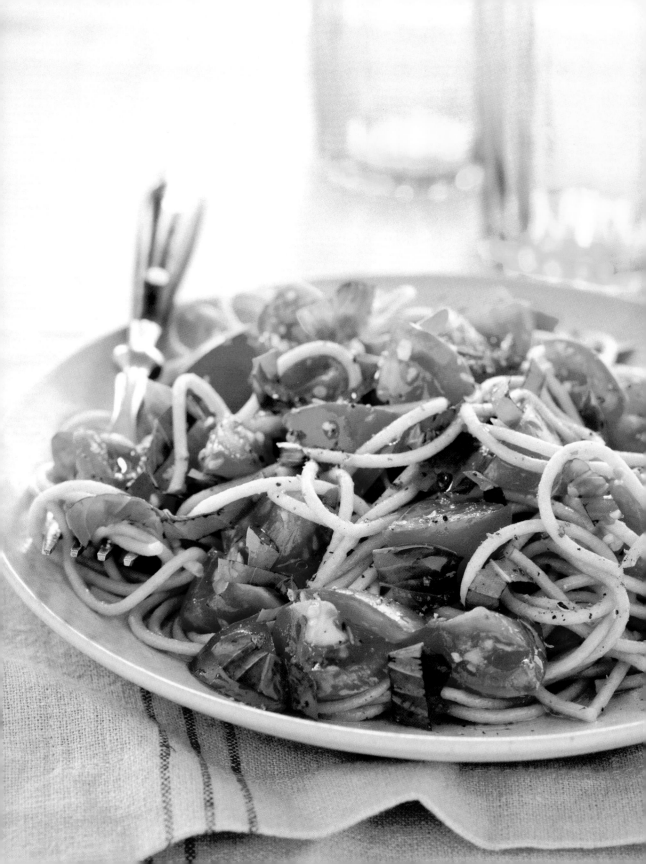

Servings: 4 x 1 cup
Prep time: 10 minutes
Cooking time:
0 minutes

NO-COOK FRESH TOMATO SAUCE

No cook – what's easier than that? This tomato sauce is fresh, fragrant and fabulous with a wide assortment of dishes. Plus it's ready in only 10 minutes! Try it on pizza, pasta, bruschetta and more.

INGREDIENTS

4 cups / 960 ml chopped tomatoes (bite-sized pieces)
1 clove garlic, grated fine or pressed through a garlic press
1 Tbsp / 15 ml extra virgin olive oil
½ tsp / 2.5 ml sea salt
¼ tsp / 1.25 ml freshly ground black pepper
Small handful fresh basil, thinly sliced

METHOD

1. In a large bowl, place all ingredients and toss to combine. Serve tossed with whole wheat pasta, or be creative and serve with cooked whole grains such as millet or wheat berries.

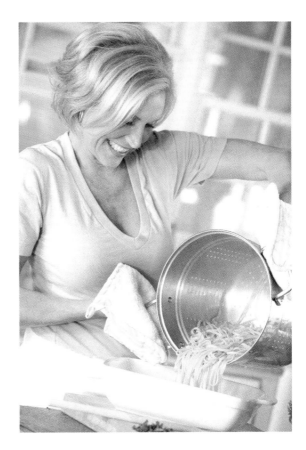

NUTRITIONAL VALUE
PER SERVING:

Calories: 63 |
Calories from Fat: 33 |
Protein: 2 g | Carbs: 7 g |
Total Fat: 4 g |
Saturated Fat: 1 g |
Trans Fat: 0 g | Fiber: 2 g |
Sodium: 205 mg |
Cholesterol: 0 mg

Servings: 14 x 2 Tbsp
Prep time: 10 minutes
Cooking time:
16 minutes
Chill time:
4 hours minimum

CHICKEN LIVER PÂTÉ

Perfect for hors d'oeuvres or appetizers, chicken liver pâté is one of the most famous party treats around. I've lightened up this version by using Yogurt Cheese and Neufchâtel cheese instead of their full-fat counterparts. Serve this pâté with sliced and toasted whole wheat French bread (crostini) or whole grain crackers, Dijon mustard and cornichons (small French pickles also known as gherkins).

Note: Yogurt Cheese must be made ahead of time.

INGREDIENTS

1 tsp / 5 ml extra virgin olive oil
½ medium yellow onion, thinly sliced
½ granny smith apple, cored and thinly sliced
10 oz / 284 g chicken livers (about 6 chicken livers)
1 clove garlic, chopped
¼ tsp / 1.25 ml smoked paprika
⅛ tsp / 0.625 ml curry powder
⅛ tsp / 0.625 ml cayenne pepper
½ tsp / 2.5 ml sea salt
⅛ tsp / 0.625 ml finely ground black pepper
2 Tbsp / 30 ml cognac
¼ cup / 60 ml Yogurt Cheese (see recipe on page 348)
¼ cup / 60 ml Neufchâtel cheese (low-fat cream cheese)

METHOD

1. Heat olive oil in a large nonstick skillet over medium-high heat. Add onion and apple and cook until soft, about 5 minutes. Add chicken livers, garlic, paprika, curry powder, cayenne, salt and pepper. Sauté until livers are cooked through and apples and onions are lightly browned, about 5 minutes. Stir in cognac and cook until absorbed, 1 minute.

2. Remove mixture from heat and scrape into a blender. Add Yogurt Cheese and Neufchâtel and blend until very smooth, at least 3 minutes. Stop blender, scrape down sides and blend for 1 minute longer to make sure all ingredients are completely incorporated. If pâté is not completely smooth at this point, use a rubber spatula to push it through a fine mesh sieve.

3. Scrape pâté into a shallow ceramic dish or a few ramekins, cover with plastic wrap, and refrigerate for at least 4 hours before serving to chill and set. If possible, refrigerate overnight. Can be refrigerated, covered, for up to five days.

NUTRITIONAL VALUE
PER SERVING:
Calories: 49 |
Calories from Fat: 21 |
Protein: 4 g | Carbs: 2 g |
Total Fat: 2 g |
Saturated Fat: 1 g |
Trans Fat: 0 g | Fiber: 0 g |
Sodium: 89 mg |
Cholesterol: 73 mg

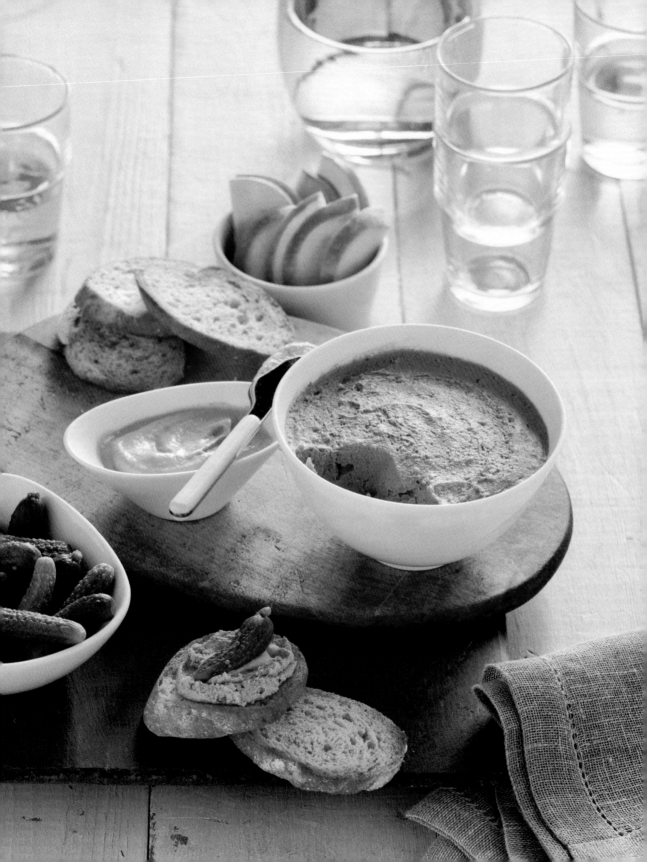

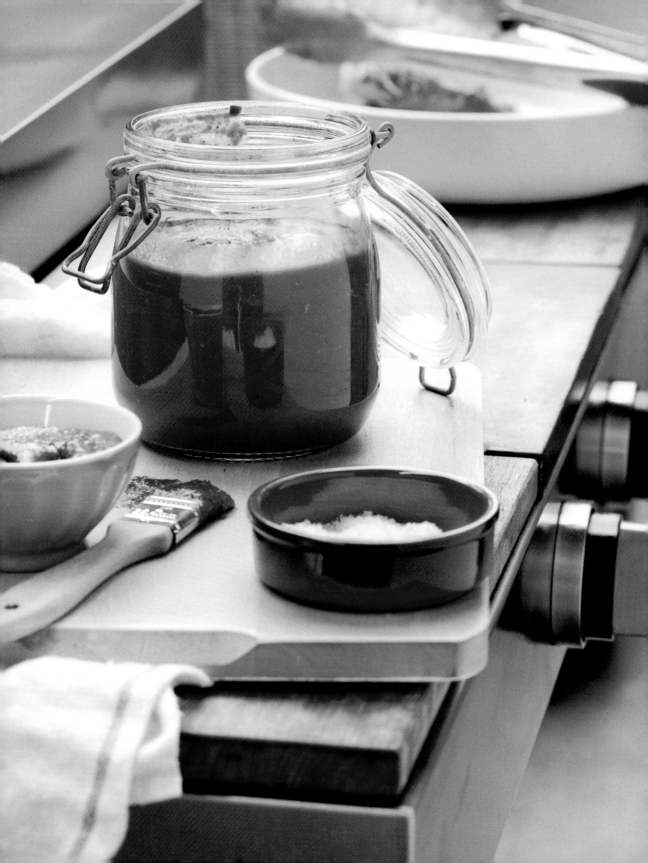

SPICY CLEAN BBQ SAUCE

Store-bought barbeque sauces are packed with added salt and sugar – two items that make it hard to reach your health and fitness goals. This Clean version is quick and easy, and packs some serious heat! For a less spicy sauce, use half the chipotle pepper.

INGREDIENTS

1 tsp / 5 ml safflower oil
½ large sweet onion, diced
2 cloves garlic, chopped
1 cup / 240 ml Clean bottled or homemade tomato sauce
1 chipotle pepper in adobo sauce, chopped
1 Tbsp / 15 ml deli mustard, or Dijon
1 Tbsp / 15 ml unfiltered cider vinegar
1 tsp / 5 ml Worcestershire sauce
2 Tbsp / 30 ml unsulfured blackstrap molasses
1 Tbsp / 15 ml honey
1 tsp / 5 ml chili powder
½ tsp / 2.5 ml smoked paprika or sweet paprika

METHOD

1. Heat safflower oil in a small saucepan over medium heat. Add onion and sauté until soft and starting to brown, 5 minutes. Add garlic and cook for 1 minute longer. Add rest of ingredients, stir to combine, and simmer for 15 minutes until slightly thickened.

2. Pour into a food processor or blender and blend until smooth. Can be stored in a sealed container in refrigerator for up to two weeks.

NUTRITIONAL VALUE
PER SERVING:
Calories: 50 |
Calories from Fat: 8 |
Protein: 1 g | Carbs: 10 g |
Total Fat: 1 g |
Saturated Fat: 0 g |
Trans Fat: 0 g | Fiber: 1 g |
Sodium: 47 mg |
Cholesterol: 0 mg

Servings: 12 x 2 Tbsp
Prep time: 10 minutes
Cooking time:
7 minutes

RAPINI PESTO

Rapini, a nutrient-rich vegetable commonly found in Italian and Chinese cuisine, has a strong and bitter flavor. It's a good match both for mild foods such as pasta, white beans and polenta, and stronger flavors such as garlic and chili spice. Try this pesto on sandwiches, pasta, salads, vegetables and potatoes.

INGREDIENTS

1 Tbsp / 15 ml pine nuts, toasted
1 bunch rapini
1 clove garlic, smashed
1 Tbsp / 15 ml white balsamic vinegar
1 Tbsp / 15 ml fresh lemon juice
2 tsp / 10 ml Dijon mustard
1 tsp / 5 ml sea salt
¼ tsp / 1.25 ml freshly ground black pepper
2 Tbsp / 30 ml extra virgin olive oil

METHOD

1. Preheat oven to 350°F / 175°C. Spread pine nuts on a baking sheet and toast in oven until golden brown, about 5 minutes. (Be careful not to burn!) Remove and set aside.

2. Bring a large pot of water to boil over high heat. Trim one inch from stalk ends of rapini. When water is at a rolling boil, submerge rapini and blanch for 2 minutes. Remove and plunge into a bowl of cold water. Drain, spin dry thoroughly in a salad spinner, or pat dry thoroughly with cloth or paper towels.

3. In a food processor, pulse garlic and toasted pine nuts until roughly chopped. Add rapini, vinegar, lemon juice, mustard, sea salt and pepper. Pulse until chopped. While processor is running, stream in olive oil until thoroughly combined. Stop processor to scrape down sides and then blend for another 10 seconds. Pesto will not be completely smooth. Can be stored, tightly covered, in refrigerator for up to one week.

NUTRITIONAL VALUE
PER SERVING:
Calories: 77 |
Calories from Fat: 54 |
Protein: 1 g | Carbs: 2 g |
Total Fat: 4 g |
Saturated Fat: 0.5 g |
Trans Fat: 0 g | Fiber: 1 g |
Sodium: 165 mg |
Cholesterol: 0 mg

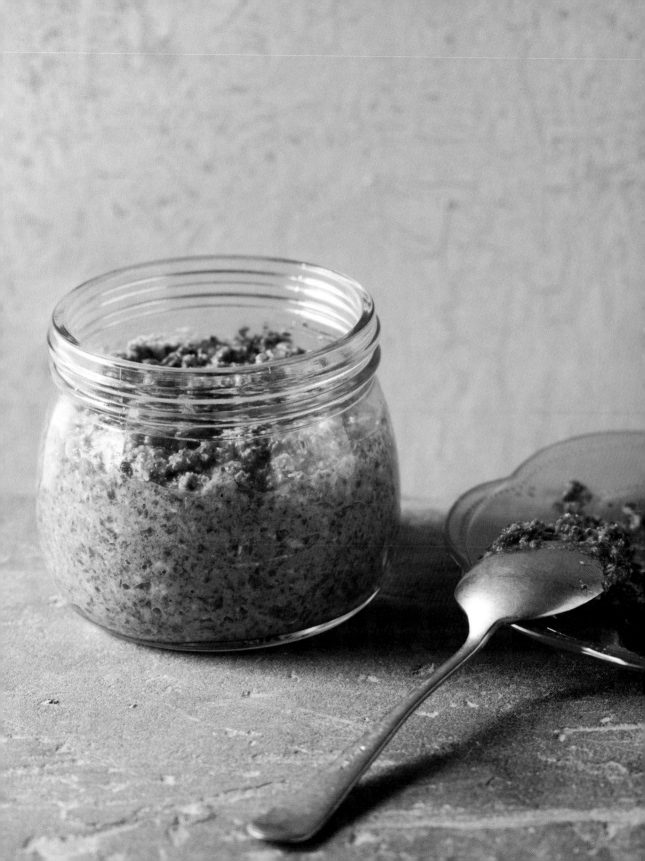

Herbs

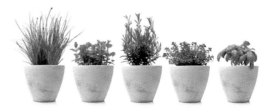

If your pantry is free of herbs then you are missing out on some of the most vibrant flavors in cooking. Herbs can add flare to your fare by boosting flavor, while also increasing the visual appeal of your meal. Additionally, they will boost the health benefits thanks to the high levels of phytonutrients, vitamins and minerals found in herbs.

I can understand if you are hesitant to introduce herbs to your cooking regimen. They can be confusing, especially when deciding which herb to pair with what dish. Let's see if I can clear that up for you here.

10 COMMON CULINARY HERBS, *Their Nutritional Benefits & How to Use:*

HERB	NUTRITIONAL BENEFIT	HOW TO USE
1 │ Arugula (Rocket)	Vitamins A & C	Salad green, in pasta, on pizza, in an omelet, arugula pesto
2 │ Basil	Vitamin K, vitamin A, calcium, iron / Antibacterial & anti-inflammatory	Basil pesto, on pizza, in pasta, in stir-fries, in tomato soup
3 │ Bay Leaves	Vitamin A, vitamin C, iron, manganese, calcium, potassium, magnesium / Anticancer & anti-inflammatory	**Use whole in slow simmering dishes such as:** soup, sauce, stew, on fish, meat or poultry. Also use as a pickling spice.
4 │ Chives	Vitamin A, vitamin C, potassium, calcium, folic acid / Digestive aid & anticancer	Use in salad, soup, stew, sauce, dips, potato dishes, meat, fish & egg dishes
5 │ Cilantro (coriander)	Vitamin C / Antioxidant, antibacterial, anxiolytic, cholesterol lowering, digestive aid	*The flavors of the leaves and seeds are very different* **Fresh leaves (cilantro):** purées, sauces and dressings, soups, salsa, salads, meat and fish dishes **Dried seeds (coriander):** breads, cakes, curry & casseroles

HERB	NUTRITIONAL BENEFIT	HOW TO USE
6 | Dill	Iron, manganese, calcium / Digestive aid	Use with fish (especially salmon and trout), soup, as a pickling spice, in dips, egg dishes & potato dishes
7 | Oregano	Vitamin K, manganese, iron, fiber / Antibacterial & antioxidant	Meat, poultry, lamb, pork and fish dishes, sauces, vegetable dishes, bread, soups, stews, on pizza & in oil infusions
8 | Parsley	Vitamin K, vitamin C, vitamin A / Anticancer, antioxidant & anti-inflammatory	Use as garnish, in egg dishes, potato dishes, soups, pasta dishes, salads, pesto, fish, lamb, meat, poultry, veal and pork dishes
9 | Rosemary	Vitamin B6, Iron, Calcium / Memory aid & antioxidant	**Fresh or dried rosemary:** lamb, stew & marinades, fish and poultry dishes, tomato sauce, vegetables (especially roasted) & potato dishes
10 | Thyme	Vitamin K, iron, manganese / Respiratory aid, antiseptic, antispasmodic & expectorant	Use in soups, sauces, meat, poultry, lamb, veal & fish dishes, egg dishes & Herbes de Provence

15 Additional Herbs:

Carraway	Horseradish	Mint
Chicory	Juniper	Mustard
Fennel	Lavender	Sage
Fenugreek	Lemongrass	Savory
Garlic chives	Marjoram	Tarragon

How to Store Your Herbs

- Most fresh herbs can be stored in a plastic bag after rinsing and placed in the fridge. They are best used within 2 days.
- To make fresh herbs last longer, consider purchasing an herb saver system. These simple gadgets store your herbs in the fridge for up to 2 weeks.
- Dried herbs should be stored in an airtight container in a cool, dry, dark place. They should be used within six months so as not to lose their excellent flavor. If you notice your dried herbs have turned brown, especially bay leaves, it's time to toss them!

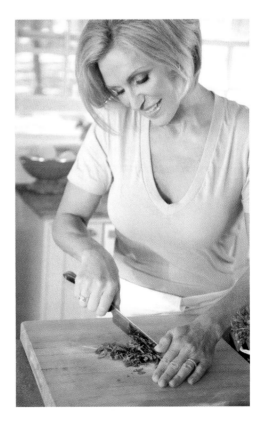

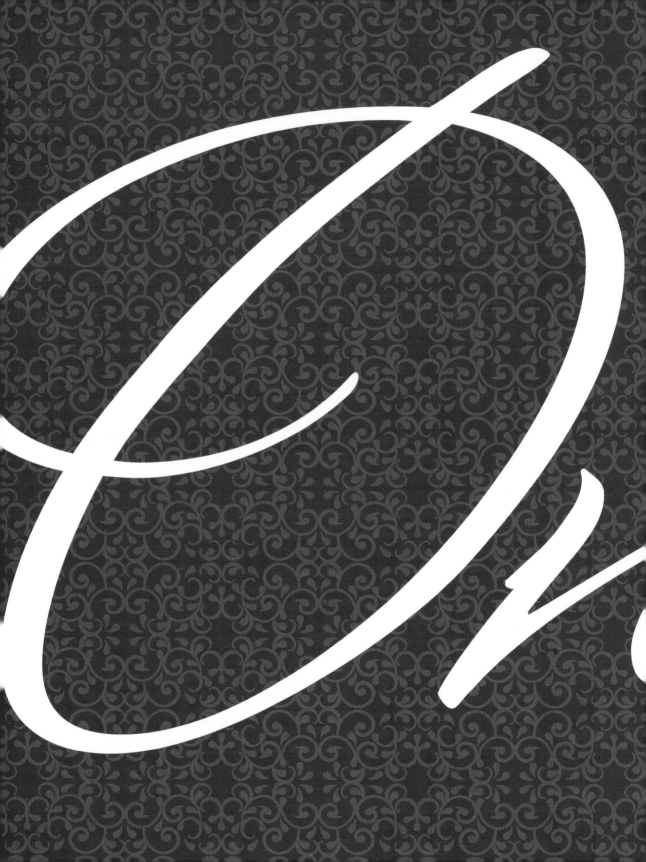

6

One Dish &
Easy Meals

140 CAMPFIRE SALMON
with Fire Roasted Peppers and Eggplant

143 ITALIAN SAUSAGE
with Sloppy Peppers

144 SHRIMP TACOS
with Grilled Pineapple Salsa

147 GREEK LAMB FLATBREAD PIZZA

148 SAUTÉED SCALLOPS
with Four Herb Pesto and Quinoa

151 PULLED PORK POBLANO VERDE

152 SWEET 'N' SPICY SHRIMP & CANTALOUPE SALAD

155 ARGENTINE COWBOY STEAK
with Grilled Onion Rings, Tomatoes and Chimichurri

156 SEAFOOD GUMBO

159 KEFIR MARINATED LAMB KEBABS
with Vegetables

160 CHICKEN AND SPINACH LASAGNA

163 BBQ CHICKEN PIZZA

164 LEFTOVER PASTA PIZZA PIE

CAMPFIRE SALMON
with Fire Roasted Peppers and Eggplant

Servings: 6 x 4 ounces
Prep time: 10 minutes (not including building campfire)
Cooking time: 15-20 minutes (depending on heat of coals and thickness of fish)

This is a fun and sophisticated way to Eat Clean when you're camping, and it sure beats hot dogs and beans! If you don't have access to a campfire and still want to "camp out," simply use a BBQ or grill. You can put up a tent in your backyard and pretend you're on a rustic vacation!

INGREDIENTS

1 ½ lbs / 681 g **wild Sockeye Salmon filet**, skin on
Eat-Clean Cooking Spray (see page 348)
1 tsp / 5 ml **sea salt**, divided
½ tsp / 2.5 ml freshly ground **black pepper**, divided
1 **eggplant**, cut into 1-inch cubes
1 **red pepper**, ribs and seeds removed, cut into 1-inch pieces
3 **jalapeños**, ribs and seeds removed, cut into 1-inch pieces
1 **lime**, cut into wedges

METHOD

1. Build a large campfire using plenty of wood. Allow fire to burn until flames are coming no more than six inches off wood, and you have enough bright red and orange coals to spread out in a 2 x 2-foot square. Place rocks around coals so that you can set roasting pans on these rocks, about six inches above hot coals.

2. Using small, clean pliers, carefully remove pin bones from salmon. If this causes flesh of salmon to tear, then leave pin bones in and remove them as you eat. Spray both skin and flesh of salmon generously with Eat-Clean Cooking Spray. Place salmon, skin-side down, on a slotted or perforated metal roasting pan. Season flesh with ½ tsp / 5 ml salt and ¼ tsp / 1.25 ml pepper.

3. Place cut vegetables on another slotted or perforated metal roasting pan and spray generously with Eat-Clean Cooking Spray. Season with remaining ½ tsp / 2.5 ml salt and ¼ tsp / 1.25 ml pepper and toss to coat.

NUTRITIONAL VALUE PER SERVING (4 OZ SALMON, ½ CUP / 120 ML VEGETABLES):
Calories: 225 |
Calories from Fat: 97 |
Protein: 25 g | Carbs: 7 g |
Total Fat: 11 g |
Saturated Fat: 2 g |
Trans Fat: 0 g | Fiber: 3 g |
Sodium: 317 mg |
Cholesterol: 70 mg

4. Cover both salmon and vegetable pans loosely with aluminum foil and place on rocks over campfire coals. Cook vegetables until soft and slightly charred in a few spots, stirring once or twice, about 15 minutes. Cook salmon until almost opaque and just barely starting to flake in thickest part of fish, about 15 minutes.

5. Remove salmon and vegetables from coals. Divide among six plates and serve with lime wedges to squeeze over top.

NOTE *The skin of salmon is edible, though you may prefer to cut fish away from skin as you are eating it.*

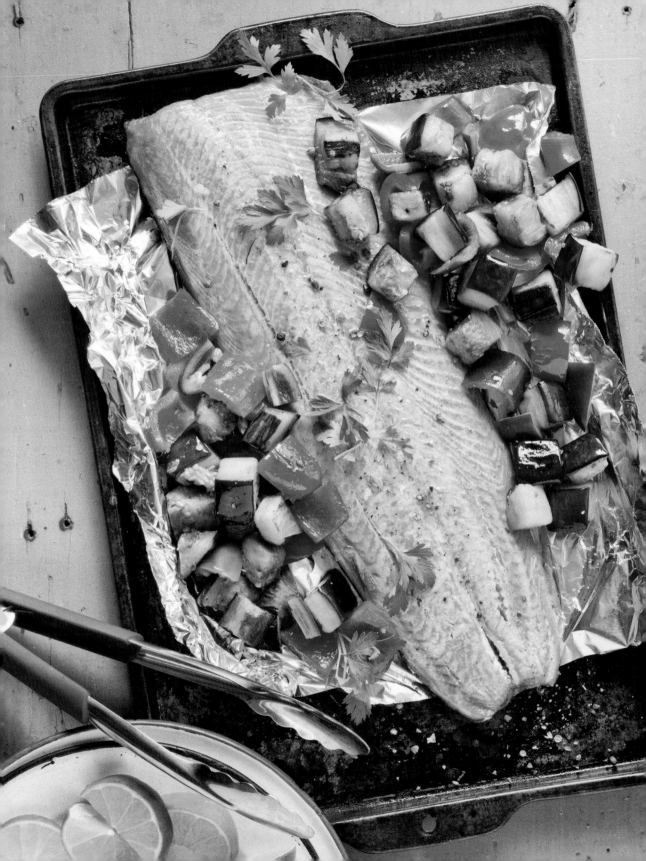

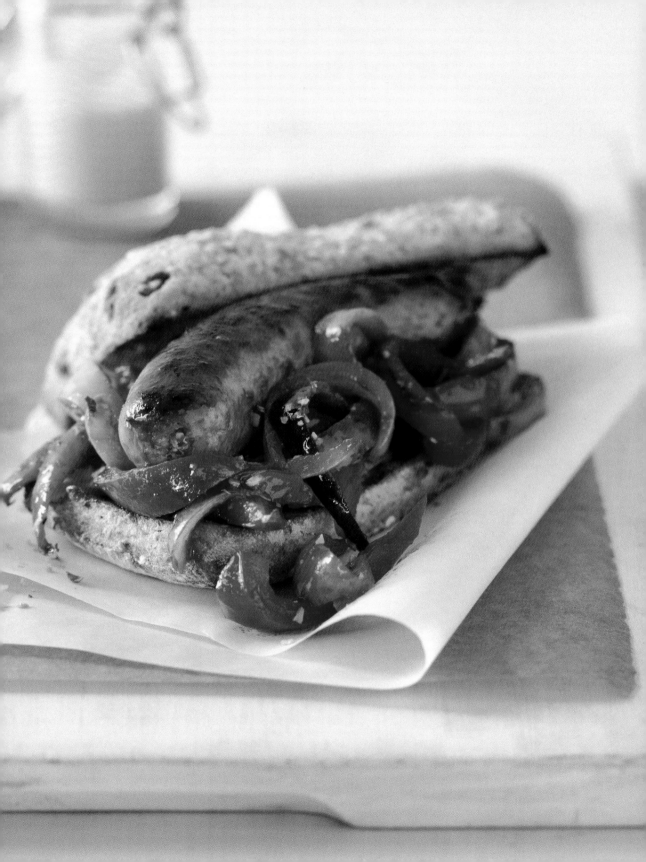

Servings: 4
Prep time: 15 minutes
Cooking time:
10-14 minutes

ITALIAN SAUSAGE
with Sloppy Peppers

This dish takes advantage of many varieties of peppers that you can find at some specialty grocery stores, ethnic grocery stores and farmers' markets. If you aren't able to find some of these varieties, you can substitute Anaheim, poblano, jalapeno or other peppers of your liking. This is a very sloppy, fun-to-eat dish!

INGREDIENTS

1 Tbsp / 15 ml + 1 tsp / 5 ml **extra virgin olive oil**, divided
6 all-natural, nitrate-free, low-fat spicy or mild **Italian chicken sausages**
½ cup / 120 ml low-sodium **chicken broth**
1 **yellow onion**, halved and thinly sliced
1 **red bell pepper**, seeded and thinly sliced
1 **Cubanelle pepper**, seeded and thinly sliced
2 **Hungarian hot wax peppers**, seeded and thinly sliced
2 **Italian griller peppers**, seeded and thinly sliced
½ tsp / 2.5 ml **fennel seeds**
½ tsp / 2.5 ml **sea salt**
¼ tsp / 1.25 ml freshly ground **black pepper**
2 cloves **garlic**, chopped
1 cup / 240 ml no-salt-added crushed **tomatoes**
Mustard, for serving
6 **whole grain hoagie rolls** or hot dog buns

METHOD

1. Heat 1 tsp / 5 ml olive oil in a large skillet over medium-high heat. Add sausages and cook, turning a few times, until browned, 3 to 5 minutes. Add chicken broth, cover, and simmer until sausages are cooked through, according to package instructions. Remove from heat and cover to keep warm.

2. Heat remaining 1 Tbsp / 15 ml olive oil over medium heat and add onion, peppers, fennel seeds, salt and pepper. Cook until soft and slightly browned, 6 to 8 minutes. (Work in batches, if necessary, to avoid overcrowding in pan.) Stir in garlic and cook for 30 seconds. Add crushed tomatoes and stir to combine.

3. To serve, squirt mustard inside hoagie rolls and add sausage. Divide pepper mixture among sausage-filled hoagies, about ⅔ cup / 160 ml for each, and serve with a big napkin!

NUTRITIONAL VALUE
PER SERVING (1 SAUSAGE-
FILLED HOAGIE WITH ⅔
CUP PEPPERS):
Calories: 308 |
Calories from Fat: 77 |
Protein: 24 g | Carbs: 34 g |
Total Fat: 8 g |
Saturated Fat: 3 g |
Trans Fat: 0 g | Fiber: 6 g |
Sodium: 869 mg |
Cholesterol: 75 mg

Servings: 4 x 2 tacos
Prep time: 10 minutes
Cooking time:
3-4 minutes

SHRIMP TACOS
with Grilled Pineapple Salsa

Fish tacos are growing in popularity, so why not try other types of seafood? These shrimp tacos are spicy, fresh and perfect for a light summer dinner on the patio.

Note: Grilled Pineapple Salsa must be made ahead of time.

INGREDIENTS

1 lb / 454 g medium **shrimp**, tails removed, peeled and deveined
¼ tsp / 1.25 ml ground **cumin**
⅛ tsp / 0.625 ml **chile chipotle powder**
¼ tsp / 1.25 ml **sea salt**
⅛ tsp / 0.625 ml freshly ground **black pepper**
Eat-Clean Cooking Spray (see page 348)
8 whole grain sprouted **corn tortillas** (about 5 inches in diameter)
1 **avocado**, pitted, peeled and thinly sliced
2 cups / 480 ml **Grilled Pineapple Salsa** (see recipe on page 355)

METHOD

1. Heat a large nonstick skillet over medium-high heat. In a medium bowl, toss together shrimp, cumin, chipotle powder, salt and pepper. Spray skillet with Eat-Clean Cooking Spray and add shrimp in an even layer. Sauté, stirring occasionally, until shrimp are cooked through, 3 to 4 minutes.

2. Divide tortillas among four plates and place ¼ cup / 60 ml cooked shrimp on each tortilla. Top each tortilla with ¼ cup / 60 ml Grilled Pineapple Salsa, and one-eighth avocado.

NUTRITIONAL VALUE
PER SERVING:
Calories: 446 |
Calories from Fat: 99 |
Protein: 22 g | Carbs: 66 g |
Total Fat: 11 g |
Saturated Fat: 1 g |
Trans Fat: 0 g | Fiber: 11 g |
Sodium: 466 mg |
Cholesterol: 103 mg

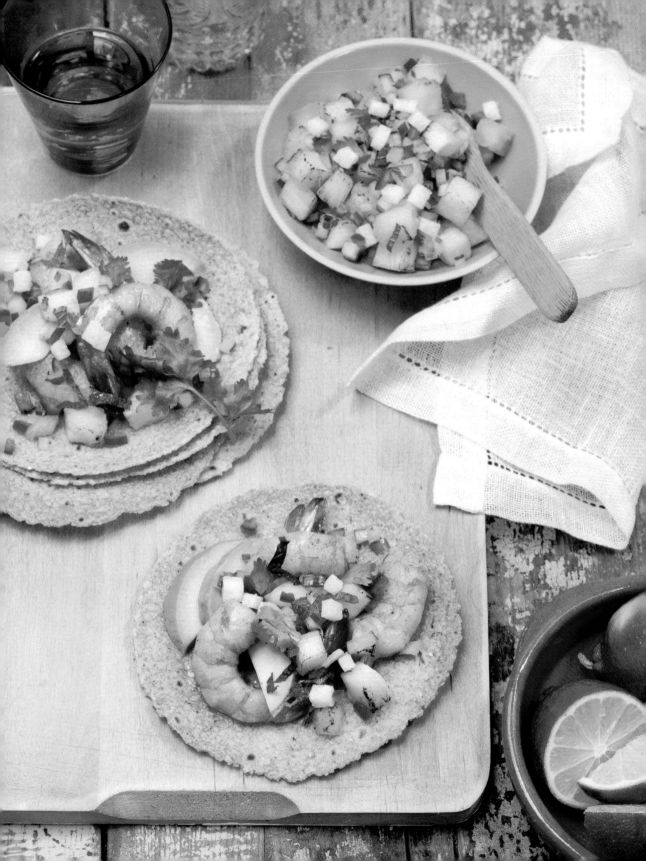

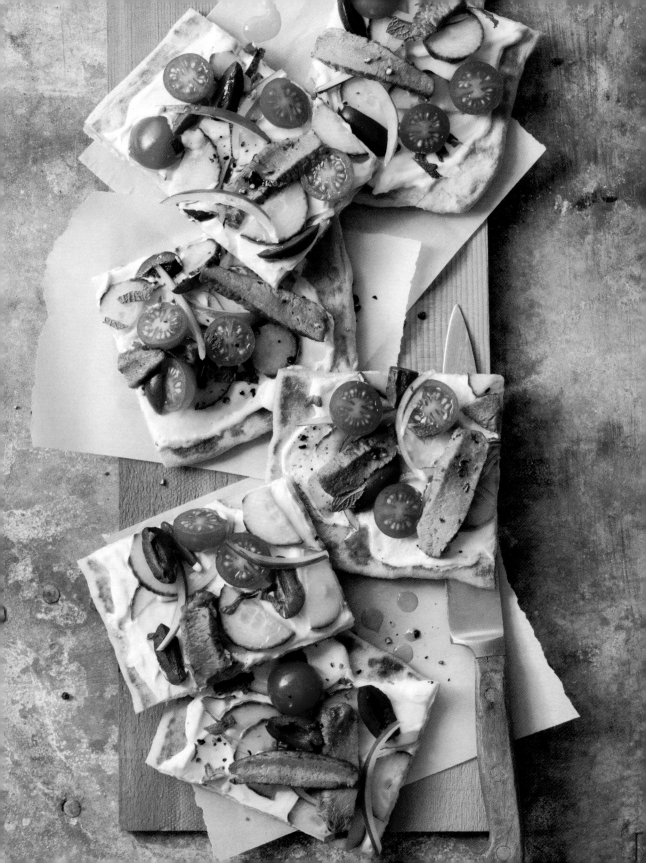

Servings: 4 x 1 pizza
Prep time: 10 minutes
Marinating time:
5 minutes
Cooking time:
10 minutes
Resting time:
5 minutes

GREEK LAMB FLATBREAD PIZZA

Everyone (especially kids!) loves pizza. Using a flatbread crust is one way to keep your pizza light and healthy without sacrificing taste. This pizza is inspired by flavors of the Mediterranean.

Note: Yogurt Cheese must be made ahead of time. If you do not have goat's yogurt, you can use regular plain, low-fat yogurt.

INGREDIENTS

1 lb / 454 g **boneless loin lamb chops**, trimmed of excess fat
1 Tbsp / 15 ml **extra virgin olive oil**
Juice of ½ **lemon**
2 cloves **garlic**, finely chopped
1 Tbsp / 15 ml finely chopped fresh **oregano**
1 tsp / 5 ml coarse **sea salt**
½ tsp / 2.5 ml freshly ground **black pepper**
Eat-Clean Cooking Spray (see page 348)
1 cup / 240 ml goat's **Yogurt Cheese** (see recipe on page 348)
4 **whole wheat flatbreads**
½ **English cucumber**, thinly sliced into disks
1 cup / 240 ml **cherry tomatoes**, halved
½ cup / 120 ml pitted **kalamata olives**, halved lengthwise
¼ medium **red onion**, thinly sliced
1 Tbsp / 15 ml chopped fresh **mint**

METHOD

1. Place lamb, olive oil, lemon juice, garlic, oregano, salt and pepper into a resealable plastic bag and close it tightly. Shake and massage ingredients to evenly distribute around lamb. Let sit at room temperature for 5 minutes.

2. Preheat a grill or grill pan to medium-high heat and coat with Eat-Clean Cooking Spray. Remove lamb from bag and allow marinade liquid to drip off. Place on grill and cook 8 to 10 minutes, turning once for medium rare. Remove to a cutting board and let rest for 5 minutes.

3. Spread ¼ cup / 60 ml Yogurt Cheese over each flatbread and lay cucumber slices on top, dividing evenly between four flatbreads. Thinly slice lamb across the grain and divide slices among pizzas. Top with tomatoes, olives, onion and then sprinkle with mint.

NUTRITIONAL VALUE
PER SERVING:
Calories: 187 |
Calories from Fat: 71 |
Protein: 7 g | Carbs: 23 g |
Total Fat: 9 g |
Saturated Fat: 1 g |
Trans Fat: 0 g | Fiber: 4 g |
Sodium: 771 mg |
Cholesterol: 0 mg

Servings: 4
Prep time: 15 minutes
Cooking time:
10 minutes

SAUTÉED SCALLOPS
with Four Herb Pesto and Quinoa

Food does not need to be drenched in fat or oil to taste good. The secret ingredient to making lively, delicious and healthy dishes is fresh herbs. They are packed with nutrients and bring so much flavor to your food without all the bad stuff. For more on what herbs can do for you, turn to page 136.

INGREDIENTS

1 cup / 240 ml **quinoa**
1 ½ cups / 360 ml **water**
1 tsp / 5 ml + pinch **sea salt**, divided
2 cloves **garlic**
1 cup / 240 ml **basil**, loosely packed
1 cup / 240 ml **tarragon**, loosely packed
½ cup / 120 ml **chives**, loosely packed
½ cup / 120 ml **mint**, loosely packed
Zest and juice of 1 **lemon**
3 heaping Tbsp / 50 ml **walnut pieces**
¼ tsp / 1.25 ml + pinch freshly ground **black pepper**
¼ cup / 60 ml + 1 tsp / 5 ml **extra virgin olive oil**, divided
3 Tbsp / 45 ml low-sodium **vegetable broth**, if needed
1 lb / 454 g **large wild scallops**
1 cup / 240 ml **cherry or grape tomatoes**, halved

METHOD

1. In a medium saucepan, combine quinoa, water and ½ tsp / 2.5 ml sea salt over high heat until boiling. Cover and reduce heat to simmer, 15 minutes. Remove from heat, fluff, cover and set aside.

2. In a food processor, add garlic, basil, tarragon, chives, mint, zest and juice of lemon, walnut pieces, ½ tsp / 2.5 ml sea salt and ¼ tsp / 1.25 ml pepper. Pulse until chopped. While processor is running, stream in olive oil. Scrape down sides of bowl. If pesto is too thick to slowly pour, place top back on processor and stream in broth while machine is running. Set aside.

3. Heat 1 tsp / 5 ml olive oil in a nonstick skillet over medium-high heat. Blot any moisture from scallops with a paper towel. Season one side with a pinch of salt and pepper and place in a single layer in skillet. Cook 2 minutes on each side until golden brown. Do not overcook. Remove and set aside.

4. In a large serving bowl, toss quinoa, pesto and cherry tomatoes until combined. Place scallops on top. Divide quinoa mixture and scallops among four plates.

NUTRITIONAL VALUE
PER SERVING (4 OZ / 113 G
SCALLOPS, 1 CUP / 240 ML
QUINOA):
Calories: 381 |
Calories from Fat: 184 |
Protein: 30 g | Carbs: 20 g |
Total Fat: 19 g |
Saturated Fat: 2 g |
Trans Fat: 0 g | Fiber: 6 g |
Sodium: 829 mg |
Cholesterol: 60 mg

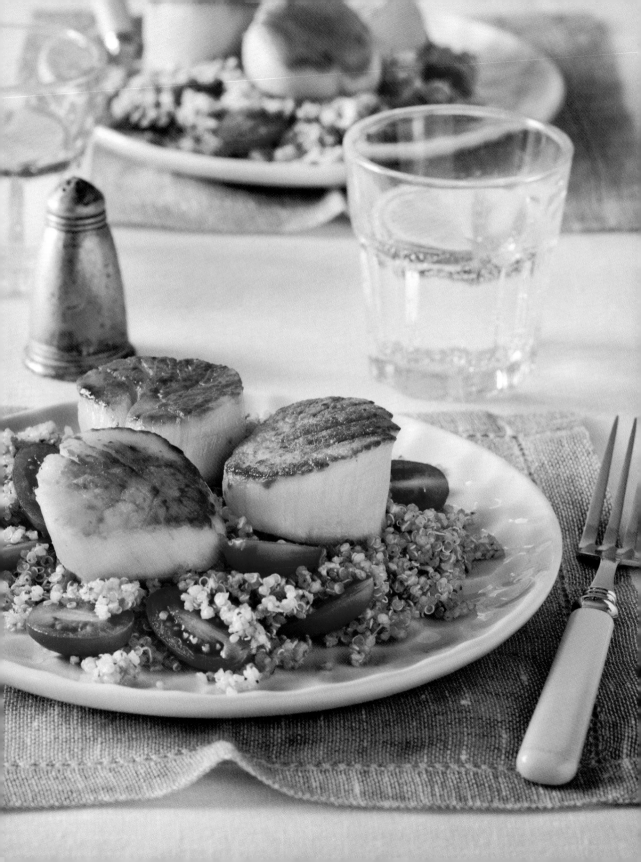

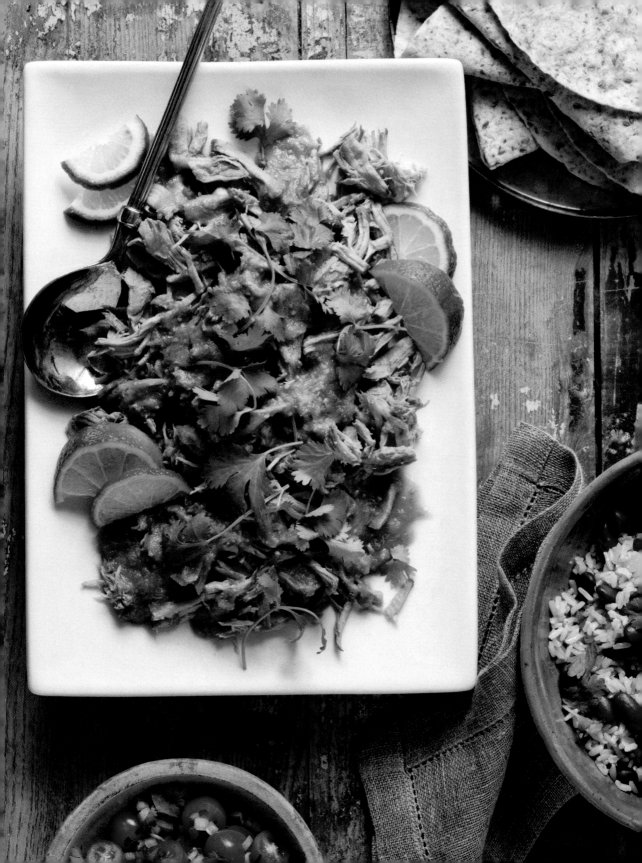

PULLED PORK POBLANO VERDE

Servings: 4 x 1 cup
Prep time: 10 minutes
Cooking time:
2 hours 10 minutes to
3 hours 15 minutes

Poblanos are chili peppers that come from Puebla, Mexico. Dried, they are called ancho chilies. They have a mild flavor but watch out! Some poblanos can be surprisingly hot. Try this dish with brown rice, black or pinto beans, vegetables or in whole grain tortillas. Garnish with fresh cilantro, if desired.

INGREDIENTS

1 tsp / 5 ml **safflower oil**

3 lbs / 1.35 kg **pork shoulder**, trimmed of excess fat and soft tissue, cut into 2-inch chunks

1 tsp / 5 ml **sea salt**, divided

1 tsp / 5 ml freshly ground **black pepper**, divided

1 lb / 454 g **tomatillos**, husked and quartered

2 **poblano peppers**, seeded, halved and sliced

2 **serrano peppers**, halved and sliced

½ large or 1 medium **yellow onion**, sliced

5 cloves **garlic**, smashed

1 Tbsp / 15 ml ground **cumin**

1 tsp / 5 ml ground **coriander**

3 to 4 cups / 720 to 960 ml low-sodium **chicken broth** (enough to almost completely cover ingredients in pot)

Juice of 1 **lime**

METHOD

1. Preheat oven to 275°F / 135°C.

1. Heat safflower oil in a Dutch oven or heavy-bottomed ovenproof pot over high heat. Add pork in a single layer, being careful not to overcrowd. Season with ½ tsp / 2.5 ml salt and ½ tsp / 2.5 ml pepper, and brown on all sides, 6 to 8 minutes. Remove to a bowl and set aside. Pour out fat and discard.

2. Return pot to burner and add tomatillos, peppers, onion and garlic. Cook, stirring occasionally, until browned, 5 to 7 minutes. Stir in cumin, coriander, and remaining ½ tsp / 2.5 ml salt and ½ tsp / 2.5 ml pepper. Return pork to pot along with any accumulated juices and pour in chicken broth until ingredients are almost covered. Bring liquid to a boil, cover pot, and transfer to oven to slowly cook for 2 to 2½ hours, until pork is tender enough to easily pull apart.

3. Remove pot from oven. Using a shallow ladle or large spoon, skim off any fat that has floated to top and discard. Then take a paper towel and lay it over surface of liquid to absorb any residual fat left on top. Discard paper towel.

4. Pull pork out of sauce and place it on a baking sheet. Using forks, pull pork apart into shreds, removing any remaining fat. Using a hand-held immersion blender, blend sauce until smooth. (You can also blend sauce in a stand blender, working in batches. Be careful if using a stand blender, as hot liquids can expand.) Return sauce in pot to stove over medium-high heat. Bring to a rapid simmer and reduce sauce by half, about 10 minutes. Stir in lime juice. Taste, and make any final adjustments to seasoning with salt and pepper.

NUTRITIONAL VALUE
PER SERVING:
Calories: 289 |
Calories from Fat: 123 |
Protein: 35 g | Carbs: 5 g |
Total Fat: 13 g |
Saturated Fat: 4 g |
Trans Fat: 0 g | Fiber: 1 g |
Sodium: 468 mg |
Cholesterol: 116 mg

Servings: 4 x 2½ cups
Prep time: 10 minutes
Cooking time:
4 minutes

SWEET 'N' SPICY SHRIMP AND CANTALOUPE SALAD

This salad is as pleasing to the eye as it is to the palate. Its bright colors just scream spring. Topped with a simple dressing, the flavors of the fruit and shrimp really shine through.

SALAD INGREDIENTS

1 Tbsp / 15 ml **olive oil**
1 lb / 454 g **large shrimp** (26 – 30 count), peeled and deveined, tails on
2 large cloves **garlic**, minced
¼ tsp / 1.25 ml **sea salt**
⅛ tsp / 0.625 ml freshly ground **black pepper**
¼ tsp / 1.25 ml smoked **paprika**
¼ tsp / 1.25 ml ground **cumin**
⅛ tsp / 0.625 ml **cayenne**
6 cups / 1.4 L **mixed greens**
3 cups / 720 ml **Tuscan-style cantaloupe**, cut into large bite-sized pieces
2 Tbsp / 30 ml toasted **pepitas** (shelled pumpkin seeds)

VINAIGRETTE INGREDIENTS

2 tsp / 10 ml **sherry vinegar**
2 tsp / 10 ml **extra virgin olive oil**
⅛ tsp / 0.625 ml **sea salt**
⅛ tsp / 0.625 ml freshly ground **black pepper**

METHOD

1. Heat olive oil in a large skillet over medium-high heat. Make sure shrimp are drained, and if necessary, pat dry with a paper towel. Add shrimp to skillet and cook, 2 minutes. Turn over and add garlic, salt, pepper and spices. Cook an additional 2 minutes until done, then toss a few times to evenly distribute seasoning on shrimp. Remove from heat and set aside.

2. In a small bowl, whisk together vinaigrette ingredients and set aside.

3. Divide greens and cantaloupe evenly among four plates. Divide shrimp among four plates, placing them on and around greens. Drizzle vinaigrette over top of each salad, and then top with toasted pepitas. Serve immediately.

NUTRITIONAL VALUE
PER SERVING:
Calories: 169 |
Calories from Fat: 64 |
Protein: 13 g | Carbs: 15 g |
Total Fat: 8 g |
Saturated Fat: 1 g | Trans
Fat: 0 g | Fiber: 3 g |
Sodium: 205 mg |
Cholesterol: 64 mg

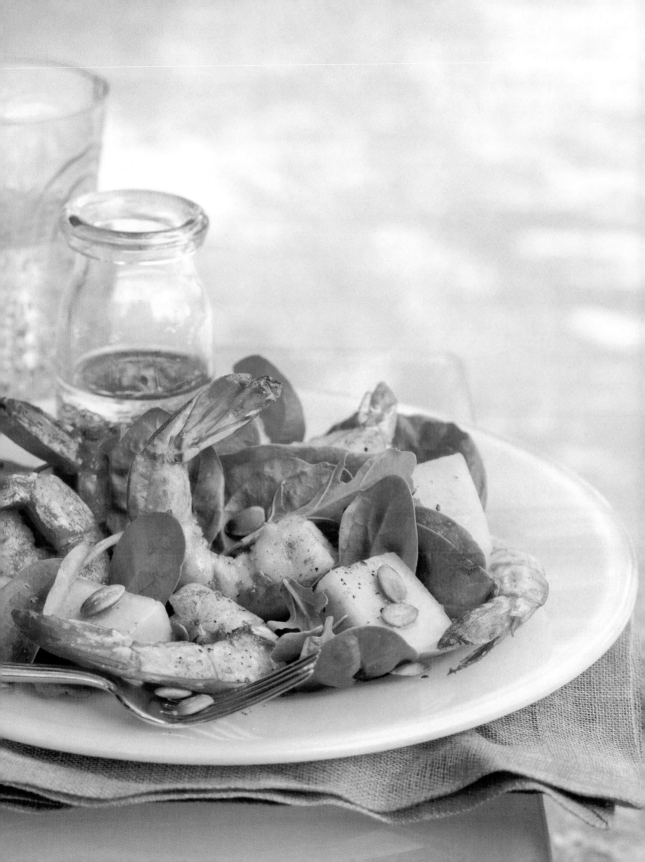

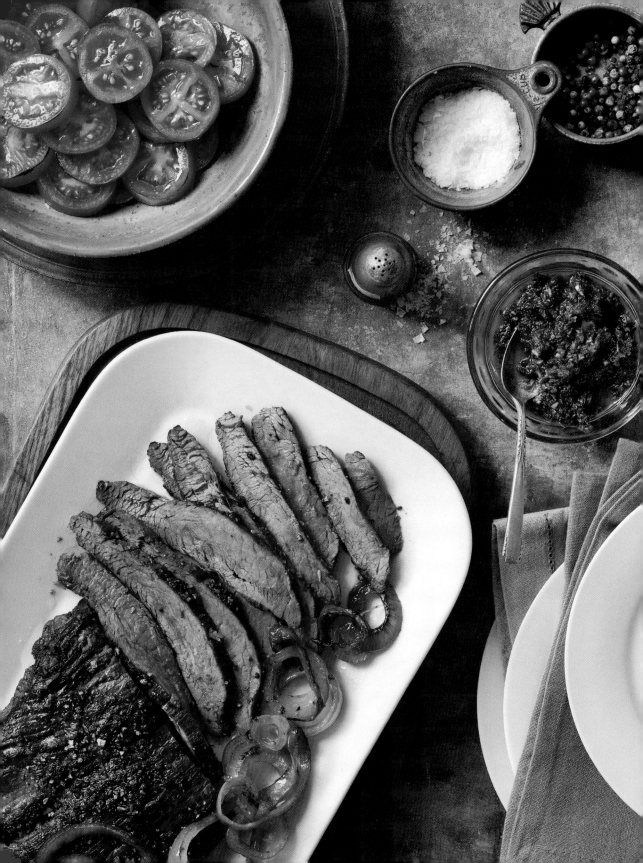

Servings: 4
Prep time: 10 minutes
Cooking time:
11-13 minutes
Resting time:
25 minutes

ARGENTINE COWBOY STEAK
with Grilled Onion Rings, Tomatoes and Chimichurri

Saddle up cowpokes! A cowboy steak is a substantial cut of meat, about two inches thick. For this recipe I've chosen flat iron steak, which is cut from the shoulder. If you purchase your steak from a butcher, it may be called "top blade" roast.

Note: Chimichurri must be made ahead of time.

INGREDIENTS

1 lb / 454 g **flat iron steak**, trimmed of excess fat
1 tsp / 5 ml smoked **paprika**
½ tsp / 2.5 ml coarse **Celtic sea salt**
¼ tsp / 1.25 ml freshly ground **black pepper**
Eat-Clean Cooking Spray (see page 348)
1 medium **red onion**, sliced into ½-inch rings
2 **tomatoes**, sliced ½-inch thick
½ cup / 120 ml **Chimichurri**, divided (see recipe on page 357)

METHOD

1. Heat a grill or grill pan to medium-high heat. Allow steak to sit at room temperature for 15 minutes to take chill off. Season both sides with smoked paprika, Celtic sea salt and pepper. Spray both sides of steak and grill with Eat-Clean Cooking Spray. Place steak on grill and cook 4 to 5 minutes on each side for medium rare. Remove and let rest, 10 minutes.

2. Spray both sides of onion and tomato slices and place in a single layer on grill. Grill tomatoes 1 minute on each side. Grill onions 2 minutes on each side. Thinly slice steak across grain and toss with ¼ cup / 60 ml chimichurri. Place steak in center of a serving platter. Place grilled onions and tomatoes on both sides of steak. Top steak, onions and tomatoes with another ¼ cup / 60 ml chimichurri and serve.

NUTRITIONAL VALUE
PER SERVING:
Calories: 228 |
Calories from Fat: 128 |
Protein: 16 g | Carbs: 9 g |
Total Fat: 14 g |
Saturated Fat: 4 g |
Trans Fat: 0 g | Fiber: 2 g |
Sodium: 441 mg |
Cholesterol: 51 mg

Servings: 10 x 1 cup
Prep time: 15 minutes
Cooking time:
40-45 minutes

SEAFOOD GUMBO

*The word "gumbo" refers to the African word "kigombo," which means okra. Gumbo is
a spicy stew that hails from the southern United States. It's typically made with seafood,
chicken, sausage and pork, but the main ingredients are broth and rice. You can change the
taste of gumbo by making it as spicy – or mild – as you like.*

INGREDIENTS

3 Tbsp / 45 ml **olive oil**
3 Tbsp / 45 ml **whole wheat flour**
1 **onion**, chopped
2 stalks **celery**, chopped
1 large **green pepper**, seeded and chopped
4 large cloves **garlic**, chopped
1½ tsp / 7.5 ml **sea salt**
1 tsp / 5 ml freshly ground **black pepper**
1 tsp / 5 ml low-sodium **Old Bay seasoning**
½ tsp / 2.5 ml **cayenne pepper** (more for spicier gumbo)
2 Tbsp / 30 ml **tomato paste**
4 cups / 960 ml low-sodium **chicken broth**
12 oz / 340 g cut **frozen** or **fresh okra** (about 3 cups / 720 ml)
1 tsp / 5 ml chopped fresh **thyme**
2 **bay leaves**
1 lb / 454 g 51-60 **count shrimp**, peeled and deveined
12 oz / 340 g low-fat all-natural fully cooked **andouille sausage**
    (or other low-fat spicy sausage), cut into ½-inch rounds
Steamed long grain **brown rice**, for serving
Hot sauce, to garnish

METHOD

1. Heat a Dutch oven or large heavy-bottomed pot over medium heat. Add olive oil
and flour, and cook, stirring occasionally, until mixture is medium brown and smells
toasty, about 8 minutes. Add onion, celery, pepper, garlic, salt, pepper, Old Bay and
cayenne. Cook vegetables until tender, stirring occasionally, about 10 minutes.

2. Add tomato paste, broth, okra, thyme and bay leaves. Bring mixture to a boil, stir
to combine ingredients, and then reduce heat to simmer, uncovered, for 20 minutes.
Increase heat to high. Add shrimp and sausage, and gently stir to submerge them in
hot liquid. Cook for 3 to 4 minutes until shrimp are cooked through and sausage is
heated through.

3. Taste, and make any final adjustments to seasoning with salt and pepper. Remove bay
leaves and discard. Serve in bowls over steamed brown rice, with hot sauce to garnish.

NUTRITIONAL VALUE
PER SERVING:
Calories: 156 |
Calories from Fat: 65 |
Protein: 14 g | Carbs: 9 g |
Total Fat: 7 g |
Saturated Fat: 1 g |
Trans Fat: 0 g | Fiber: 2 g |
Sodium: 603 mg |
Cholesterol: 65 mg

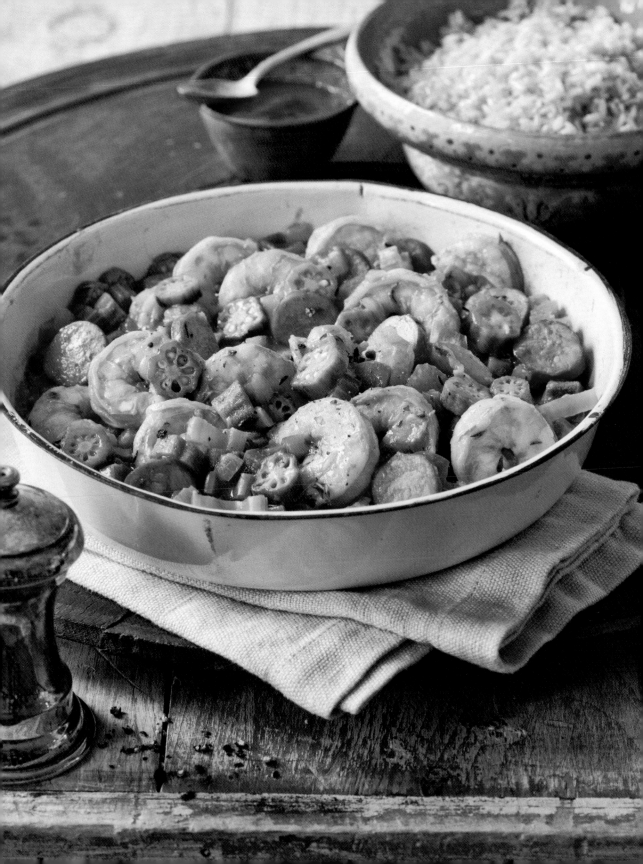

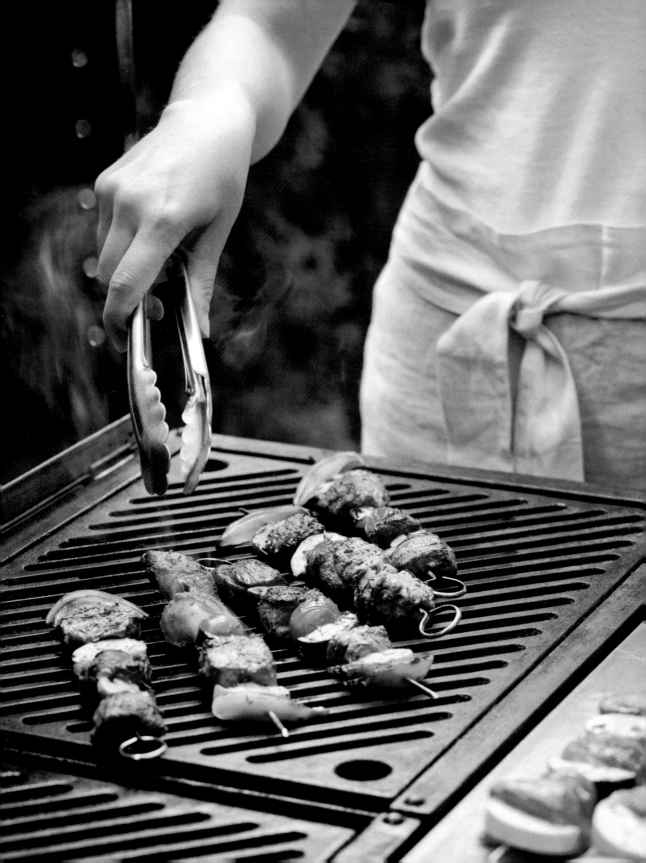

Servings: 4
Prep time: 20 minutes
Cooking time:
7-10 minutes
Marinating time:
3 hours

KEFIR MARINATED LAMB KEBABS
with Vegetables

I get a lot of questions about kefir, a cultured milk beverage that is popular in the Middle East and Eastern Europe, although it's growing in popularity in North America. It looks like liquid yogurt, tastes tangy and rich, and it's chock full of healthful bacteria that aid digestion.

INGREDIENTS

1 lb / 454 g **boneless leg of lamb**, trimmed of fat, cut into 1½-inch cubes
1 cup / 240 ml plain low-fat **kefir**
2 cloves **garlic**, minced
2 tsp / 10 ml fresh whole **rosemary leaves**
Zest and juice of ½ **lemon**
½ tsp / 2.5 ml ground **cumin**
¼ tsp / 1.25 ml ground **turmeric**
⅛ tsp / 0.625 ml **cayenne pepper**
¼ tsp / 1.25 ml **sea salt**, plus more to taste
⅛ tsp / 0.625 ml freshly ground **black pepper**, plus more to taste
1 cup / 240 ml **white button mushrooms**, halved
1 **baby zucchini**, halved lengthwise and sliced into ½-inch moons (about 1 cup / 240 ml)
1 cup / 240 ml **cherry tomatoes**
¼ **red onion**, cut into 1½-inch pieces and separated into single layers (about ¼ cup / 60 ml)
Eat-Clean Cooking Spray (see page 348)

METHOD

1. In a glass container, place lamb, kefir, garlic, rosemary, lemon zest and juice, cumin, turmeric, cayenne, salt and pepper, and stir to thoroughly combine. Make sure lamb cubes are completely submerged in kefir marinade. Cover tightly and refrigerate for at least three hours, or overnight.

2. Heat a grill or grill pan to medium-high heat. Remove lamb from marinade and thread onto skewers, alternating with mushrooms, zucchini, tomatoes and onion, until all ingredients are threaded. Discard marinade. Brush grill with a little olive oil to prevent lamb and vegetables from sticking. Spray skewered ingredients lightly with Eat-Clean Cooking Spray, and season with a pinch of sea salt and freshly ground black pepper. Place on grill and cook, turning two or three times, until lamb is cooked to medium-rare, and vegetables are slightly charred and soft, 7 to 10 minutes total. Remove from grill and divide among four plates.

NUTRITIONAL VALUE
PER SERVING:
Calories: 226 |
Calories from Fat: 81 |
Protein: 28 g | Carbs: 8 g |
Total Fat: 9 g |
Saturated Fat: 3 g |
Trans Fat: 0 g | Fiber: 2 g |
Sodium: 193 mg |
Cholesterol: 76 mg

NOTE *This recipe requires skewers. If you are using wooden or bamboo skewers, soak them in water for 20 minutes before using.*

CHICKEN AND SPINACH LASAGNA

This lasagna recipe is a great way to sneak extra greens into your diet – each serving packs two cups of fresh spinach!

Note: Yogurt Cheese and Clean Marinara Sauce must be made ahead of time.

INGREDIENTS

1½ tsp / 7.5 ml + pinch **sea salt**, divided
8 oz / 227 g **whole wheat lasagna noodles** (about 12)
Eat-Clean Cooking Spray (see page 348)
1 lb / 454 g **boneless skinless chicken breasts**
¼ tsp / 1.25 ml + pinch freshly ground **black pepper**
½ tsp / 2.5 ml **extra virgin olive oil**
12 cups / 2.9 L **spinach**
1 large clove **garlic**, minced

1 cup / 240 ml reduced-fat **ricotta**
½ cup / 120 ml **Yogurt Cheese** (see recipe on page 348)
2 **egg whites**
1 Tbsp / 15 ml chopped fresh **oregano**
2 Tbsp / 30 ml chopped fresh **basil**
3 cups / 720 ml **Clean Marinara Sauce** (see recipe on page 122)
6 Tbsp / 90 ml freshly grated **Parmigiano Reggiano**

METHOD

1. Bring a large pot of water to boil. Add 1 tsp / 5 ml salt and lasagna noodles a few at a time. Undercook noodles, until they're soft enough to bend but not soft enough to eat without further cooking, about 5 to 7 minutes. Drain, and as soon as they're cool enough to handle, spread out in a single layer on one or more baking sheets. Set aside.

2. Preheat oven to 350°F / 175°C. Heat an ovenproof skillet over medium-high heat and spray with cooking spray. Season both sides of chicken breasts with a pinch of salt and pepper. Place chicken in pan and cook until browned on one side, about 5 minutes. Turn over and place in oven to finish cooking, about 5 minutes. Remove and let rest for 5 minutes. Slice chicken a quarter-inch thick against grain and set aside.

3. Heat ½ tsp olive oil in a large skillet over medium-high heat. Add spinach and garlic, and season with a pinch of salt and pepper. Cook until spinach is wilted, about 2 to 3 minutes. Remove from heat and set aside. Combine thoroughly in a large bowl, ricotta, Yogurt Cheese, oregano and basil.

4. Spray bottom of a 12 x 10-inch baking dish with Eat-Clean Cooking Spray. Spread ½ cup / 120 ml Clean Marinara sauce on bottom of dish. Spread out four noodles, then half cheese mixture, half spinach, half sliced chicken breast and 1 cup / 240 ml of marinara. Repeat layer. Lay remaining four noodles on top and spread out remaining marinara. Cover dish and bake for 1 hour. Remove, uncover, and cut into six 4 x 5-inch servings. Top each serving with 1 Tbsp / 15 ml freshly grated Parmigiano Reggiano.

NUTRITIONAL VALUE
PER SERVING:
Calories: 392 |
Calories from Fat: 88 |
Protein: 35 g | Carbs: 10 g |
Total Fat: 13 g |
Saturated Fat: 6 g |
Trans Fat: 0 g | Fiber: 3 g |
Sodium: 1444 mg |
Cholesterol: 10 mg

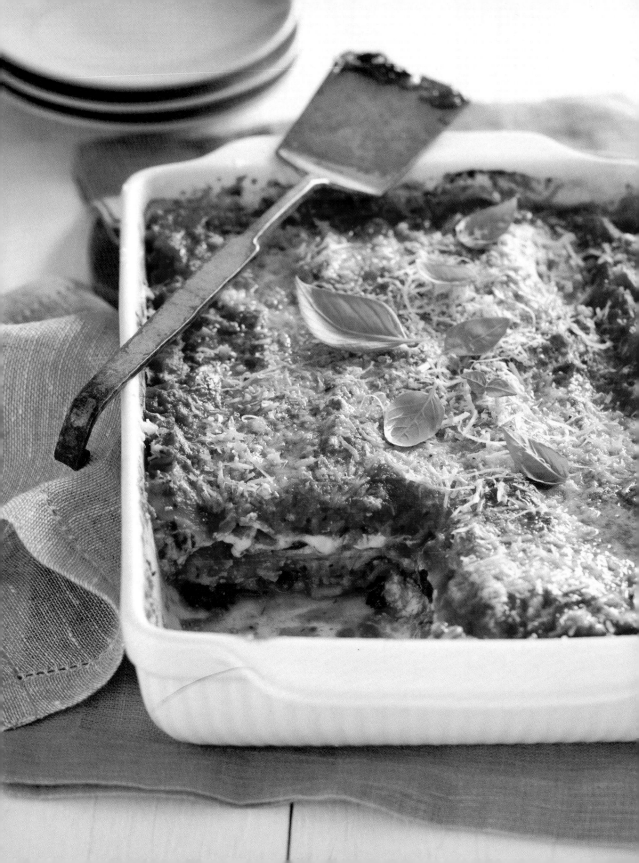

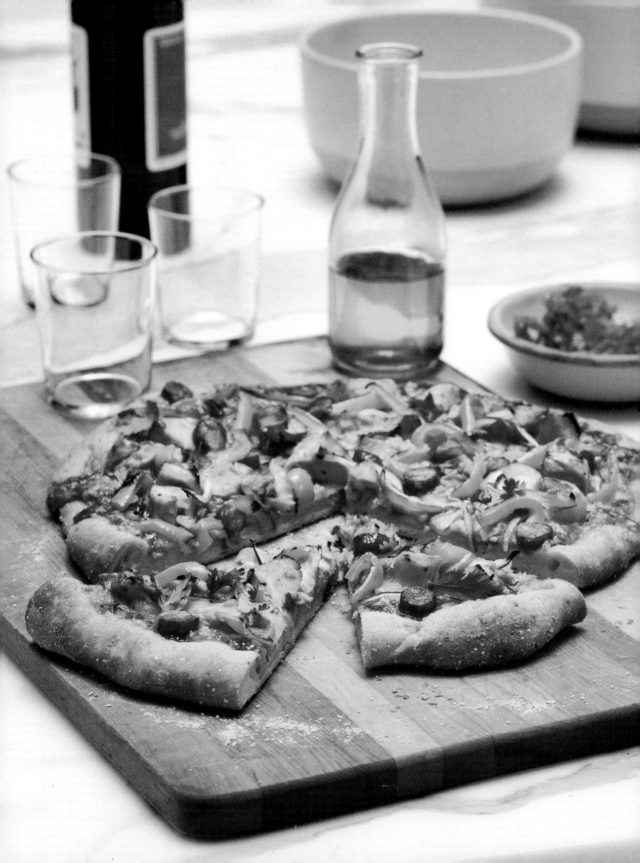

BBQ CHICKEN PIZZA

Servings: 8
Prep time: 20 minutes
Cooking time:
50-60 minutes

If you are a fan of the taste of barbeque, you'll love this pizza! I love experimenting with different sauce bases and this one is a great alternative to traditional tomato sauce.

INGREDIENTS

2 split **chicken breast** halves, bone-in, skin removed and fat trimmed (1 ½ to 2 lbs / 681 to 908 g)

¼ tsp / 1.25 ml **sea salt**

Pinch freshly ground **black pepper**

Eat-Clean Cooking Spray (see page 348)

1 lb / 454 g **whole wheat pizza dough**

1 Tbsp / 15 ml stone ground **100% whole grain cornmeal** (more if needed to prevent dough from sticking)

1 Tbsp / 15 ml **whole wheat flour**

⅔ cup / 160 ml **Spicy Clean BBQ Sauce** (see recipe on page 133) or other clean BBQ sauce

½ **red** or **orange pepper**, seeded and thinly sliced

⅛ **red onion**, thinly sliced

¼ cup / 60 ml **golden Greek pepperoncini**, drained

½ cup / 120 ml grated reduced-fat **sharp** or **medium cheddar**

½ cup / 120 ml roughly chopped **cilantro**

METHOD

1. Heat a grill to medium-high heat. Season meat side of chicken with salt and pepper, and coat lightly with Eat-Clean Cooking Spray. Grill chicken with a closed lid until grill marks form, 5 to 8 minutes. Turn chicken a quarter turn, close again and cook, undisturbed, 5 to 8 more minutes. Turn chicken over, close lid, and cook until internal temperature reads between 163°F to 165°F / 73°C to 74°C when a thermometer is inserted into thickest part of breast meat, avoiding touching any bone, 15 to 25 minutes longer. Remove chicken from grill to a baking sheet and let rest until cool enough to handle. Transfer to a cutting board and cut meat into bite-sized pieces, removing bones.

2. Preheat oven to 425°F / 220°C. If you have a pizza stone, place it on a rack in center of oven and close door.

3. Let pizza dough sit at room temperature for 15 minutes before you roll it out. Spread cornmeal on a clean work surface, and place dough on top. Lightly coat your hands and a rolling pin with whole wheat flour. Press dough into a disk and stretch it out into a 15-inch disk using your hands and rolling pin. If you are using a pizza baking sheet, sprinkle a little cornmeal on baking sheet and transfer pizza dough onto sheet.

4. Spread ⅓ cup / 80 ml BBQ sauce on dough, leaving a half-inch border without sauce. Place cut chicken in a bowl and toss to coat with remaining BBQ sauce, and then spread out chicken evenly over top of pizza. Add peppers, red onions and pepperoncini. Sprinkle grated cheddar over top. Spray the half-inch border with Eat-Clean Cooking Spray. If using a pizza stone, carefully slide prepared pizza onto preheated stone in oven. If using a baking sheet, place in oven on middle rack. Cook pizza until vegetables are soft and crust is lightly browned, 15 to 20 minutes. Remove from oven and top with fresh cilantro. Cut into eight slices and serve.

NUTRITIONAL VALUE
PER SERVING
(5-INCH SLICE):
Calories: 259 |
Calories from Fat: 55 |
Protein: 15 g | Carbs: 35 g |
Total Fat: 6 g |
Saturated Fat: 2 g |
Trans Fat: 0 g | Fiber: 4 g |
Sodium: 506 mg |
Cholesterol: 27 mg

LEFTOVER PASTA PIZZA PIE

This pasta pizza pie is a cross between a pizza pie, a pasta dish and an omelet, which means it works for breakfast, lunch or dinner! Tasty hot or cold, it's perfect for brown-bag meals.

INGREDIENTS

2 whole **eggs**
4 **egg whites**
⅓ cup / 80 ml chopped fresh **basil**
¼ cup / 60 ml reconstituted **sun-dried tomatoes**,
    drained and julienne-cut into thin strips (see note)
¼ cup / 60 ml freshly grated **Parmigiano Reggiano**
½ tsp / 2.5 ml **sea salt**
¼ tsp / 1.25 ml freshly ground **black pepper**
3 cups / 720 ml cooked **whole grain long strand pasta** (spaghetti, linguini or fettuccini)
Eat-Clean Cooking Spray (see page 348)

METHOD

1. Heat a 10-inch ovenproof nonstick skillet over medium heat. Place rack at second highest position in oven and turn broiler on high.

2. In a large bowl, beat eggs and egg whites. Add basil, sun-dried tomatoes, Parmigiano Reggiano, salt and pepper, and stir to combine. Add pasta and stir to combine well. Spray skillet with Eat-Clean Cooking Spray and pour in pasta mixture. Using a rubber spatula, pat it down a little so ingredients are level. Cook 5 minutes until browned on bottom. Transfer to rack under broiler and cook until eggs are cooked through and top is lightly browned, about 3 minutes. (Keep an eye on pizza pie to make sure it doesn't burn.)

3. Use a hot pad or oven mitt to remove skillet from broiler because it will be very hot. Let cool for 2 minutes, then shake pan a little to loosen pizza pie. If it doesn't move, use a rubber spatula to carefully loosen edges. To unmold, invert a large plate on top of skillet, and turn pizza pie on top of pan. Then invert another large plate on pizza pie and turn it over. (Top of pizza pie should now be facing up.) Cut into four slices and serve. Can be refrigerated for up to three days.

NUTRITIONAL VALUE
PER SERVING
(5-INCH SLICE):
Calories: 224 |
Calories from Fat: 52 |
Protein: 15 g | Carbs: 30 g |
Total Fat: 6 g |
Saturated Fat: 2 g |
Trans Fat: 0 g | Fiber: 4 g |
Sodium: 188 mg |
Cholesterol: 110 mg

NOTE *To reconstitute sun-dried tomatoes, soak in water for 30 minutes.*

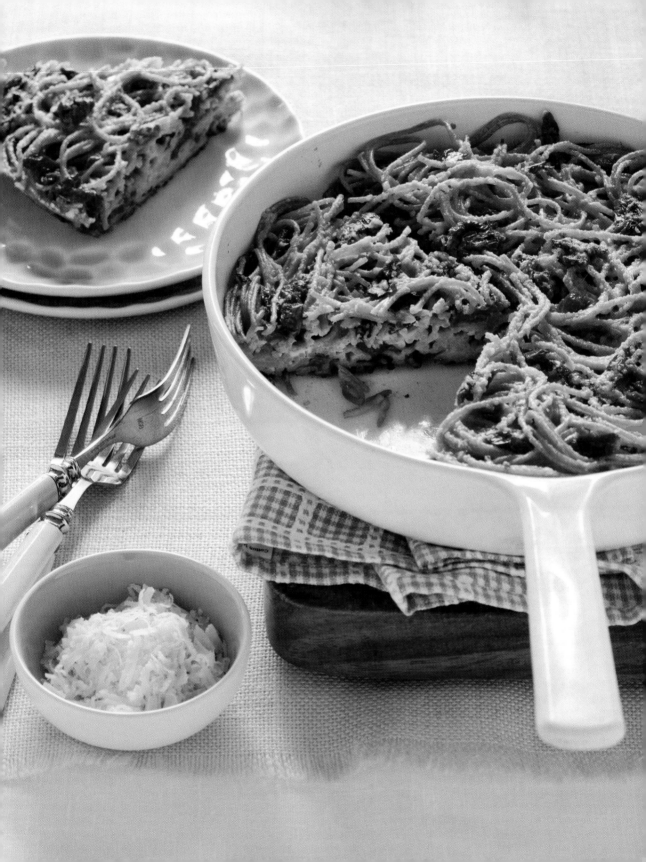

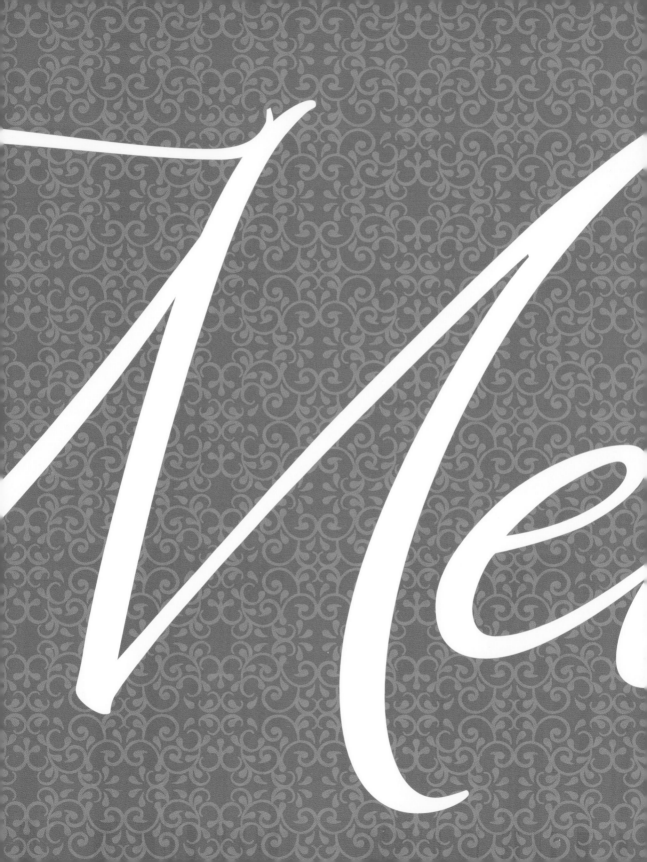

7

Vegetarian Meals

168   VENICE BEACH ROASTED VEGETABLE AND AVOCADO SUB

171   FRENCH GREEN LENTIL SALAD
with Easter Egg Radishes and Mache

172   PESTO STUFFED PORTOBELLO PIZZAS

175   PERSIAN COUSCOUS AND CHICKPEAS
with Kumquats

176   CURRY SPICED LENTIL FALAFEL
with Tahini Sauce

179   TOFU FAJITAS
with Peppers

180   ROASTED VEGETABLE EGGPLANT PARMESAN

183   QUINOA RISOTTO
with Garlic Herb Creminis

184   LONG-LIFE VEGETABLE STIR-FRY

187   ROASTED RED POTATOES, ASPARAGUS AND FRISÉE
with Crispy Croutons

188   *Vegetarian Done Right*

Servings: 2
Prep time: 10 minutes
Cooking time:
25 minutes

VENICE BEACH ROASTED VEGETABLE AND AVOCADO SUB

When I think of Venice Beach I think of sand, surf and muscles! This sandwich is fun and fresh, perfect for a day at the beach.

Note: Yogurt Cheese must be made ahead of time.

INGREDIENTS

3 slices eggplant, ½-inch thick and sliced crosswise into disks
½ baby zucchini, sliced ¼-inch thick lengthwise into planks
Eat-Clean Cooking Spray (see page 348)
⅛ tsp / 0.625 ml sea salt
⅛ tsp / 0.625 ml freshly ground black pepper
3 Tbsp / 45 ml Yogurt Cheese (see recipe on page 348)
8 inches of whole grain baguette, halved lengthwise
½ avocado, pitted and smashed
3 large or 6 small tomato slices

METHOD

1. Place oven rack in top third of oven and preheat to 425°F / 220°C. Place eggplant and zucchini on a baking sheet. Spray both sides of vegetables with Eat-Clean Cooking Spray, and season with salt and pepper. Place in oven and roast until zucchini is soft and slightly browned on bottom, 10 minutes. Using a metal spatula, remove zucchini and set aside. Place sheet with eggplant back in oven and cook for 15 minutes longer, turning once.

2. Spread yogurt cheese on one half of baguette, and smashed avocado on other half. Layer eggplant, zucchini and tomato slices on bottom half of baguette. Place other half of baguette on top. Using a serrated knife, slice sandwich in half and serve.

NUTRITIONAL VALUE
PER SERVING:
Calories: 221 |
Calories from Fat: 91 |
Protein: 8 g | Carbs: 25 g |
Total Fat: 11 g |
Saturated Fat: 2 g |
Trans Fat: 0 g | Fiber: 7 g |
Sodium: 184 mg |
Cholesterol: 1 mg

TIP *Try adding some fresh herbs such as chopped basil to Yogurt Cheese for extra flavor!*

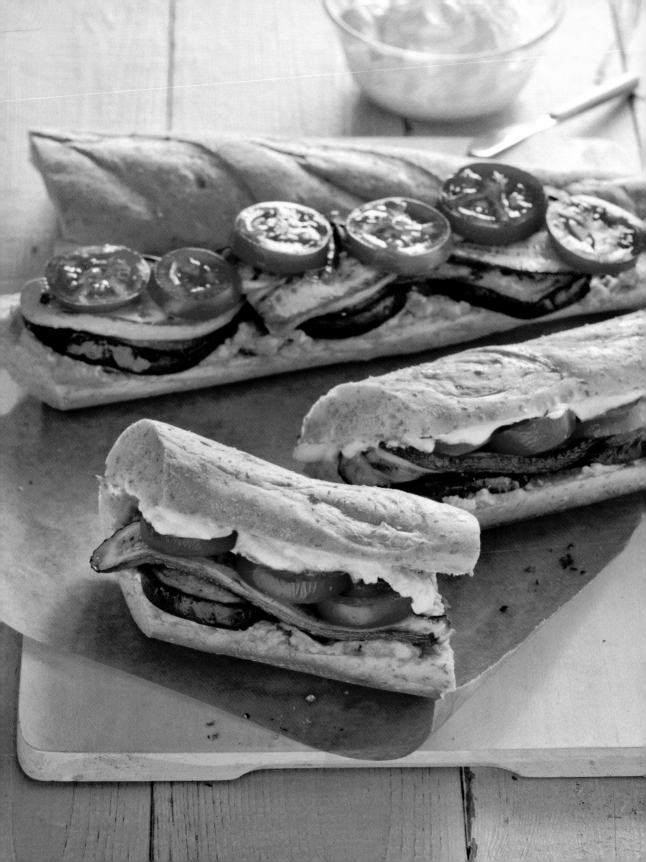

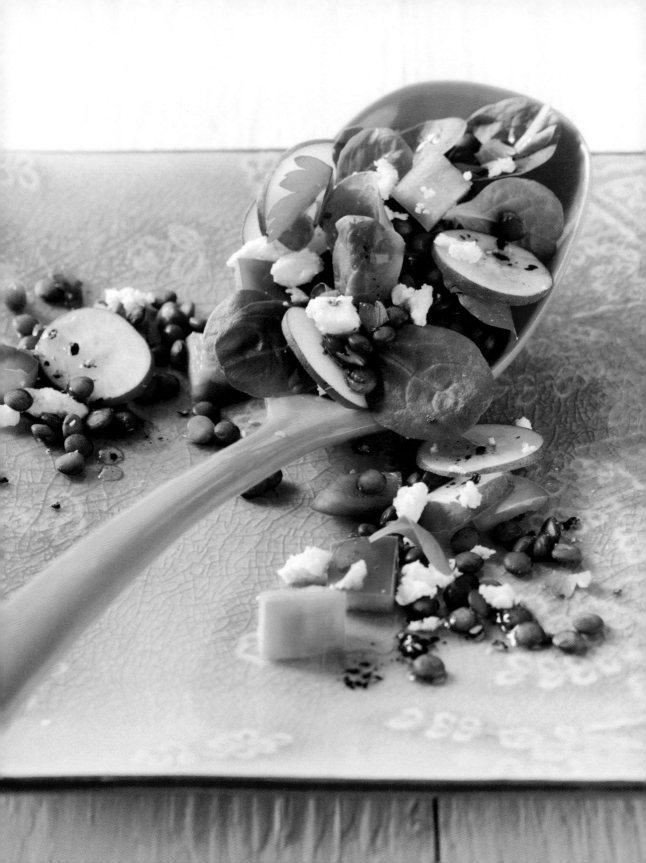

Servings: 4 x 1 cup
Prep time: 15 minutes
Cooking time:
20-25 minutes

FRENCH GREEN LENTIL SALAD
with Easter Egg Radishes and Mache

French green lentils, or lentilles du Puy, are a special sort of lentil grown in the south of France on a rugged mountain. The word "puy" actually refers to an isolated volcanic hill. These lentils grow without water or fertilization, and retain their shape even when fully cooked.

INGREDIENTS

SALAD
½ cup / 120 ml French green lentils (lentilles du Puy)
1 bay leaf
1 sprig fresh thyme
Healthy pinch sea salt
1 bunch Easter egg radishes (red, white, pink, and purple radishes),
    trimmed and thinly sliced (about 1 cup / 240 ml)
½ green pepper, diced
2 cups / 480 ml mache, or similar green such as spinach or arugula
2 oz / 57 g low-fat feta (about a 2-inch cube), crumbled
1 Tbsp / 15 ml freshly chopped basil
1 Tbsp / 15 ml freshly chopped parsley

VINAIGRETTE
1 Tbsp / 15 ml fresh lemon juice
1 Tbsp / 15 ml white balsamic vinegar
¼ tsp / 1.25 ml sea salt
⅛ tsp / 0.625 ml freshly ground black pepper
1 Tbsp / 15 ml extra virgin olive oil

METHOD

1. Add lentils to a small pot and cover with 2 inches of cold water. Add bay leaf, sprig of thyme and salt. Bring to a boil over high heat, and then reduce heat to simmer, covered, until tender but still intact, 20 to 25 minutes. Drain, and discard bay leaf and thyme sprig. Transfer lentils to a large bowl.

2. In a small bowl, whisk together all vinaigrette ingredients and pour over lentils. Add radishes, green pepper, mache or other green, feta, basil and parsley, and toss to combine. Serve immediately.

NUTRITIONAL VALUE
PER SERVING:
Calories: 146 |
Calories from Fat: 40 |
Protein: 8 g | Carbs: 19 g |
Total Fat: 5 g |
Saturated Fat: 1 g |
Trans Fat: 0 g |
Fiber: 5 g | Sodium: 285 mg |
Cholesterol: 3 mg

Servings: 4 x 1 pizza
Prep time: 10 minutes
Cooking time:
10 minutes

PESTO STUFFED PORTOBELLO PIZZAS

This dish is so speedy and simple to make, yet tastes like you've spent much longer in the kitchen. The large meaty Portobello mushrooms replace standard pizza dough, which makes this a wonderful low-carb, vegetarian pizza dish.

INGREDIENTS

4 Portobello mushroom caps, stems removed
½ cup Basil Lemon Pesto (see recipe on page 126) or other Clean pesto sauce
4 oz / 170 g fresh mozzarella, drained and sliced ¼-inch thick
4 campari tomatoes or other vine-ripened tomatoes, sliced ¼-inch
    thick (enough to almost cover top of four pizzas)

METHOD

1. Preheat oven to 425°F / 220°C.

2. Using a soup spoon, scrape out gills from underside of portobello caps and discard. Spread 2 Tbsp / 30 ml pesto in scraped-out hollow of each mushroom cap. Top with mozzarella and tomato slices, enough to cover top of each mushroom.

3. Place pizzas on a baking sheet and bake in oven until mozzarella is melted and portobello mushrooms are cooked, but still hold their shape, about 10 minutes.

NUTRITIONAL VALUE
PER SERVING:
Calories: 201 |
Calories from Fat: 121 |
Protein: 12 g | Carbs: 10 g |
Total Fat: 14 g |
Saturated Fat: 4 g |
Trans Fat: 0 g | Fiber: 4 g |
Sodium: 434 mg |
Cholesterol: 20 mg

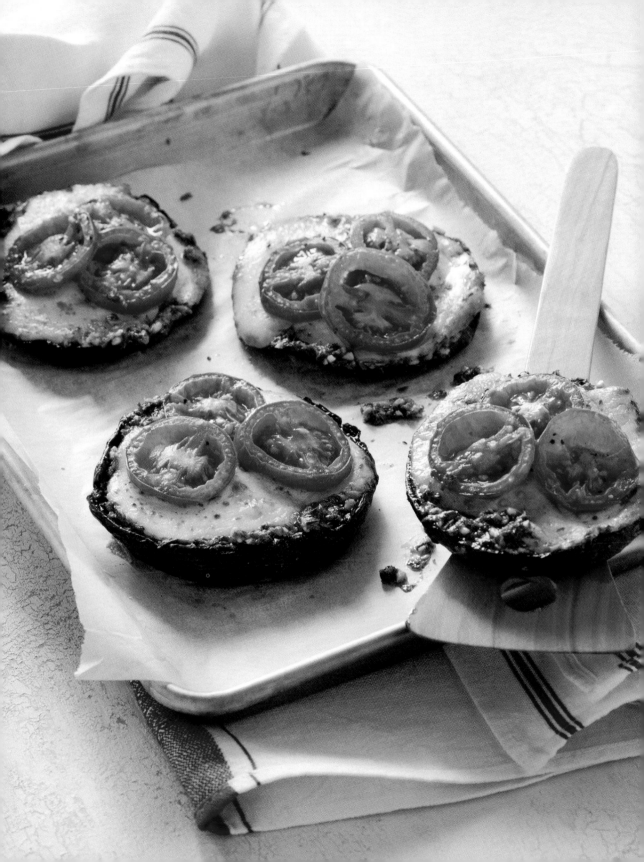

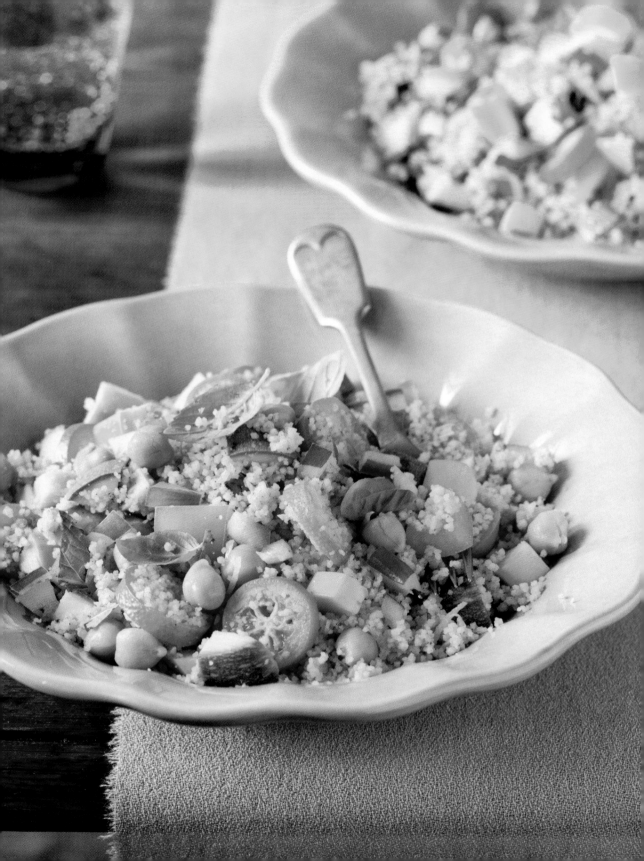

Servings: 7 x 1 cup
Prep time: 15 minutes
Cooking time:
5 minutes

PERSIAN COUSCOUS AND CHICKPEAS
with Kumquats

Kumquats are fruit that look like tiny oranges. They are not citrus fruit, but they are indeed sour. The skin is sweet and the flesh is tart – a refreshing addition to this Middle Eastern couscous dish.

INGREDIENTS

COUSCOUS

1 cup / 240 ml whole wheat couscous
1 cup / 240 ml cooked chickpeas
1 cup / 240 ml diced baby zucchini
½ yellow bell pepper, diced
½ cup / 120 ml sliced kumquats
¼ cup / 60 ml diced red onion
2 Tbsp / 30 ml chopped fresh basil
1 Tbsp / 15 ml chopped fresh mint

DRESSING

Zest and juice of 1½ lemons
½ tsp / 2.5 ml ground cumin
⅛ tsp / 0.625 ml ground allspice
⅛ tsp / 0.625 ml ground cinnamon
⅛ tsp / 0.625 ml cayenne pepper
½ tsp / 2.5 ml sea salt
¼ tsp / 1.25 ml freshly ground black pepper

METHOD

1. Bring 1¼ cups / 300 ml water to boil in a small saucepan over high heat. Stir in couscous, cover, and remove from heat. Let sit to hydrate and plump up, about 5 minutes. Fluff and add to a large bowl. Add rest of ingredients up to, but not including, basil and mint. Toss to combine and allow heat of couscous to warm veggies.

2. Whisk together all dressing ingredients in a small bowl. Pour dressing over couscous and chickpea mixture. Add basil and mint and toss to combine.

NUTRITIONAL VALUE
PER SERVING:
Calories: 148 |
Calories from Fat: 12 |
Protein: 6 g | Carbs: 29 g |
Total Fat: 1 g |
Saturated Fat: 0 g |
Trans Fat: 0 g | Fiber: 6 g |
Sodium: 119 mg |
Cholesterol: 0 mg

CURRY SPICED LENTIL FALAFEL
with Tahini Sauce

Traditional falafels are made from spiced chickpeas and fava beans ground into a paste, rolled into balls and fried. Using brown lentils and chickpea flour, and lightly sautéing the balls before baking them is a new and healthier take on this popular Middle Eastern dish.

INGREDIENTS

2/3 cup / 160 ml brown lentils
2 cups / 480 ml water
3 Tbsp / 45 ml extra virgin
    olive oil, divided
1 onion, finely chopped
2 ribs celery, finely chopped
1 carrot, finely chopped
3 cloves garlic, minced
1 Tbsp / 15 ml ground cumin

1/2 tsp / 2.5 ml curry powder
1/4 tsp / 1.25 ml cayenne
1 tsp / 5 ml sea salt
1/2 tsp / 2.5 ml freshly ground
    black pepper
1/2 cup / 120 ml chickpea flour
1/2 cup / 120 ml finely chopped parsley
3/4 cup / 175 ml Tahini Sauce
    (see recipe on page 352), divided

METHOD

1. Combine lentils and water in a medium saucepan over high heat. Bring to a boil, and then reduce heat to simmer for 25 to 30 minutes until tender, but not falling apart. Drain.

2. Preheat oven to 350°F / 175°C. Heat 1 Tbsp / 15 ml olive oil in a large skillet over medium heat. Add onion, celery and carrot, and cook vegetables until tender, but not brown, 5 to 7 minutes. Add garlic and cook for 1 minute longer. Add cooked and drained lentils to pan, along with cumin, curry powder, cayenne, salt and pepper. Stir to combine. Remove from heat.

3. Add half of lentil mixture to a food processor and pulse chop until fairly smooth. Scrape mixture into a large bowl and add rest of lentils. Add flour and parsley, and mix well. Using a small ice cream scoop about the size of a large golf ball, or a soup spoon, scoop out equal-sized portions of lentil mixture and shape into falafel rounds two inches in diameter and half an inch thick, and place on a baking sheet or tray.

4. Working in batches, heat remaining olive oil in a skillet over medium heat. Add falafel rounds and cook until browned, 2 minutes on each side. Transfer to a baking sheet and continue cooking falafel rounds until they are all browned. Transfer them to preheated oven to finish cooking for 15 minutes. Remove and serve warm with Tahini Sauce.

NUTRITIONAL VALUE
PER SERVING:
Calories: 398 |
Calories from Fat: 275 |
Protein: 11 g | Carbs: 26 g |
Total Fat: 31 g |
Saturated Fat: 4 g |
Trans Fat: 0 g | Fiber: 7 g |
Sodium: 584 mg |
Cholesterol: 0 mg

TIP

Leftover falafel can be reheated in oven to retain crispiness. Also delicious wrapped in an Ezekiel sprouted whole grain tortilla or pita, with tomato slices and shredded lettuce.

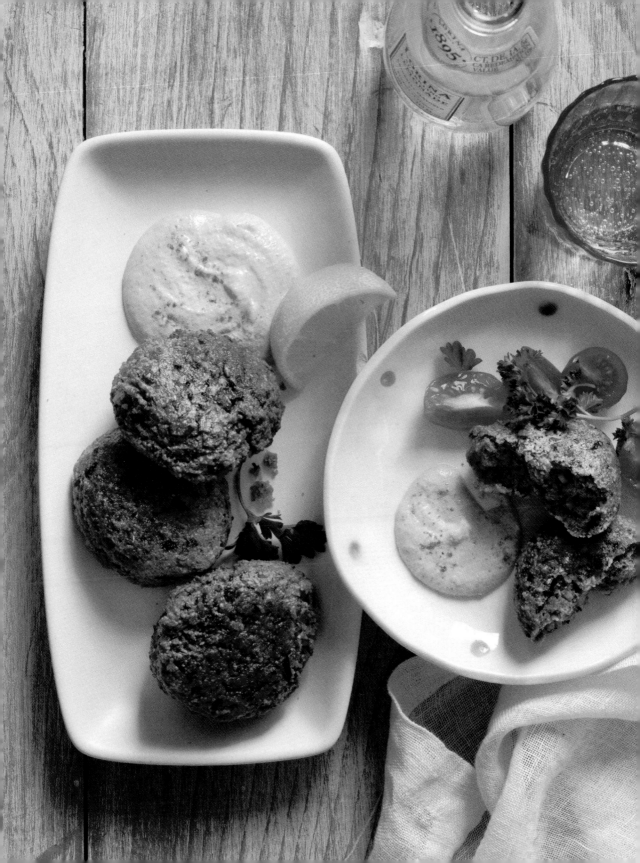

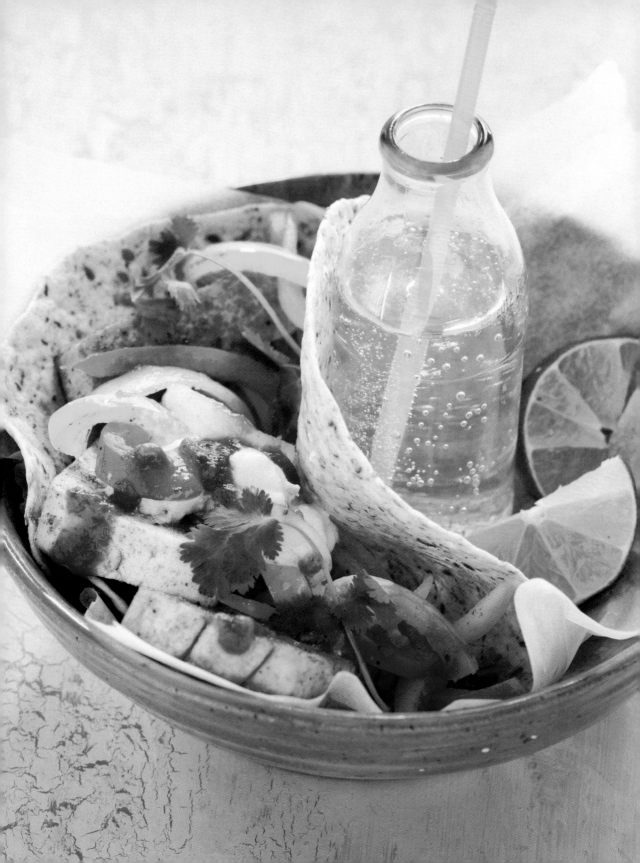

Servings: 4
Prep time: 20 minutes
Cooking time:
12 minutes

TOFU FAJITAS
with Peppers

Tofu is one of those magical foods with the ability to transform into whatever you need it to be. It can be blended into pudding, scrambled into eggs and now, stuffed into fajitas – it's about time!

Note: Yogurt Cheese and Salsa Roja must be made ahead of time.

INGREDIENTS

1½ tsp / 7.5 ml ground cumin
1½ tsp / 7.5 ml chili powder
¾ tsp / 3.75 ml ground coriander
¾ tsp / 3.75 ml sea salt
¼ tsp / 1.25 ml freshly ground
   black pepper
Eat-Clean Cooking Spray (see page 348)
12 oz / 340 g extra-firm tofu, drained
   and patted dry with a paper or tea
   towel, cut into 8 equal slices
½ red pepper, seeded and thinly sliced
½ yellow pepper, seeded and thinly sliced

1 Anaheim pepper, seeded
   and thinly sliced
½ yellow onion, thinly sliced
4 all-natural whole wheat tortillas
   (7 to 8 inches in diameter)
8 Tbsp / 120 ml Salsa Roja (see recipe
   on page 118) or other Clean salsa
8 Tbsp / 120 ml Yogurt Cheese (see
   recipe on page 348), to garnish
Fresh cilantro, to garnish

METHOD

1. In a small bowl, mix together cumin, chili powder, coriander, salt and pepper. Heat a large nonstick skillet over medium-high heat and spray with Eat-Clean Cooking Spray. Sprinkle one-third spice mixture on one side of tofu slices and add them to skillet, seasoned side down, in a single layer, working in batches if necessary. Sprinkle other side of tofu slices with another third of spice mixture and spray with more Eat-Clean Cooking Spray. Cook until brown on one side, about 3 minutes, then flip and cook until brown on the other side, another 3 minutes. Remove and set aside.

2. Return skillet to stove and reduce heat to medium. Spray with Eat-Clean Cooking Spray and add peppers and onions in a single layer, working in batches if necessary. Sprinkle with remaining third of spice mixture and toss to coat. Spread out peppers in a single layer and let cook without stirring until browned on underside, about 3 minutes. Stir or toss and continue to cook for an additional 2 to 3 minutes until soft and browned in spots. Remove skillet from heat.

3. To serve, divide tortillas among four plates and top each with two slices tofu. Divide sautéed peppers and onions among four tortillas. Top each with 2 Tbsp / 30 ml Salsa Roja, 2 Tbsp / 30 ml Yogurt Cheese and a few sprigs of cilantro.

NUTRITIONAL VALUE
PER SERVING:
Calories: 243 |
Calories from Fat: 60 |
Protein: 16 g | Carbs: 25 g |
Total Fat: 7 g |
Saturated Fat: 2 g |
Trans Fat: 0 g | Fiber: 5 g |
Sodium: 636 mg |
Cholesterol: 1 mg

Servings: 6
Prep time: 15 minutes
Cooking time:
50-60 minutes
Cooling time:
10 minutes

ROASTED VEGETABLE EGGPLANT PARMESAN

Packed with vegetables, this dish is more of an eggplant-based vegetarian lasagna than a Parmesan, which typically calls for breadcrumbs. Whatever it is, it's sure to impress your dinner guests – vegetarian or not.

Note: Clean Marinara must be made ahead of time.

INGREDIENTS

1 eggplant, sliced crosswise into ¼-inch-thick disks
1 baby zucchini, halved crosswise and sliced into ¼-inch-thick planks
1 red bell pepper, seeded and quartered
1 yellow bell pepper, seeded and quartered
3 Tbsp / 45 ml extra virgin olive oil, divided
½ tsp / 2.5 ml sea salt
¼ tsp / 1.25 ml freshly ground black pepper
3 cups / 720 ml Clean Marinara (see recipe on page 122)
4 oz / 114 g fresh mozzarella, sliced ¼-inch thick
2 Tbsp / 30 ml grated real Parmigiano Reggiano cheese

METHOD

1. Preheat oven to 425°F / 220°C. Place eggplant on one baking sheet, and zucchini, red and yellow peppers on another baking sheet. Using a pastry brush, coat both sides of eggplant slices with 2 Tbsp / 30 ml oil. Drizzle remaining oil over rest of veggies. Sprinkle all vegetables with salt and pepper and spread out in a single layer. Place in oven to roast until soft and starting to brown, 12 to 15 minutes. (You want vegetables almost completely cooked through.) Remove and set aside.

2. Lower heat in oven to 350°F / 175°C. In a three-quart baking dish, spread ½ cup / 120 ml marinara over bottom. Begin layering vegetables, starting with eggplant, completely covering bottom of pan. Spread a layer of sauce over eggplant and add a layer of another vegetable, then sauce. Repeat until all vegetables and sauce have been used, making sure to reserve enough sauce to top last layer of vegetables. To finish assembling dish, lay sliced mozzarella over top, and then spread out an even layer of Parmigiano Reggiano. Bake, uncovered, in oven until cheese is bubbly and lightly browned, 35 to 45 minutes. Remove, and let sit to cool slightly before serving, 10 minutes.

NUTRITIONAL VALUE
PER SERVING:
Calories: 231 |
Calories from Fat: 125 |
Protein: 13 g | Carbs: 19 g |
Total Fat: 14 g |
Saturated Fat: 3 g |
Trans Fat: 0 g | Fiber: 6 g |
Sodium: 487 mg |
Cholesterol: 21 mg

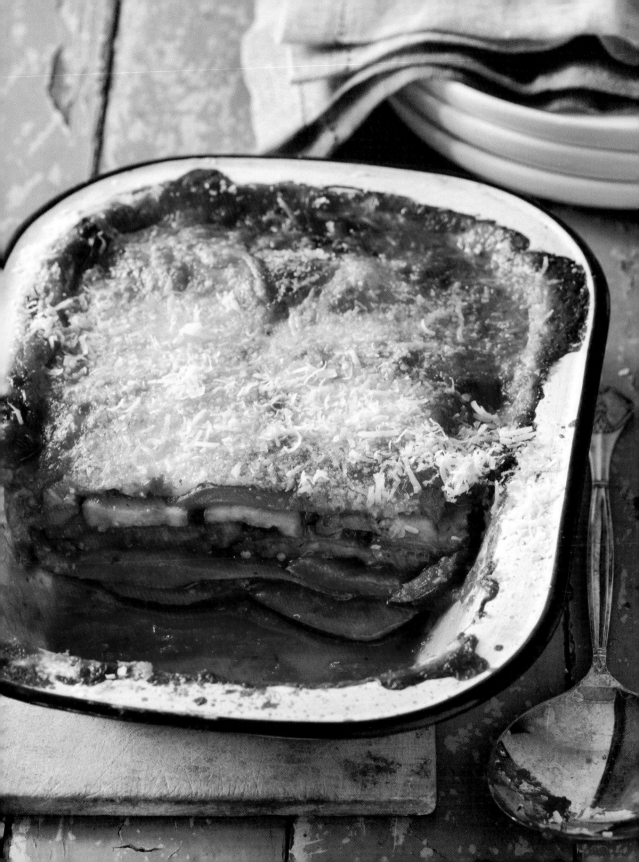

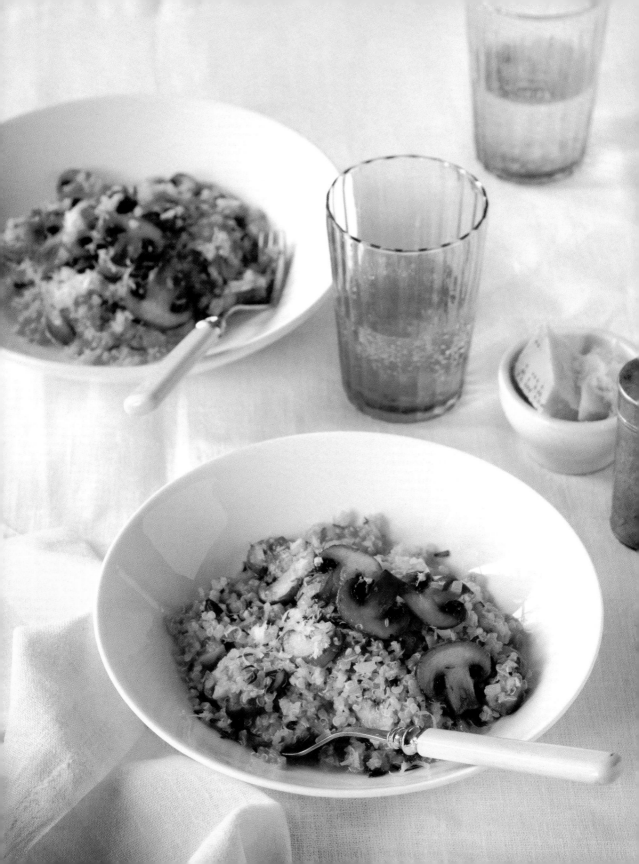

Servings: 4 x 1 cup
Prep time: 10 minutes
Cooking time:
25 minutes

QUINOA RISOTTO
with Garlic Herb Creminis

Quinoa is one of those foods that should be a staple in every vegetarian's (and meat eater's, for that matter!) diet. It usually has a crunchy, grainy texture, but is softened by the cheese in this recipe, which makes it an ideal choice for a protein-packed risotto.

INGREDIENTS

3 cups / 720 ml low-sodium
  vegetable broth
2 Tbsp / 30 ml extra virgin
  olive oil, divided
4 cups / 960 ml sliced cremini mushrooms
2 cloves garlic, chopped
1 tsp / 5 ml finely chopped fresh thyme
½ tsp / 2.5 ml finely chopped
  fresh rosemary

¾ tsp / 3.75 ml + pinch sea salt, divided
¼ tsp / 1.25 ml + pinch freshly
  ground black pepper, divided
2 Tbsp / 30 ml chopped shallots
1 cup / 240 ml white quinoa
¼ cup / 60 ml dry white wine
2 Tbsp / 30 ml finely grated
  Parmigiano Reggiano cheese

METHOD

1. Heat vegetable broth in a saucepan until just simmering. Reduce heat to low to keep hot.

2. Heat 1 Tbsp / 15 ml olive oil in a large skillet over medium-high heat. Add cremini mushrooms in a single layer and let cook, undisturbed, 2 minutes. Stir in garlic, thyme and rosemary, and season with a pinch of salt and pepper. Continue cooking until mushrooms are browned and garlic is fragrant and soft, but not burnt, about 2 minutes longer. Remove from heat and set aside.

3. Heat remaining 1 Tbsp / 15 ml olive oil in a large skillet over medium heat. Add shallots and sauté until soft but not brown, about 2 minutes. Stir in quinoa, remaining salt and pepper, and let cook for 1 minute. Stir in white wine and cook until absorbed, about 1 minute. Ladle ½ cup / 120 ml hot vegetable broth into quinoa. Stir quinoa frequently and allow broth to be absorbed into quinoa as it cooks. When broth is almost completely absorbed, add another ½ cup / 120 ml hot broth, and repeat. Continue adding hot broth, ½ cup / 120 ml at a time, stirring frequently, until quinoa is cooked through, about 20 minutes. It will be plump and translucent.

4. Stir in reserved cooked cremini mushrooms and Parmigiano Reggiano. Risotto should be loose enough to slowly pour. If it's too tight, add more broth to loosen. Spoon risotto into four shallow bowls and serve immediately, topped with a little more grated Parmigiano, if desired.

NUTRITIONAL VALUE
PER SERVING:
Calories: 293 |
Calories from Fat: 93 |
Protein: 10 g | Carbs: 37 g |
Total Fat: 10 g |
Saturated Fat: 1 g |
Trans Fat: 0 g | Fiber: 3 g |
Sodium: 456 mg |
Cholesterol: 3 mg

LONG-LIFE VEGETABLE STIR-FRY

This dish is packed with vegetables, and therefore contains the nutrients you need to stay slim, healthy and strong. The ingredient list may look long, but cooking goes very fast! Be sure to have all ingredients prepared before you start tossing them into wok.

INGREDIENTS

1 Tbsp / 15 ml high-heat safflower oil
1 Tbsp / 15 ml sesame oil
4 dried arbol chiles, stems removed
2 Tbsp / 30 ml grated fresh ginger
1 cup / 240 ml sliced cremini or white button mushrooms
1 cup / 240 ml shredded carrots
½ red bell pepper, seeded and thinly sliced
¼ head green cabbage, cored and thinly sliced
1 x 5.5-oz / 160 ml can whole baby sweet corn, drained
1 x 8-oz / 240 ml can sliced bamboo shoots, drained
1 x 8-oz / 240 ml can sliced peeled water chestnuts, drained
4 large cloves garlic, chopped
2 scallions, thinly sliced on diagonal
1 Tbsp / 15 ml low-sodium soy sauce
1 Tbsp / 15 ml rice wine vinegar
1 tsp / 5 ml sea salt
¼ tsp / 1.25 ml freshly ground black pepper
4 cups / 960 ml cooked quinoa
1 tsp / 5 ml toasted sesame seeds

METHOD

1. Heat a very large dry wok, cast iron skillet, or sauté pan over medium-high heat. Do not add oils until wok or pan is thoroughly heated. Add safflower oil and sesame oil and swirl to coat wok. Add arbol chiles and ginger, and using a metal spatula or tongs, stir into oil for only a few seconds. Immediately add mushrooms, carrots, red pepper and cabbage, and cook until soft, about 4 minutes. Add corn, bamboo shoots and chestnuts, and cook for 1 to 2 minutes. Stir in garlic and cook for one minute longer. Stir in scallions, soy sauce, vinegar, salt and pepper until combined well.

2. Serve immediately with cooked quinoa and garnish with sesame seeds.

NUTRITIONAL VALUE
PER SERVING (1 CUP /
240 ML VEGGIES AND
1 CUP / 240 ML QUINOA):
Calories: 350 |
Calories from Fat: 80 |
Protein: 12 g | Carbs: 58 g |
Total Fat: 9 g |
Saturated Fat: 0.5 g |
Trans Fat: 0 g | Fiber: 10 g |
Sodium: 645 mg |
Cholesterol: 0 mg

NOTE *Unless you are tolerant of very spicy foods, do not eat arbol chiles. They are for flavoring the dish, but are generally not consumed. You may wish to remove them before serving.*

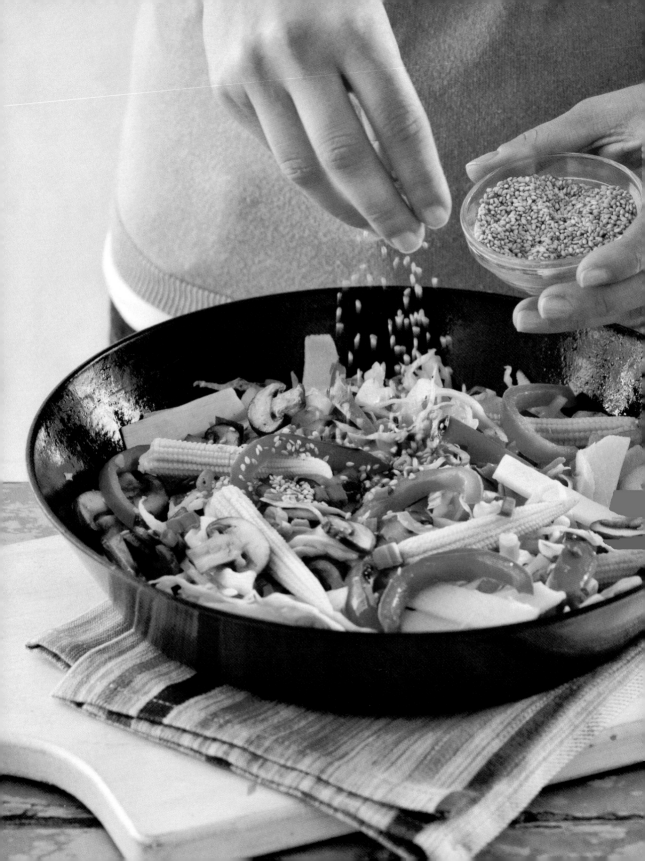

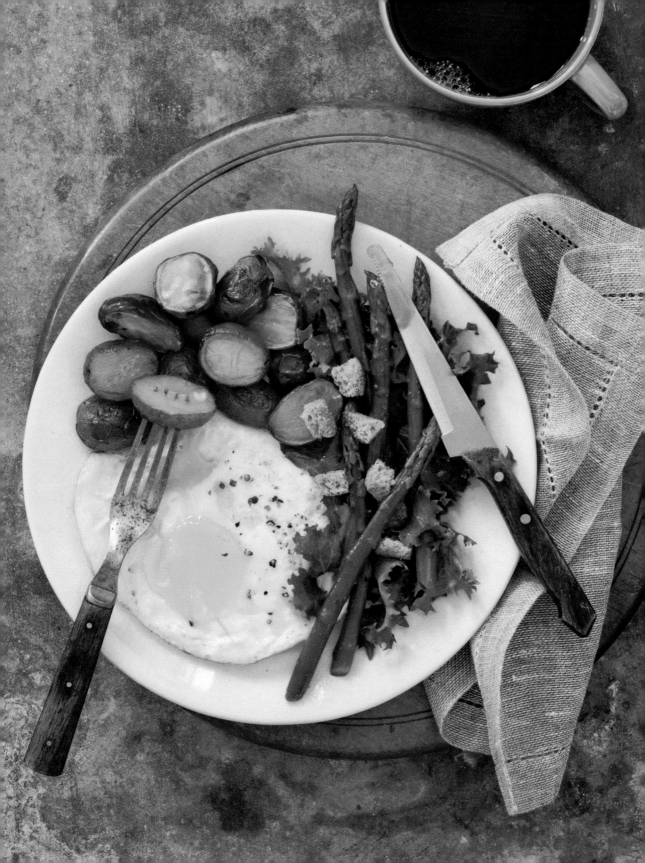

ROASTED RED POTATOES, ASPARAGUS AND FRISÉE
with Crispy Croutons

This dish is like breakfast for dinner with a twist. The potatoes are crispy, the asparagus is tender, the salad is refreshing and the eggs bring it all together.

INGREDIENTS

1 lb / 454 g baby red potatoes, halved (about 4 cups / 960 ml)

3½ tsp / 17.5 ml extra virgin olive oil, divided

¼ tsp / 1.25 ml sea salt, plus a few pinches, divided

⅛ tsp / 0.625 ml freshly ground black pepper, plus a few pinches, divided

1 bunch baby asparagus (about 30 stalks), tough ends trimmed

1 head frisée lettuce, torn into bite-sized pieces (about 6 cups / 1.5 L)

Juice of ½ lemon

Eat-Clean Cooking Spray (see page 348)

4 whole eggs

4 egg whites

8 Tbsp / 120 ml Crispy Herb and Garlic Croutons (see recipe on page 354)

METHOD

1. Preheat oven to 425°F / 220°C. Place potatoes on a baking sheet and toss with 2 tsp / 10 ml olive oil, ¼ tsp / 1.25 ml sea salt and ⅛ tsp / 0.625 ml black pepper. Turn potatoes cut side down and place in oven. Roast until soft when pierced with a skewer, and lightly browned, about 15 minutes.

2. In the meantime, place asparagus on a baking sheet and toss with 1 tsp / 5 ml olive oil and a pinch of sea salt and freshly ground black pepper. Roast in oven until slightly soft and lightly browned, about 7 minutes.

3. Toss frisée with lemon juice, remaining ½ tsp / 2.5 ml olive oil, and a small pinch of sea salt and freshly ground black pepper.

4. Heat a nonstick skillet over medium-low heat and coat with Eat-Clean Cooking Spray. Add eggs and egg whites, and season with a small pinch of sea salt and freshly ground black pepper. Cook until whites are set and opaque, about 2 minutes. If you like your egg sunny side up, slide egg out of pan onto a plate. If you prefer your egg cooked over easy, medium or hard, gently flip egg, and cook until yolk reaches desired doneness. (You can test doneness of egg yolk by gently pressing on it with your finger – the firmer it gets, the more cooked it is.)

5. Divide asparagus among four plates, and put 1½ cups / 360 ml frisée on top of each pile of asparagus. Place 1 cup / 240 ml potatoes on side of frisée on each plate, and place cooked egg on side opposite potatoes. Sprinkle 2 Tbsp / 30 ml Crispy Herb and Garlic Croutons over each plate.

NUTRITIONAL VALUE
PER SERVING:
Calories: 270 |
Calories from Fat: 94 |
Protein: 16 g | Carbs: 29 g |
Total Fat: 10 g |
Saturated Fat: 3 g |
Trans Fat: 0 g | Fiber: 7 g |
Sodium: 307 mg |
Cholesterol: 211 mg

Vegetarian Done Right

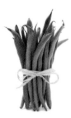

The choice to adopt a vegetarian lifestyle is brilliant as long as it is done correctly. Vegetarians can well exceed the recommended intake of vegetables each day and in general significantly reduce their chances of suffering from cardiovascular disease and developing diabetes or cancer. However, they also run the risk of developing iron deficiencies, vitamin B12 deficiencies, osteoporosis and more. It's all about balance!

How to Be a Healthy Vegetarian:

Whether you're a man, woman (even pregnant or breastfeeding), teenager or child, you can follow a healthy vegetarian diet. Educate yourself as much as possible on this lifestyle choice. The key is ensuring you get enough of the right kind of foods in the best combinations to get the most nutrients.

Getting Complete Protein:

You will meet your needs by consuming the recommended portions in the correct combinations.

ON THEIR OWN:

Egg whites, Soy protein isolate, Whey protein isolate, Quinoa*, Hempseeds*, Soy products (edamame, tofu, tempeh, miso)*, Spirulina*

* The bioavailability of these options is lower than pure egg whites.

IN COMBINATION:

Legumes + whole grains, nuts and seeds + legumes, grains + nuts and seeds, corn + legumes

SOME EXAMPLES OF EACH:

Grains (oats, millet, buckwheat, quinoa, amaranth, brown rice), Legumes (black beans, chickpeas, kidney beans, lentils, pinto beans, puy lentils), Nuts and seeds (sunflower seeds, pumpkin seeds, almonds, walnuts, cashews)

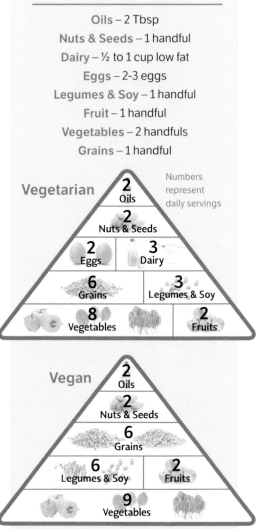

Portion Sizes

Oils – 2 Tbsp

Nuts & Seeds – 1 handful

Dairy – ½ to 1 cup low fat

Eggs – 2-3 eggs

Legumes & Soy – 1 handful

Fruit – 1 handful

Vegetables – 2 handfuls

Grains – 1 handful

Vegetarian

Numbers represent daily servings

2 Oils
2 Nuts & Seeds
2 Eggs | 3 Dairy
6 Grains | 3 Legumes & Soy
8 Vegetables | 2 Fruits

Vegan

2 Oils
2 Nuts & Seeds
6 Grains
6 Legumes & Soy | 2 Fruits
9 Vegetables

NUTRIENT	WHAT IT SUPPORTS	VEGETARIAN SOURCES	NOTES
Calcium	Strong teeth and bones, Muscle maintenance, Hormone function	Dairy, Dark green vegetables, Almonds, Broccoli Fortified tofu and soy milk	
Iodine	Thyroid health, Metabolism	Green, leafy vegetables, Asparagus, Kelp, Iodized sea salt	
Iron	Red blood cell function	Green, leafy vegetables, Beans, Lentils, Tofu, Pumpkin seeds, Millet, Dried figs, Apricots and Dates	Pair with foods high in Vitamin C and avoid caffeine consumption in order to get best absorption.
Omega-3 Fatty Acids	Healthy heart, eyes and skin, Brain development	Flax, chia and hemp seeds, Eggs, Walnuts, Soybeans	Supplement may be indicated especially for vegetarians avoiding fish.
Protein	Tissue growth and repair, Hormone and enzyme function	Whole grains, Nuts, Seeds, Bean sprouts, Hummus, (see Getting Complete Protein on page 188)	
Vitamin B12	Nerve formation, Cell production (especially red blood cells)	Fortified soy milk and cereals	Supplement may be indicated since it is found primarily in animal products.
Vitamin D	Strong teeth and bones, Healthy immunity	Sunlight exposure, Fortified cereals, Soy and cow's milk	Supplement may be indicated if you are not getting enough sunlight.
Zinc	Healthy immunity, Wound healing, Cell division, Enzyme function	Green, leafy vegetables, Whole grains, Soy products, Avocados, Bananas, Apricots, Apples, Cashews, Almonds, Wheat germ	Supplement may be indicated since zinc from plant sources is less bioavailable than from animal sources.

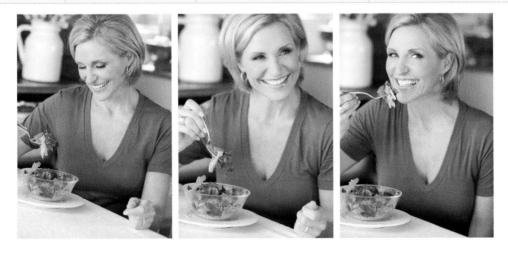

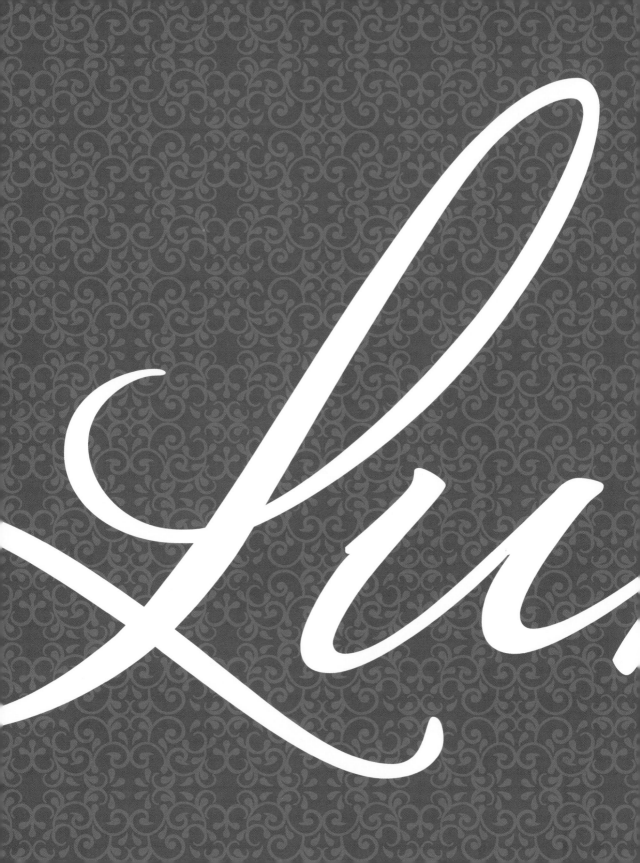

8

Lunch Outside the Lunchbox

192 BISON BURGER DOGS

195 SPANISH-STYLE TUNA SANDWICH

196 GARDEN VEGGIE STUFFED PITA POCKETS

199 QUINOA AND BLACK BEAN LUNCH BOWL

200 FRESH FIG CANAPÉS
with Mint and Balsamic Syrup

203 VANISHING PARTY NUTS

204 SCATTERED SUSHI BOWL
with Ginger Glazed Salmon (Chirashizushi)

207 SPICY ITALIAN TEMPEH SAUSAGE AND SPINACH
with Rotini

208 EGG SALAD WITH A TWIST

211 GRILLED CHICKEN CAESAR SALAD
with Spicy Kefir Caesar Dressing and Grilled Mini Pita Bread

212 JAMAICAN JERK STEAK
with Pineapple Lettuce Wraps

215 BBQ CHICKEN CHOP CHOP SALAD

Servings: 4
Prep time: 10 minutes
Cooking time:
7-12 minutes

BISON BURGER DOGS

Hot dogs remind me of the summer barbeques of my youth. Now as an adult, I'm cautious of eating store-bought wieners. I don't know what's in them – what a scary thought! Now you can bring hot dogs back to the table by making your own.

INGREDIENTS

1 lb / 454 g lean ground bison
¼ medium yellow onion, grated
1 clove garlic, put through a garlic press or finely minced
1 Tbsp / 15 ml yellow mustard
1 Tbsp / 15 ml tomato paste
2 Tbsp / 30 ml fresh basil, chopped
1 tsp / 5 ml sea salt, divided
½ tsp / 2.5 ml freshly ground black pepper
Eat-Clean Cooking Spray (see page 348)
4 whole grain hot dog buns
Fixin's, such as mustard, tomato slices, shredded lettuce, pickles and red onion

METHOD

1. Heat a grill or grill pan to medium-high heat. Mix together bison, onion, garlic, mustard, tomato paste, ½ tsp / 2.5 ml salt and all pepper until just combined. Don't over mix. Score meat into four equal sections and roll each into shape of a hot dog about five inches long. Place dogs on a baking sheet or plate and season with remaining ½ tsp / 2.5 ml salt.

2. Wash your hands well. Spray grill with Eat-Clean Cooking Spray and place dogs on grill. Cook 7 to 12 minutes until desired doneness, turning two or three times. Remove and serve in hot dog buns with your favorite fixins!

NUTRITIONAL VALUE
PER SERVING:
Calories: 296 |
Calories from Fat: 141 |
Protein: 21 g | Carbs: 21 g |
Total Fat: 16 g |
Saturated Fat: 0 g |
Trans Fat: 0 g | Fiber: 4 g |
Sodium: 682 mg |
Cholesterol: 59 mg

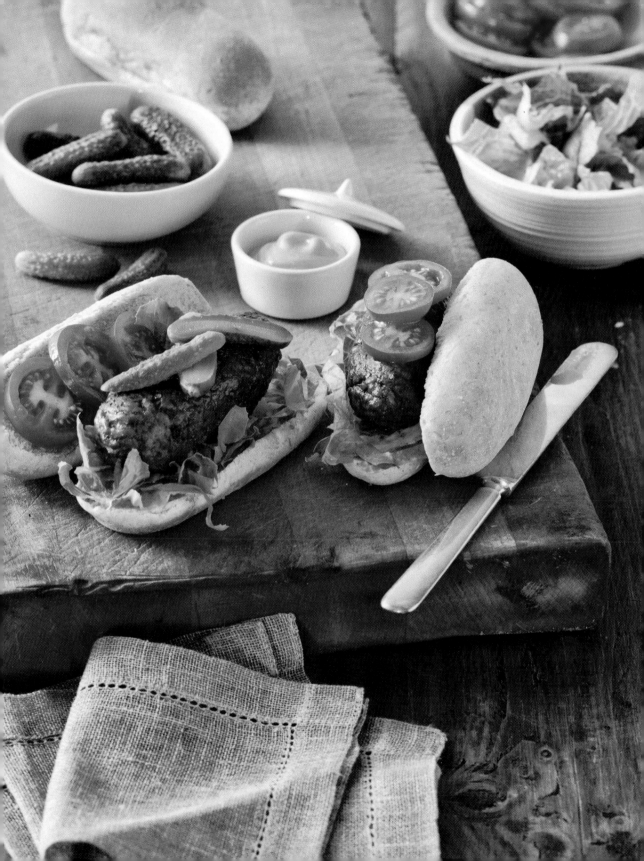

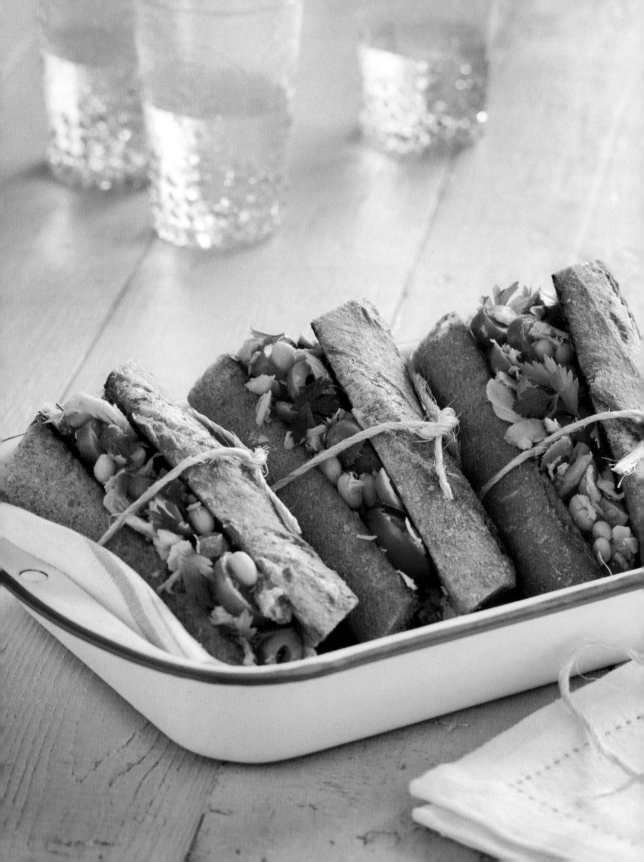

Servings: 4
Prep time: 10 minutes
Cooking time:
0 minutes

SPANISH-STYLE TUNA SANDWICH

This sandwich is inspired by Spanish cuisine. In Las Ramblas, a part of Spain popular with both tourists and locals, these tuna sandwiches are served in little stands. Try one as a late lunch before a satisfying siesta.

INGREDIENTS

1 x 5-oz can low-sodium dolphin-safe solid white **albacore tuna**, packed in water, drained
1 cup / 240 ml cooked **white beans**
½ cup / 120 ml sliced **cherry tomatoes**
¼ cup / 60 ml chopped **pimentos**
¼ cup / 60 ml pitted **green olives**, sliced
2 Tbsp / 30 ml fresh **lemon juice**
2 Tbsp / 30 ml **extra virgin olive oil**
¼ tsp / 1.25 ml **sea salt**
⅛ tsp / 0.625 ml freshly ground **black pepper**
16 inches **whole grain baguette**, cut in half lengthwise and toasted

METHOD

1. Place tuna and white beans in a small bowl and, using a fork, break up tuna into bite-sized pieces and slightly mash beans. Add rest of ingredients and mix well. Place tuna mixture on bottom half of toasted baguette and place top half of baguette on tuna. Cut long sandwich into four equal sections and serve. Or wrap up and take it to go!

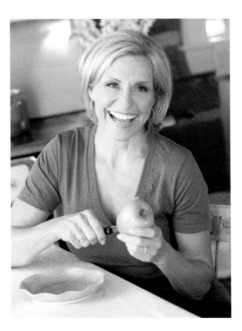

NUTRITIONAL VALUE
PER SERVING:
Calories: 297 |
Calories from Fat: 60 |
Protein: 19 g | Carbs: 42 g |
Total Fat: 7 g |
Saturated Fat: 1 g |
Trans Fat: 0 g | Fiber: 6 g |
Sodium: 707 mg |
Cholesterol: 15 mg

Servings: 1
Prep time: 10 minutes
Cooking time:
0 minutes

GARDEN VEGGIE STUFFED PITA POCKETS

Eating a lunch full of fresh vegetables gives me enough energy to tackle the afternoon without stopping. This pita pocket is packed with vegetables and nutrients. To prevent the bread from getting soggy, assemble your pita right before you eat it.

Note: Yogurt Cheese and Zesty Hummus must be made ahead of time.

INGREDIENTS

1 whole wheat pita, about 6 inches in diameter
2 Tbsp / 30 ml Zesty Hummus (see recipe on page 357)
2 Tbsp / 30 ml Yogurt Cheese (see recipe on page 348)
¼ cup / 60 ml shredded or grated carrot
¼ cup / 60 ml sliced mushrooms
¼ cup / 60 ml sliced radishes
¼ cup / 60 ml deli sprouts (such as clover, lentil, radish and fenugreek)
1 Tbsp / 15 ml unsalted sunflower seeds

METHOD

1. Cut pita in half. Divide hummus between two pita halves and spread on inside of each. Repeat with Yogurt Cheese. Divide veggies between two pita halves and stuff inside each. Sprinkle sunflower seeds inside each pita half. Serve immediately, or wrap up and take to go!

NUTRITIONAL VALUE
PER SERVING:
Calories: 331 |
Calories from Fat: 103 |
Protein: 16 g | Carbs: 45 g |
Total Fat: 7 g |
Saturated Fat: 2 g |
Trans Fat: 0 g | Fiber: 9 g |
Sodium: 397 mg |
Cholesterol: 1 mg

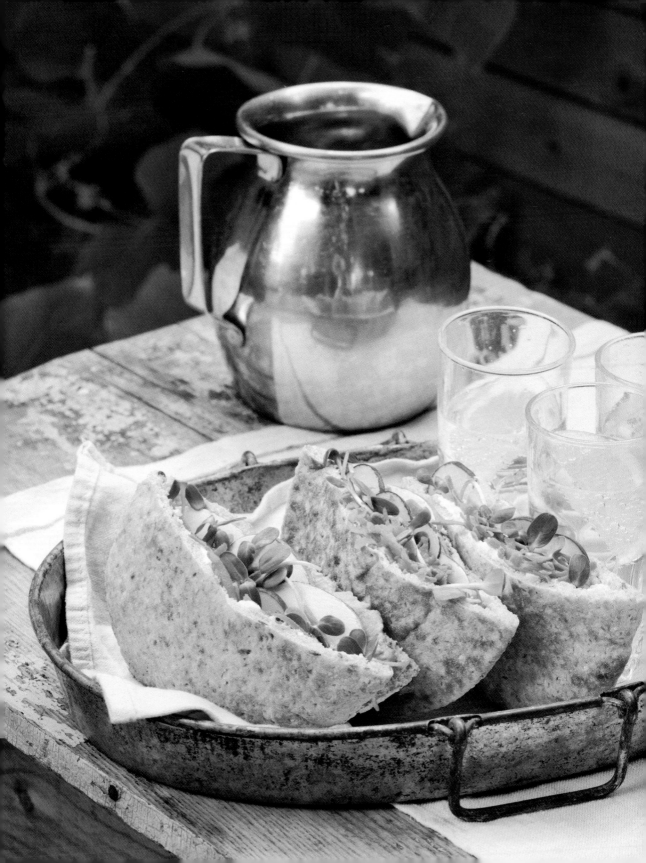

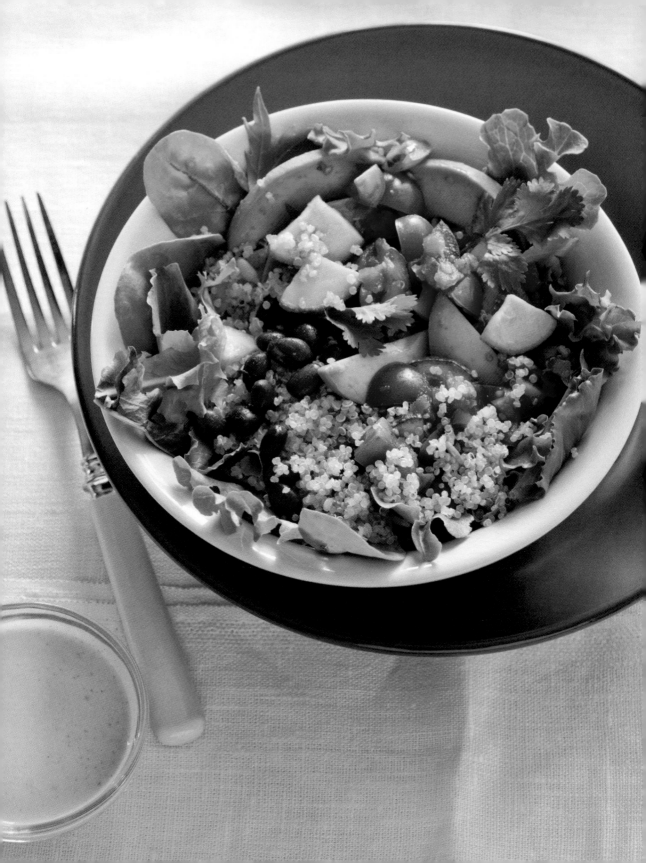

Servings: 4 x 2 cups
Prep time: 10 minutes
Cooking time:
10-15 minutes

QUINOA AND BLACK BEAN LUNCH BOWL

This midday munch is a new take on your typical rice and beans dish. With quinoa it still feels and tastes like a grain-based dish, but is packed with muscle-building protein.

Note: Zesty Hummus must be made ahead of time.

INGREDIENTS

½ cup / 120 ml quinoa
½ cup / 120 ml cooked black beans
1 small baby zucchini, quartered lengthwise and sliced crosswise
¼ cup / 60 ml Zesty Hummus (see recipe on page 357) or store-bought
Juice of ½ lemon
3 cups / 720 ml mixed greens
¼ cup / 60 ml fresh salsa
1 avocado, pitted and sliced
2 Tbsp / 30 ml chopped cilantro

METHOD

1. In a small saucepan, bring 1 cup / 240 ml water to boil over high heat. Add quinoa. Cover, reduce heat and simmer until most of water is absorbed, 10 to 12 minutes. Remove from heat, fluff, cover and let sit 5 more minutes.

2. In a small sauté pan, heat black beans and zucchini over medium-high heat. Add a splash of water and cook until water is evaporated and zucchini is slightly soft.

3. To make dressing, combine hummus and lemon juice.

4. Divide mixed greens between two bowls and add quinoa, and black bean and zucchini mixture. Pour dressing over top, and add salsa, avocado and cilantro to each bowl.

NUTRITIONAL VALUE
PER SERVING:
Calories: 200 |
Calories from Fat: 94 |
Protein: 6 g | Carbs: 22 g |
Total Fat: 9 g |
Saturated Fat: 1 g |
Trans Fat: 0 g | Fiber: 8 g |
Sodium: 193 mg |
Cholesterol: 0 mg

Servings:
4 x 2 canapés
Prep time: 10 minutes
Cooking time:
2 minutes

FRESH FIG CANAPÉS
with Mint and Balsamic Syrup

Canapés are cute little appetizers in which a thin piece of bread, toast or a cracker is topped with caviar, anchovies, cheese or another savory food. For this recipe I've used endive instead of toast and fresh figs for the topping. Fig trees produce figs twice a year, in May and June, and also in December and January.

Note: Yogurt Cheese must be made ahead of time. If goat yogurt is unavailable, use plain, low-fat yogurt.

INGREDIENTS

1 head Belgian endive (yielding at least 8 leaves)
3 Tbsp / 45 ml goat Yogurt Cheese (see recipe on page 348)
2 fresh figs, each sliced into four rounds
¼ cup / 60 ml balsamic vinegar
¼ tsp / 1.25 ml walnut oil
1 tsp / 5 ml thinly sliced fresh mint (chiffonade – see note)

METHOD

1. Trim stalk end of Belgian endive a quarter-inch and remove outside leaves. Continue trimming end by quarter-inches and peeling leaves until you have eight leaves. Place leaves on a small serving plate and place 1 tsp / 5 ml Yogurt Cheese in middle of each. Place a slice of fig on top of each spoonful of Yogurt Cheese. (If making recipe in advance of serving, stop at this point. Balsamic syrup should be made right before serving, as it has a tendency to thicken as it cools, which makes it difficult to drizzle.)

2. To make balsamic syrup, bring balsamic vinegar to a gentle boil over medium-high heat in a small saucepan. Reduce heat and simmer, whisking, until slightly thickened but still pourable, about 2 minutes. If syrup gets too thick to pour, whisk in a few drops of water until the right consistency is achieved. Remove from heat.

3. Drip walnut oil over sliced figs. Drizzle balsamic syrup over canapés and sprinkle with mint. Serve immediately.

NUTRITIONAL VALUE
PER SERVING:
Calories: 60 |
Calories from Fat: 8 |
Protein: 3 g | Carbs: 12 g |
Total Fat: 1 g |
Saturated Fat: 0 g |
Trans Fat: 0 g | Fiber: 5 g |
Sodium: 37 mg |
Cholesterol: 0 mg

NOTE *Stack mint leaves, placing larger mint leaves on bottom. Roll them up and thinly slice using a sharp chef's knife. This is called a chiffonade cut, meaning "cut into rags."*

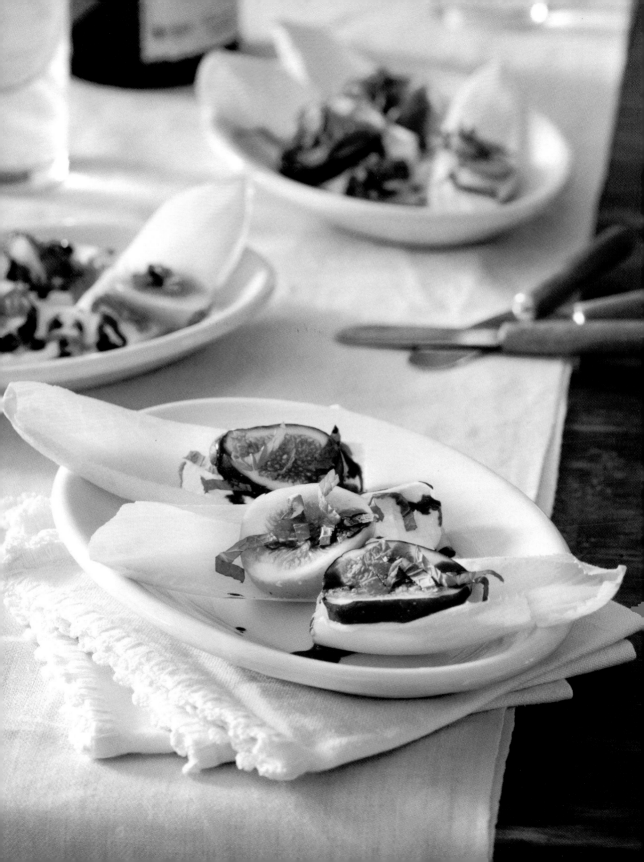

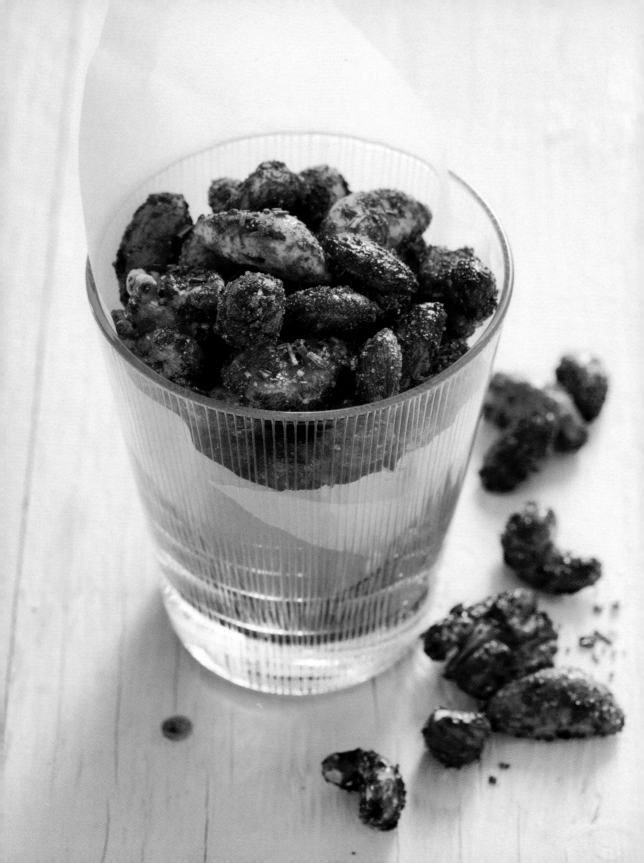

VANISHING PARTY NUTS

Servings: 16 x 1/8 cup
Prep time: 5 minutes
Cooking time:
5 minutes

Nuts for lunch? That's nuts ... or is it? I'm not suggesting you eat just nuts for your midday meal, but they make the perfect brown bag accompaniment to a fresh salad or simple sandwich.

INGREDIENTS

2 Tbsp / 30 ml raw turbinado sugar or other unrefined sugar, divided
1 tsp / 5 ml coarse sea salt
1/4 tsp / 1.25 ml cayenne pepper
2 cups / 480 ml of your favorite unsalted mixed nuts, such as
   almonds, walnuts, cashews, Brazil nuts and hazelnuts
1 Tbsp / 15 ml organic unsulfured molasses
1 heaping Tbsp / 15 ml fresh rosemary leaves

METHOD

1. Preheat oven to 350°F / 175°C. Mix 1 Tbsp / 15 ml turbinado sugar, salt and cayenne in a small bowl. Spread out nuts on a baking sheet and roast in oven until hot, about 5 minutes.

2. Transfer nuts to a medium-sized bowl. Add sugar mixture, molasses and rosemary to bowl. Stir well to combine. (Heat from nuts will cause seasonings to melt slightly and adhere.) Add remaining 1 Tbsp / 15 ml turbinado sugar and stir again to evenly distribute over nuts. Serve warm. Store leftover nuts at room temperature in a sealed container.

NUTRITIONAL VALUE
PER SERVING:
Calories: 109 |
Calories from Fat: 69 |
Protein: 3 g | Carbs: 7 g |
Total Fat: 8 g |
Saturated Fat: 1 g |
Trans Fat: 0 g | Fiber: 1 g |
Sodium: 100 mg |
Cholesterol: 0 mg

Servings: 6 x 1½ cups
Prep time: 25 minutes
Cooking time:
45-50 minutes

SCATTERED SUSHI BOWL
with Ginger Glazed Salmon (Chirashizushi)

Think of your favorite sushi roll. Now deconstruct it and throw everything into a bowl – that's a sushi bowl!

INGREDIENTS

1 cup / 240 ml **brown calrose sushi rice**
2 to 2½ cups / 480 to 600 ml **water**
¼ cup / 60 ml **rice wine vinegar**
2 tsp / 10 ml **honey** or **agave nectar**
½ tsp / 2.5 ml **sea salt**
1 lb / 454 g **wild-caught salmon**, skin on
1 Tbsp / 15 ml low-sodium **soy sauce**
½ tsp / 2.5 ml **brown sugar**
½ tsp / 2.5 ml **grated ginger**
½ **English cucumber**, thinly
  sliced into quarter rounds

1 cup / 240 ml **daikon radish**, peeled
  and thinly sliced into quarter rounds
1 medium **carrot**, peeled and thinly
  sliced into quarter rounds
2 **scallions**, finely chopped
Nori (dried seaweed), torn or
  chopped fine, to garnish
Black and white **sesame seeds**, to garnish
Low-sodium **soy sauce** and
  wasabi paste, to garnish

METHOD

1. Preheat oven to 450°F / 230°C.

2. Cook brown calrose rice according to package directions if you are using a rice cooker. For stove top, rinse rice well, then combine with 2 to 2½ cups / 480 to 600 ml water. Bring to a boil, then cover and reduce heat to simmer until all water is absorbed, 45 to 50 minutes. Fluff with a fork.

3. Meanwhile, in a small bowl, combine rice wine vinegar, honey and salt, and pour over cooked rice. Stir to combine, and set aside.

4. Cover a baking sheet with aluminum foil and place salmon on foil. Use your finger to feel for any pin bones. They will be small and sharp, barely poking out of the flesh as you press with your finger. Use food-safe pliers or tweezers to remove them, or have your butcher or fishmonger do it for you. (Alternatively, you can leave them in while cooking salmon, but you will have to remove them before serving.) In a small bowl, whisk together soy sauce, brown sugar and grated ginger, and pour it over top of salmon to coat. Place it in oven and cook until almost done, 12 to 14 minutes. If you prefer your salmon well done, cook it for a few minutes longer, but it will not be as tender or moist. Remove and let salmon rest for a few minutes. Using a metal spatula, separate salmon from skin. Break salmon into bite-sized pieces. If you did not remove pin bones before, you will need to do so now.

5. To assemble sushi bowls, divide sushi rice among bowls. Scatter chopped vegetables and salmon over top. Garnish with nori and sesame seeds. Serve with low-sodium soy sauce and wasabi paste for your guests to mix together and drizzle over top.

NUTRITIONAL VALUE
PER SERVING:
Calories: 242 |
Calories from Fat: 51 |
Protein: 15 g | Carbs: 25 g |
Total Fat: 8 g |
Saturated Fat: 2 g |
Trans Fat: 0 g | Fiber: 1 g |
Sodium: 280 mg |
Cholesterol: 39 mg

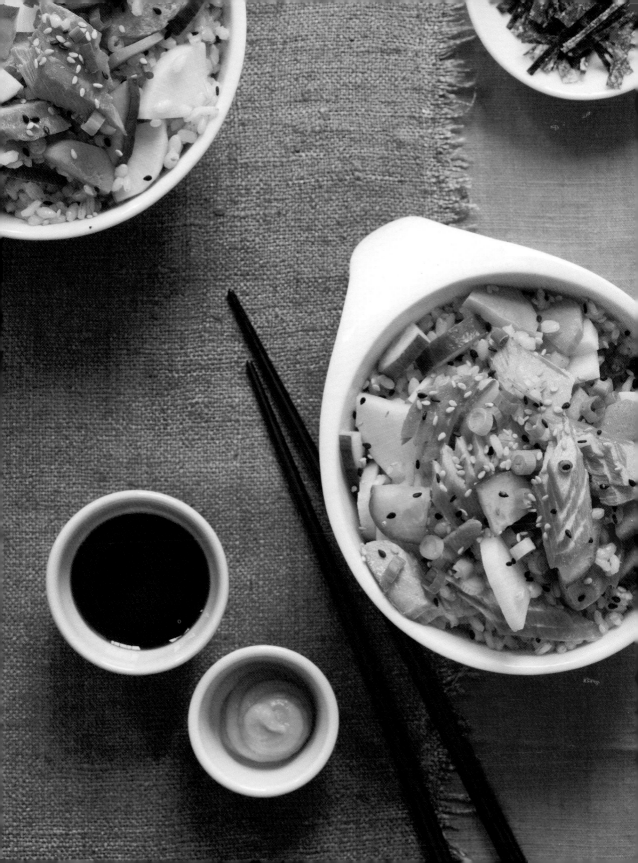

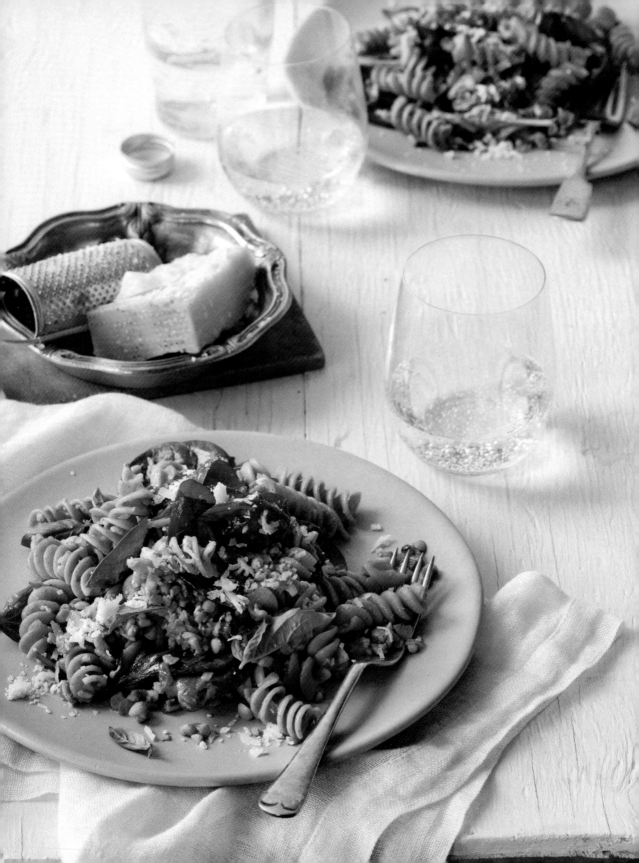

Servings: 4 x 1½ cup
Prep time: 15 minutes
Cooking time:
25 minutes

SPICY ITALIAN TEMPEH SAUSAGE AND SPINACH
with Rotini

Tempeh is a fermented food made from soybeans. It's high in protein, vegan and can be adapted to suit many types of dishes. Tempeh can be sliced thin, cut into chunks, grilled, baked, broiled and even crumbled as is the case for this recipe.

INGREDIENTS

4 oz whole wheat rotini (or penne, or similar pasta)

2 Tbsp / 30 ml extra virgin olive oil

1 medium yellow onion, finely chopped

1 x 8-oz / 225 g package organic tempeh, crumbled into small pieces

1 tsp / 5 ml fennel seeds

½ tsp / 2.5 ml red pepper flakes

2 Tbsp / 30 ml chopped fresh oregano

1 tsp / 5 ml sea salt

½ tsp / 2.5 ml freshly ground black pepper

4 large cloves garlic, chopped

1 cup / 240 ml low-sodium vegetable stock

8 cups / 2 L fresh baby spinach, loosely packed

¼ cup / 60 thinly sliced basil leaves

4 tsp / 20 ml grated Pecorino Romano or Parmigiano Reggiano (divided), if desired

METHOD

1. Bring a large pot of salted water to boil over high heat. Add pasta and cook according to package directions until al dente. Drain pasta and set aside.

2. Heat olive oil in a large skillet over medium-high heat. Add onion and sauté until soft and translucent, 3 to 5 minutes. Add tempeh, fennel seeds, red pepper flakes, oregano, salt and pepper. Cook until tempeh begins to brown, about 5 minutes. Add garlic and cook for 1 minute longer.

3. Add vegetable stock, reduce heat to low, and cook until broth is almost completely absorbed, 2 to 3 minutes. Add reserved pasta to pan and fold in spinach. Divide among four plates and top with sliced basil and 1 tsp / 5 ml grated cheese per plate, if desired.

NUTRITIONAL VALUE
PER SERVING:

Calories: 312 |

Calories from Fat: 100 |

Protein: 17 g | Carbs: 37 g |

Total Fat: 10.5 g |

Saturated Fat: 1.5 g |

Trans Fat: 0 g | Fiber: 14 g |

Sodium: 312 mg |

Cholesterol: 0 mg

EGG SALAD WITH A TWIST

Servings: 3 ·
Prep time: 10 minutes
Cooking time:
15 minutes

Traditional egg salad sandwiches may be delicious, but they won't help you fit into your skinny jeans! By using mostly egg whites and swapping the mayonnaise for Yogurt Cheese, you can enjoy this classic favorite any day of the week – guilt free.

Note: Yogurt Cheese must be made ahead of time.

INGREDIENTS

6 free range eggs
1 tsp / 5 ml Dijon mustard
2 Tbsp / 30 ml Yogurt Cheese (see recipe on page 348)
¼ tsp / 1.25 ml white wine vinegar
½ tsp / 2.5 ml sea salt
¼ tsp / 1.25 ml freshly ground black pepper
¼ cup / 60 ml diced celery
3 pieces whole grain bread, lightly toasted
1 medium tomato, thinly sliced
1 tsp / 5 ml snipped chives
¾ tsp / 3.75 ml white truffle-infused olive oil, divided (If you cannot find, skip this part of step 5.)

METHOD

1. Place eggs in a small pot or saucepan and cover with cold water. Place on stove over high heat and bring to a boil. As soon as water is boiling, cover and remove from heat. Set timer for exactly 15 minutes.

2. While eggs are cooking, mix together mustard, Yogurt Cheese, vinegar, salt and pepper, and set aside.

3. When timer goes off after 15 minutes, drain hot water from eggs and fill pot with cold water to cool eggs. Drain water as it warms and refill with cold water, repeating until water stays cool. (You can speed up this process by adding ice to cold water.) When eggs have cooled, drain water and peel eggs. Transfer to a cutting board.

4. Cut eggs in half and pop out yolks. Put two yolks in Dijon mixture and discard rest. Using a fork, mash yolks and stir them in with other ingredients.

5. Dice egg whites and add them to Dijon mixture. Add celery and stir to combine. Scoop out half a cup of egg salad and place it on one slice of toast, and repeat with remaining two slices of toast. Top egg salad with tomato slices and snipped chives. Drizzle ¼ tsp / 1.25 ml truffle oil over each sandwich.

NUTRITIONAL VALUE
PER SERVING (1 OPEN-
FACED SANDWICH):
Calories: 237 |
Calories from Fat: 112 |
Protein: 16 g | Carbs: 17 g |
Total Fat: 11 g |
Saturated Fat: 3 g |
Trans Fat: 0 g | Fiber: 4 g |
Sodium: 511 mg |
Cholesterol: 430 mg

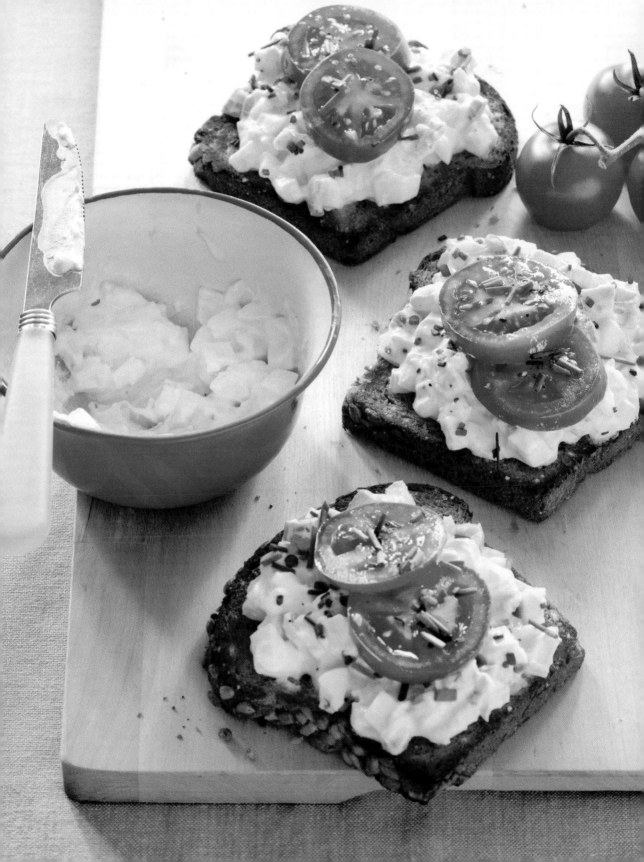

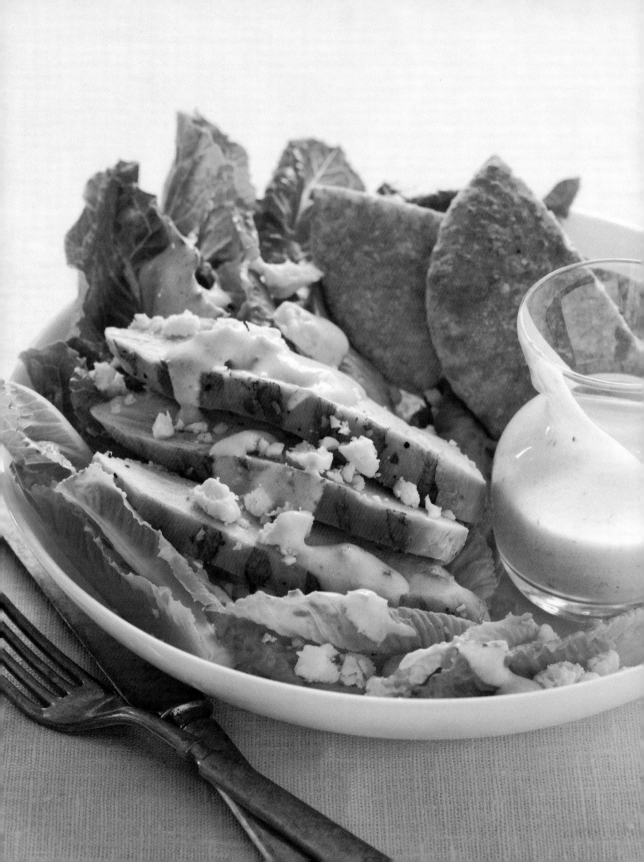

GRILLED CHICKEN CAESAR SALAD
with Spicy Kefir Caesar Dressing and Grilled Mini Pita Bread

It may surprise you to learn that Caesar salad was the brainchild of Caesar Cardini, an Italian-born Mexican who came up with the dish in the 1920s, and not the infamous Roman general Julius Caesar. Regardless of where it originated, I have a feeling both Caesars would approve of this salad!

INGREDIENTS
DRESSING
1 chipotle pepper in adobo sauce
1 large clove garlic
½ tsp / 2.5 ml anchovy paste
2 Tbsp / 30 ml fresh lime juice
½ cup / 120 ml low-fat kefir
2 Tbsp / 30 ml extra virgin olive oil
¼ tsp / 1.25 ml sea salt
⅛ tsp / 0.625 ml freshly
    ground black pepper

SALAD
1.5 lbs / 680 g boneless skinless
    chicken breasts
Eat-Clean Cooking Spray (see page 348)
½ tsp / 2.5 ml + pinch sea salt
¼ tsp / 1.25 ml + pinch freshly
    ground black pepper
6 mini whole wheat pitas, about
    4 inches in diameter
2 hearts of romaine, halved and
    cut into 1½-inch strips
6 tsp / 30 ml cotija cheese, crumbled
Lime wedges, for garnish

METHOD

1. Preheat a grill or grill pan to medium-high heat.

2. Spray both sides of chicken breasts with Eat-Clean Cooking Spray, and season with salt and pepper. Place on grill and cook until cooked through, 5 to 6 minutes on each side. Remove cooked chicken to a cutting board to rest.

3. In a blender, place all dressing ingredients and blend on high speed until smooth and thoroughly combined, about 1 minute. Set aside.

4. Spray top side of pitas with Eat-Clean Cooking Spray and season with a small pinch of salt and pepper. Place on grill until marks appear, for 1 to 2 minutes. Remove and set aside.

5. Place cut romaine hearts in a large bowl and toss with ½ cup / 120 ml Caesar Dressing. Divide salad among six plates, about two cups per serving. Thinly slice chicken breasts across grain and divide among plates, fanning out on side of lettuce. Drizzle remaining ¼ cup / 60 ml dressing over chicken and sprinkle 1 tsp / 5 ml cheese over each salad. Serve with grilled pitas and lime wedges, for squeezing over top of salad.

NUTRITIONAL VALUE
PER SERVING:
Calories: 246 |
Calories from Fat: 44 |
Protein: 31 g | Carbs: 19 g |
Total Fat: 5 g |
Saturated Fat: 1 g |
Trans Fat: 0 g | Fiber: 3 g |
Sodium: 456 mg |
Cholesterol: 70 mg

Servings: 4 x 2 wraps
Prep time: 15 minutes
Cooking time:
8-10 minutes
Chill time:
1-24 hours

JAMAICAN JERK STEAK
and Pineapple Lettuce Wraps

Lettuce wraps are the perfect vehicle for sandwich fillings and stuffing because they are crisp, light and don't weigh you down. These wraps are spicy… if you can't handle the heat, get out of the kitchen!

Note: Jerk Seasoning must be made ahead of time.

INGREDIENTS

1 lb / 454 g **beef flank steak**, trimmed of excess fat
2 Tbsp / 30 ml **Jerk Seasoning** (see recipe on page 358)
½ **red bell pepper**, seeded and diced
1 cup / 240 ml diced fresh **pineapple**
¼ cup / 60 ml thinly sliced **green onion**
Eat-Clean Cooking Spray (see page 348)
½ head **iceberg lettuce**, separated into 8 large leaves

METHOD

1. Spread half of Jerk Seasoning on each side of flank steak. Wash your hands thoroughly afterward. Cover steak and refrigerate for at least an hour, and up to 24 hours.

2. In a small bowl, combine red bell pepper, pineapple and green onion. Cover and refrigerate until ready to use.

3. When you are ready to cook steak, remove it from refrigerator and let sit at room temperature 15 minutes to take the chill off. Heat a grill or grill pan to medium-high heat. Spray both sides of steak with Eat-Clean Cooking Spray and place on grill. Cook to desired doneness, 4 to 5 minutes on each side for medium rare. Remove to a cutting board and let rest 5 minutes.

4. Divide lettuce leaves among four plates. Thinly slice steak across grain and divide among lettuce cups. Place 2 Tbsp / 30 ml of pineapple pepper mixture in each lettuce cup.

5. Roll lettuce around steak, pineapple and pepper mixture to eat.

NUTRITIONAL VALUE
PER SERVING:
Calories: 240 |
Calories from Fat: 93 |
Protein: 26 g | Carbs: 10 g |
Total Fat: 10 g |
Saturated Fat: 4 g |
Trans Fat: 0 g | Fiber: 2 g |
Sodium: 466 mg |
Cholesterol: 45 mg

TIP *Use a toothpick or bamboo skewer to hold wraps closed, if desired.*

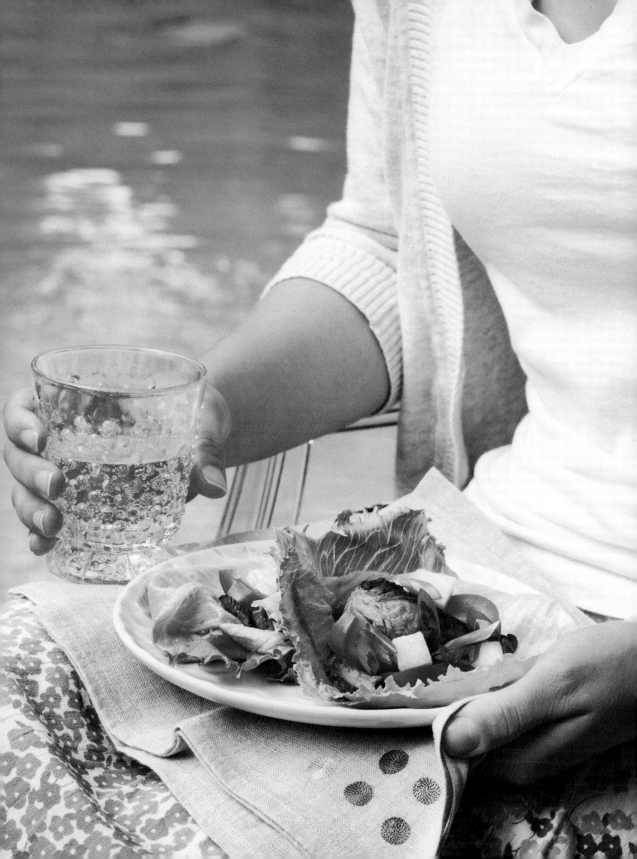

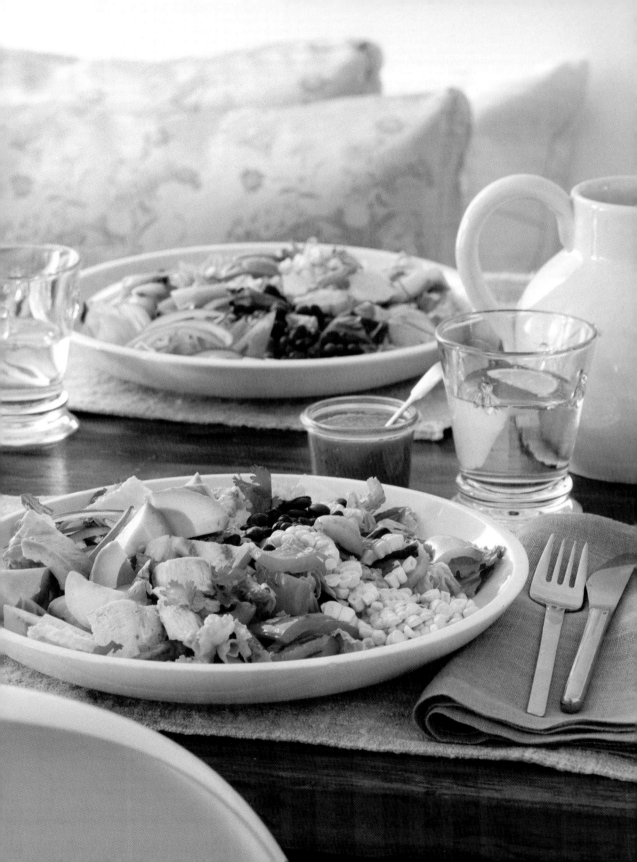

Servings: 5 x 1 cup
Prep time: 20 minutes
Cooking time:
15 minutes

BBQ CHICKEN CHOP CHOP SALAD

This recipe is called a "Chop Chop Salad" because, well, there's a whole lot of chopping involved! Some people find the process of chopping vegetables to be soothing – I'm one of them. Try this salad the next time you're in the mood for some kitchen therapy!

Note: Spicy Clean BBQ Sauce must be made ahead of time.

INGREDIENTS

¼ cup / 60 ml Spicy Clean BBQ
Sauce (see recipe on page 133)
1 clove garlic, minced
½ tsp / 2.5 ml Dijon mustard
Juice of 1 lime
1 Tbsp / 15 ml red wine vinegar
¼ tsp / 1.25 ml freshly ground pepper
1 Tbsp / 15 ml extra virgin olive oil
16 oz / 454 g chicken breasts
2 ears corn, husked
1 red pepper, seeded and quartered
1 yellow pepper, seeded and quartered

1 baby zucchini, halved lengthwise
Eat-Clean Cooking Spray (see page 348)
Sea salt, to taste
Freshly ground black pepper, to taste
1 head romaine, halved
lengthwise and chopped
2 cups / 480 ml cooked black beans
(if using canned, use BPA-free cans)
¼ red onion, thinly sliced
1 avocado, pit removed and cut
into bite sized pieces
¼ cup / 60 ml chopped cilantro

METHOD

1. In a small bowl, whisk together BBQ sauce, garlic, mustard, lime juice, vinegar and black pepper. Whisk in olive oil and set aside.

2. Heat a grill or grill pan to medium-high heat. Lightly spray chicken breasts, corn, peppers and zucchini with Eat-Clean Cooking Spray and season with sea salt and freshly ground black pepper. Cook chicken and vegetables on grill, turning once, until marks appear and vegetables are slightly softened but not cooked through, about 2 minutes each side. Continue cooking chicken until cooked through, about 5 minutes on each side. Remove and set aside until cool enough to handle.

3. In a very large bowl, add romaine, black beans and onion. Cut corn from cobs (see tip) and add to bowl. Cut peppers, zucchini and chicken into bite sized pieces, and add to bowl. Pour reserved BBQ dressing over top and toss to combine. Add avocado and cilantro, and very gently toss to combine. Serve immediately.

NUTRITIONAL VALUE
PER SERVING:
Calories: 367 |
Calories from Fat: 110 |
Protein: 30 g | Carbs: 36 g |
Total Fat: 11 g |
Saturated Fat: 2 g |
Trans Fat: 0 g | Fiber: 11 g |
Sodium: 160 mg |
Cholesterol: 54 mg

TIP

To keep corn from going all over your counter when cutting it off the cob, place a bundt pan in a large bowl and place the stalk end of the corn in the hole of the pan. Holding the tip of the corn, slice down the ear and the large bowl will collect kernels. No mess!

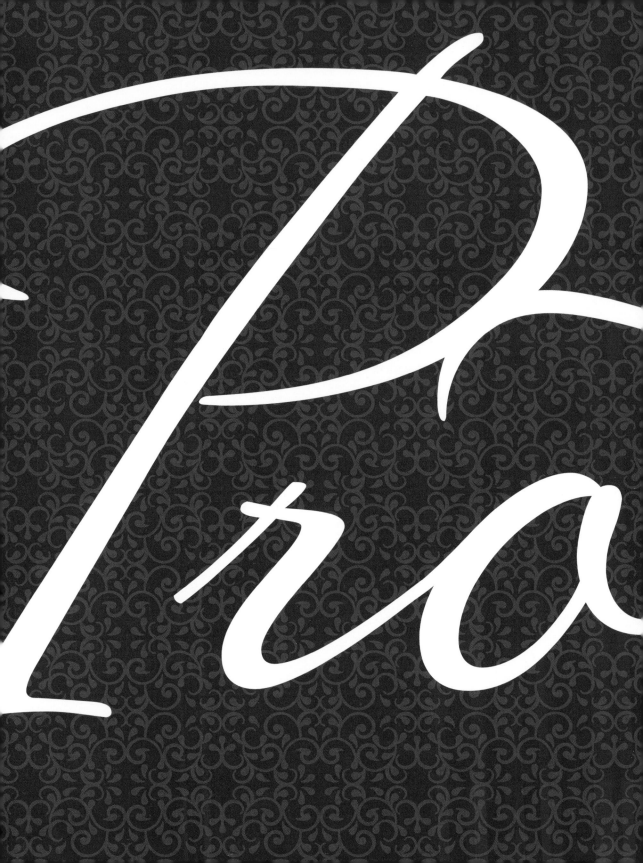

9

Proteins

218 HAZELNUT CRUSTED VENISON MEDALLIONS
with Herb Roasted Carrots and Parsnips

221 DOVER SOLE WRAPPED ASPARAGUS
with Dijon Blanc Sauce

222 BBQ PORK RIBS

225 BAKED CHICKEN TENDERS

226 HALIBUT *with Minted Lima Bean Purée*

229 FILET MIGNON *with Fig Demi-Glace*

230 MEDITERRANEAN LAMB & BISON MEATBALLS

233 SPICY AHI POKE *with Avocado*

234 OLIVE TAPENADE STUFFED SOLE

237 YELLOWFIN TUNA *with Cashew Sauce*

238 BLACKENED SOLE

241 COCONUT SHRIMP *with Spicy Orange Dipping Sauce*

242 GRILLED BLUE MARLIN
with Strawberry Nectarine Salsa

245 CRUNCHY BAKED GINGER DILL SALMON

246 PUERCO PIBIL *(Braised Boar in Mexican Achiote Sauce)*

249 CHILI RUBBED GRILLED OSTRICH TENDERLOIN

250 SALMON *with Sun-Dried Tomato Tapenade in Parchment*

253 VENISON BOURGUIGNON

254 *A "How-To" for Fish*

HAZELNUT-CRUSTED VENISON MEDALLIONS
with Herb Roasted Carrots and Parsnips

Looking for something different for Thanksgiving this year? What about a simple swap for Sunday dinner? This dish has it all – moist meat, roasted root vegetables ... basically the best of the fall season on a plate.

INGREDIENTS

2 large **carrots**, halved and sliced ½-inch thick
2 large **parsnips**, halved and sliced ½-inch thick
2 tsp / 10 ml **olive oil**, divided
1 tsp / 5 ml chopped fresh **chives**
1 tsp / 5 ml chopped fresh **thyme**
¼ tsp / 1.25 ml **sea salt**, divided
¼ tsp / 1.25 ml freshly ground **black pepper**, divided
½ lb / 227 g **venison tenderloin**, cut into ½-inch medallions
⅓ cup / 80 ml finely chopped **hazelnuts**

METHOD

1. Preheat oven to 400°F / 200°C.

2. On a baking sheet, combine carrots, parsnips, 1 tsp / 5 ml olive oil, chives, thyme and half of salt and pepper. Roast in oven until soft and lightly browned, stirring once, about 25 minutes.

2. In the meantime, place venison medallions between two layers of plastic wrap and, using flat side of a meat tenderizer, pound until they are a quarter-inch thick. Pulse hazelnuts in a food processor until finely chopped, then pour into a dish. Season venison on one side with remaining salt and pepper, and place in dish of chopped hazelnuts one at a time, pressing nuts into both sides. Set aside.

3. Heat 1 tsp / 5 ml olive oil in a large cast iron skillet over low heat. Place venison in skillet in a single layer and cook 1 minute on each side until browned.

4. Fan out venison on a serving platter with roasted vegetables.

NUTRITIONAL VALUE
PER SERVING
(4 OZ VENISON, 1½ CUPS /
360 ML VEGETABLES):
Calories: 469 |
Calories from Fat: 167 |
Protein: 38 g | Carbs: 37 g |
Total Fat: 22 g |
Saturated Fat: 2 g |
Trans Fat: 0 g | Fiber: 8 g |
Sodium: 413 mg |
Cholesterol: 0 mg

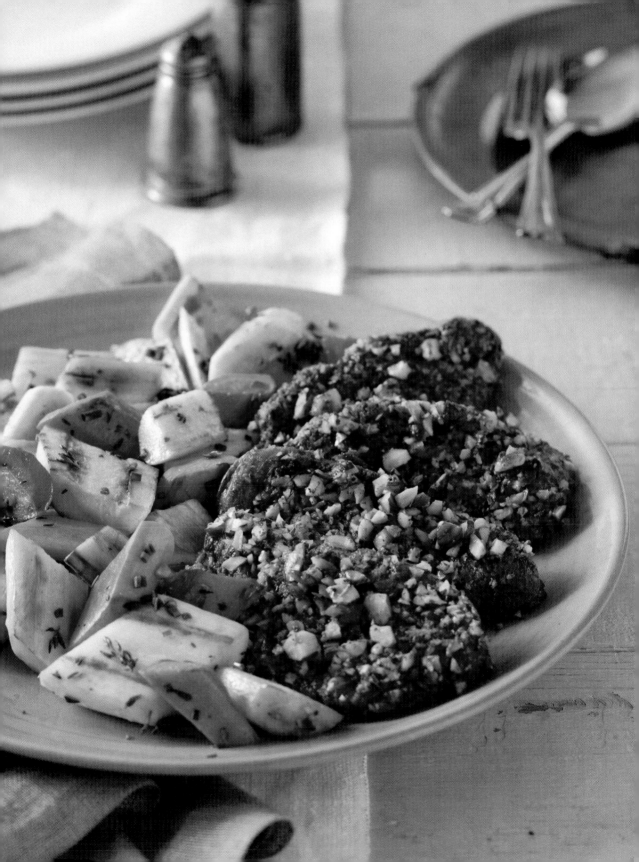

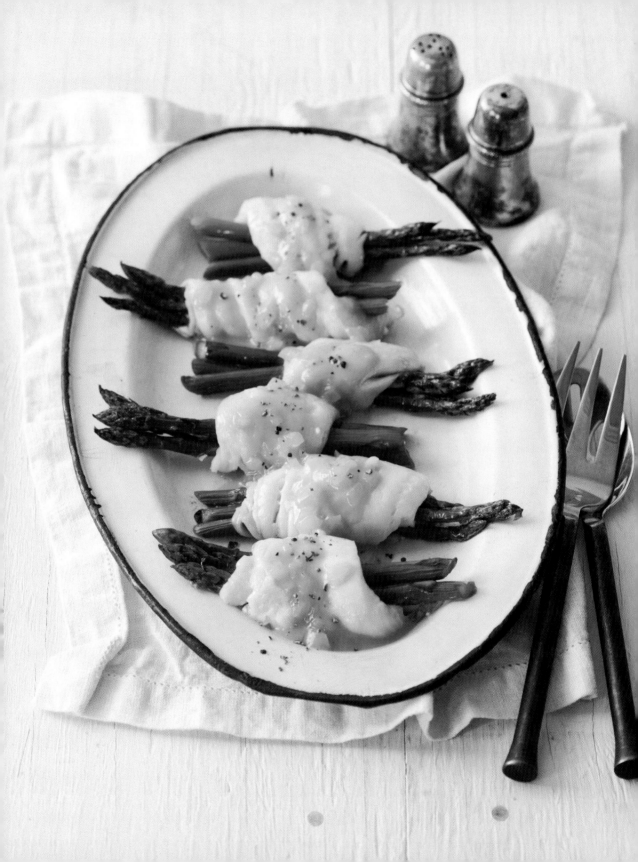

DOVER SOLE WRAPPED ASPARAGUS
with Dijon Blanc Sauce

Dover sole actually refers to two types of fish: the common sole, fished in Europe, and the flatfish of the Pacific Ocean, which strongly resembles the former. Both fish typically have a light taste that is popular with those who prefer mild-tasting sea fare.

INGREDIENTS

Eat-Clean Cooking Spray (see page 348)
4 filets wild caught **Dover sole** (about ¾ lb / 340 g)
12 **asparagus spears**, stalk ends trimmed 1 inch
¼ tsp / 1.25 ml **sea salt**
⅛ tsp / 0.625 ml freshly ground **black pepper**
2 Tbsp / 30 ml **Dijon Blanc Sauce** (see recipe on page 358)

METHOD

1. Preheat oven to 425°F / 220°C. Spray a baking sheet lightly with Eat-Clean Cooking Spray. Lay sole fillets on baking sheet and place three asparagus spears in center of each filet cross-wise. Take ends of one filet and wrap around asparagus. Repeat with remaining three filets. Spray top of sole and asparagus bundles with Eat-Clean Cooking Spray, and season each with salt and pepper.

2. Bake in oven for 10 minutes until fish is opaque and firm and asparagus is tender-crisp. Remove from oven and, using a metal spatula, carefully transfer to a serving plate. Spoon 1½ tsp / 7.5 ml Dijon Blanc Sauce over each bundle. Serve immediately.

NUTRITIONAL VALUE
PER SERVING:

Calories: 110 |
Calories from Fat: 34 |
Protein: 16 g | Carbs: 4 g |
Total Fat: 4 g |
Saturated Fat: 1 g |
Trans Fat: 0 g | Fiber: 0 g |
Sodium: 243 mg |
Cholesterol: 45 mg

Servings:
4 x 3 or 4 ribs
Prep time: 10 minutes
Cooking time:
3 hours 10 minutes

BBQ PORK RIBS
so tender you won't believe it!

They say the way to a man's heart is through his stomach. I'm not sure if that's true, however, I do know that if you make these ribs, you're sure to win his culinary respect.

Note: Spicy Clean BBQ Sauce must be made ahead of time.

INGREDIENTS

3 lbs / 1.36 kg **bone-in pork back ribs**, trimmed of extra fat,
     membrane removed (see directions below)
1 clove **garlic**, minced
½ tsp / 2.5 ml **sea salt**
¼ tsp / 1.25 ml freshly ground **black pepper**
2 cups / 480 ml low-sodium **beef broth** (or enough to come ⅓ up side of ribs)
½ cup / 120 ml **Spicy Clean BBQ Sauce** (see recipe on page 133)

METHOD

1. Preheat oven to 275°F / 135°C.

2. To remove rib membrane, turn rib side up. Starting on one end, use a knife or kitchen shears to loosen white membrane and pull it away. If membrane is slippery, use a paper towel to grab onto it. You may have to repeat this process a few times to completely remove it from ribs. Removing membrane will produce more tender ribs.

3. Cut ribs into two equal sections by cutting through meat between two bones. Place ribs meat side up in a metal or ceramic pan large enough to accommodate them in a single layer. Spread garlic, salt and pepper evenly over both sections of meat. Pour beef broth around ribs until it comes a third of the way up the side of the ribs. Cover tightly with a lid or use aluminum foil, and place in oven to braise until tender, about 3 hours.

4. Remove ribs from oven and transfer to a baking sheet. Discard braising liquid. (If making ahead, you can prepare them up until this point, and then store them in fridge, covered, for up to three days until ready to BBQ.)

5. Heat a grill or grill pan to medium-high heat. Using a pastry brush, coat ribs on both sides with Spicy Clean BBQ Sauce and place on grill, meat side down, in a single layer. Cook just long enough to caramelize sauce on both sides, 5 to 10 minutes. Remove ribs from grill, divide into four portions and add extra BBQ sauce if desired … and napkins!

NUTRITIONAL VALUE
PER SERVING:
Calories: 428 |
Calories from Fat: 207 |
Protein: 31 g | Carbs: 11 g |
Total Fat: 22 g |
Saturated Fat: 6 g |
Trans Fat: 0 g | Fiber: 1 g |
Sodium: 658 mg |
Cholesterol: 79 mg

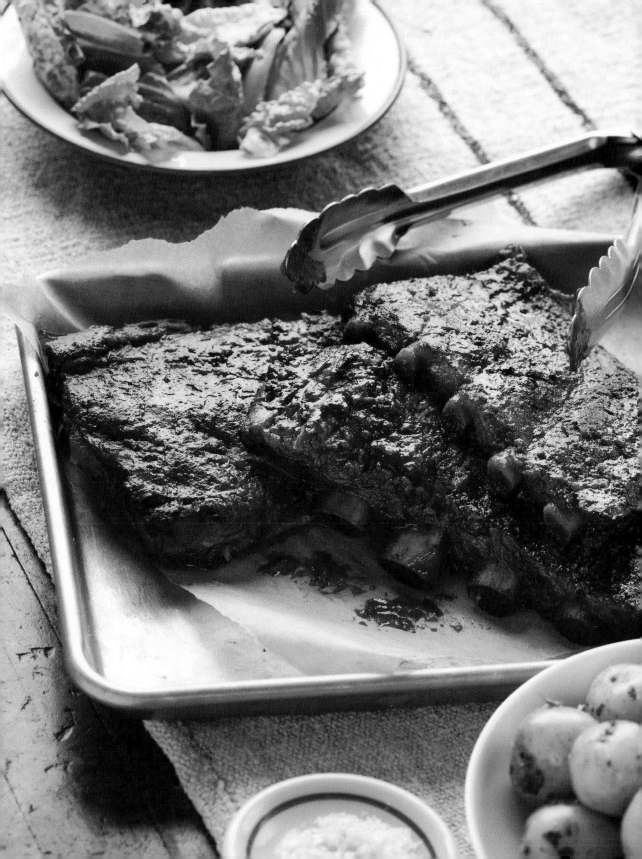

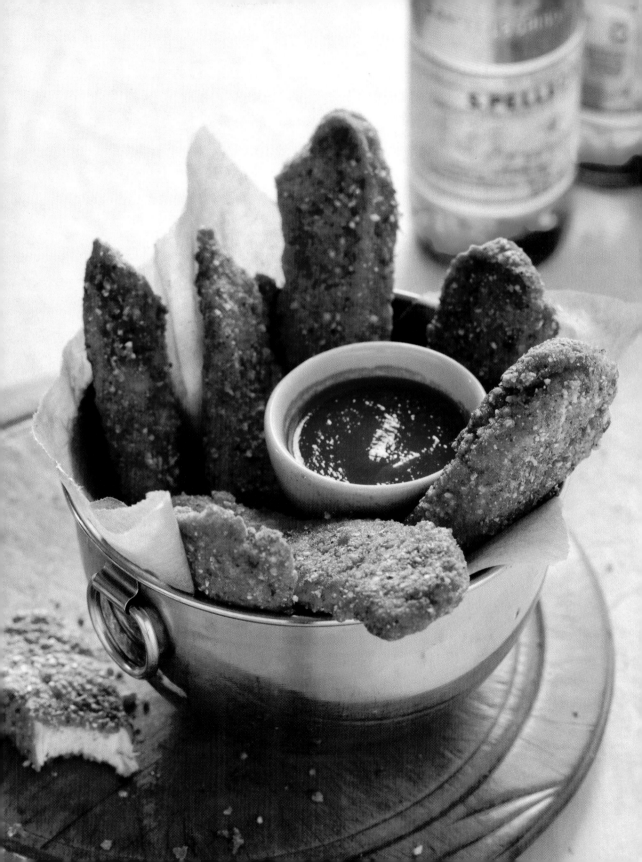

Servings: 4 x 4 oz
Prep time: 10 minutes
Cooking time:
15 minutes

BAKED CHICKEN TENDERS

This recipe brings pub food right into your kitchen ... the Eat-Clean Diet *way of course! The secret is in the spice coating – it makes these tenders come alive on your plate. Serve alongside fresh greens or homemade baked fries for a more traditional take.*

INGREDIENTS

½ cup / 120 ml whole grain **corn flour**
¼ cup / 60 ml whole grain **cornmeal**, medium or finely ground
¼ cup / 60 ml **wheat germ**
1½ tsp / 7.5 ml **chili powder**
1½ tsp / 7.5 ml **garlic powder**
½ tsp / 2.5 ml **onion powder**
½ tsp / 2.5 ml **sweet paprika**
½ tsp / 2.5 ml ground **mustard**
½ tsp / 2.5 ml **white pepper**
½ tsp / 2.5 ml ground **cumin**
½ tsp / 2.5 ml dried ground **Mexican oregano**
¼ tsp / 1.25 ml **cayenne**
1 tsp / 5 ml **sea salt**, divided
3 **egg whites**
3 Tbsp / 45 ml low-fat **milk**
1 lb / 454 g **chicken breast tenders**
Eat-Clean Cooking Spray (see page 348)

METHOD

1. Preheat oven to 450°F / 230°C. In a medium bowl, whisk together all ingredients from corn flour to cayenne. Add ½ tsp / 2.5 ml sea salt. In a small bowl, whisk together egg whites and milk until thoroughly combined. Pour coating and egg mixture into two separate shallow dishes, such as pie pans or low-sided casserole dishes.

2. Season chicken with ½ tsp / 2.5 ml sea salt. To create your "breading station," place two shallow dishes and a baking sheet sprayed with Eat-Clean Cooking Spray close together. To create crunchy coating, dredge a chicken breast tender in dry coating mixture, coating both sides well. Gently shake off any excess coating and dip both sides in egg mixture. Allow any excess to drip off and place tender back in dry coating mixture, and coat both sides. Gently shake off any excess and place on baking sheet. Repeat with remaining chicken tenders until all are coated. There will be extra coating mixture and egg wash, which you will need to discard after using.

3. Spray top of chicken tenders lightly with Eat-Clean Cooking Spray. Bake in oven, turning once, until golden brown and cooked through, about 15 minutes. Serve with your favorite dipping sauce, such as Clean ketchup or BBQ sauce.

NUTRITIONAL VALUE
PER SERVING
(4 OZ TENDERS):
Calories: 453 |
Calories from Fat: 197 |
Protein: 20 g | Carbs: 40 g |
Total Fat: 20 g |
Saturated Fat: 5 g |
Trans Fat: 0 g | Fiber: 4 g |
Sodium: 1042 mg |
Cholesterol: 45 mg

HALIBUT
with Minted Lima Bean Purée

Lima bean purée is a quick and easy base for your fish that is sure to impress dinner guests – from your next-door neighbors to the city mayor. Think of it as a healthier, tastier alternative to mashed potatoes.

INGREDIENTS

12 oz / 336 g frozen **baby lima beans** (about 2 cups / 480 ml)
1 clove **garlic**, chopped
¾ tsp / 3.75 ml **sea salt**
¼ tsp / 1.25 ml freshly ground **black pepper**
¼ cup / 60 ml fresh **lemon juice**
2 Tbsp / 30 ml **extra virgin olive oil**
½ tsp / 2.5 ml fresh **lemon zest**
1 heaping Tbsp / 15 ml chopped fresh **mint**
1 heaping Tbsp / 15 ml chopped fresh **basil**
20 oz / 560 g wild-caught **halibut filet**, skin removed
½ tsp / 2.5 ml **sea salt**
¼ tsp / 1.25 ml freshly ground **black pepper**
Eat-Clean Cooking Spray (see page 348)

METHOD

1. In a small saucepan, bring 2 cups / 480 ml water to boil over high heat. Add lima beans and simmer, covered, until tender, about 5 minutes. Drain and place in a food processor. Add garlic, salt, pepper and lemon juice. Pulse until combined but still chunky. While processor is running, slowly stream in olive oil. Stop processor to scrape down sides, and then process for one minute longer until purée is smooth and all ingredients are well blended. Stop processor, and add lemon zest, mint and basil. Process for one minute longer. Scrape into a bowl and set aside.

2. Heat a nonstick skillet over medium-high heat. Season both sides of halibut with salt and pepper. Spray skillet with Eat-Clean Cooking Spray, place halibut presentation side down (the side the skin was removed from will be facing up) and cook until golden brown on bottom, 3 to 4 minutes. Carefully turn over and continue cooking until almost opaque at thickest part of fish, 3 to 4 minutes longer.

3. Serve fish with bean purée on the side, as shown, or spread the purée in a circle on the plate and place the filet on top.

NUTRITIONAL VALUE
PER SERVING
(5 OZ HALIBUT, ½ CUP /
120 ML PURÉE):
Calories: 296 |
Calories from Fat: 94 |
Protein: 27 g | Carbs: 23 g |
Total Fat: 17 g |
Saturated Fat: 2 g |
Trans Fat: 0 g | Fiber: 5 g |
Sodium: 826 mg |
Cholesterol: 33 mg

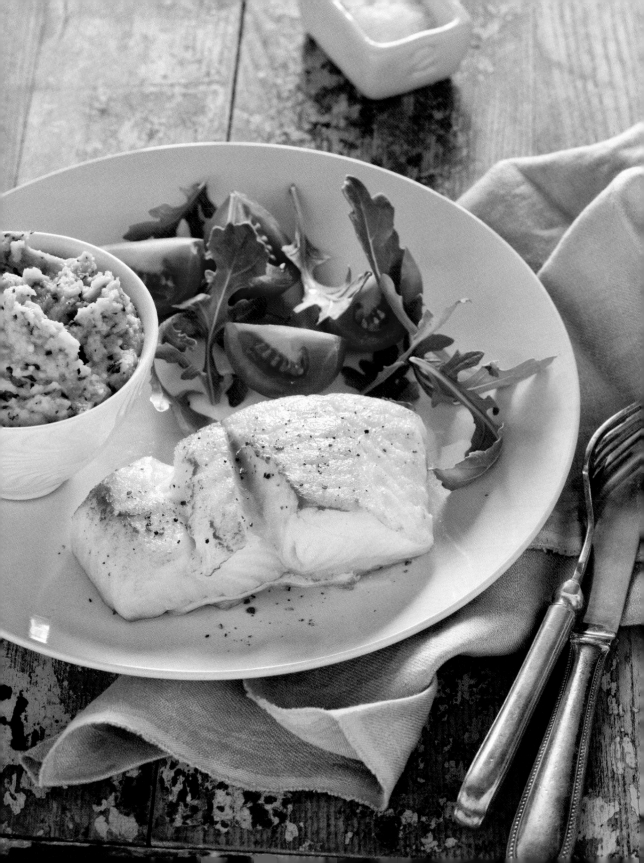

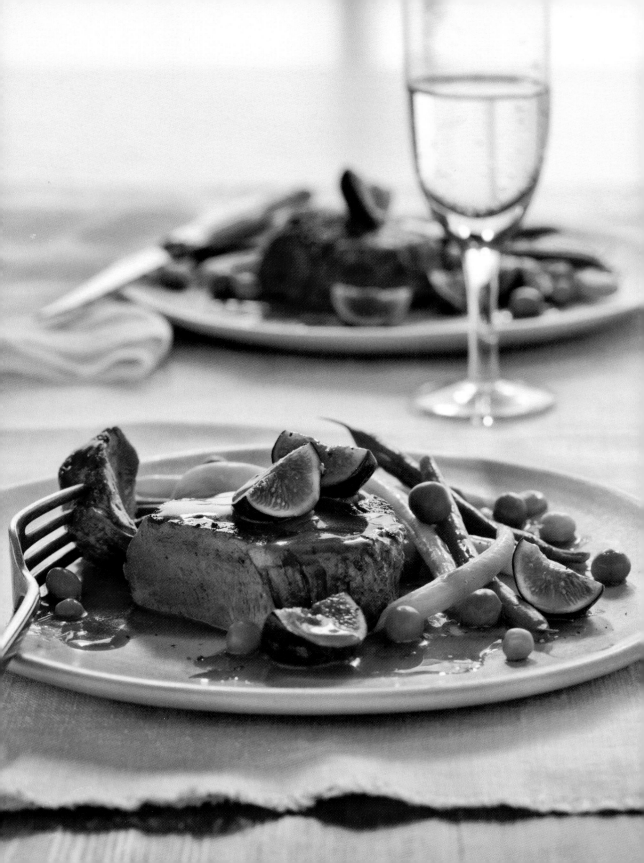

Servings: 4 x 4 oz
Prep time: 15 minutes
Cooking time:
10 minutes
Resting time:
5 minutes

FILET MIGNON
with Fig Demi-Glace

Mignon is French for "dainty" or "cute," which is a perfect description for your palm-sized portion of steak. It pairs beautifully with the Fig Demi-Glace.

Note: Fig Demi-Glace must be made ahead of time.

INGREDIENTS

1 tsp / 5 ml **safflower oil**
1 lb / 454 g **filet mignon**, also known as beef tenderloin steak (4 filets)
½ tsp / 2.5 ml **sea salt**
¼ tsp / 1.25 ml freshly ground **black pepper**
Fig Demi-Glace (see recipe on page 359)

METHOD

1. Preheat oven to 400°F / 200°C. Heat safflower oil in a large ovenproof skillet over medium-high heat until oil is starting to shimmer. Season both sides of filets evenly with salt and pepper. Place filets in hot pan carefully, so oil doesn't splatter. Cook on stove until well browned on bottom, 3 to 5 minutes. Turn filets, then place skillet in oven to finish, about 5 minutes for medium rare with a two-inch-thick filet. (A thinner-cut filet will take less time to cook.) To test doneness of steak, press on top with your finger. If it is still soft, but not as soft as it was uncooked, it is rare. The firmer it is when you press on it, the more done it is. Since filet mignon is the most tender cut of beef, it is best to eat it rare to medium rare.

2. When filet is cooked to your desired doneness, remove from oven and set on stove on a cold burner to rest for 5 minutes. This will allow meat to relax and juices to redistribute, rather than run all over the cutting board or your plate. Divide filets among four plates and top each with ¼ cup / 60 ml Fig Demi-Glace.

NUTRITIONAL VALUE
PER SERVING (4 OZ FILET):
Calories: 411 |
Calories from Fat: 234 |
Protein: 25 g | Carbs: 17 g |
Total Fat: 23 g |
Saturated Fat: 8 g |
Trans Fat: 0 g | Fiber: 2 g |
Sodium: 584 mg |
Cholesterol: 75 mg

TIP *If beef tenderloin comes whole, cut tenderloin into filets or have butcher do it for you.*

MEDITERRANEAN LAMB & BISON MEATBALLS

Although Italian spaghetti first comes to mind when meatballs are mentioned, they are popular in many different cultures and regions of the world, flavored by different and sometimes exotic spice mixtures. Here I've mixed up the meat, choosing lean lamb and bison as the base.

Note: Clean Marinara Sauce must be made ahead of time.

INGREDIENTS

1 medium **yellow** or **white onion**, quartered
3 large cloves **garlic**
½ cup / 120 ml fresh **basil**
½ cup / 120 ml fresh **mint**
½ cup / 120 ml fresh **parsley**
3 to 4 slices **100% whole grain bread**
1 **egg white**
2 Tbsp / 30 ml **tomato paste**
½ tsp / 2.5 ml **red pepper flakes**

½ tsp / 2.5 ml ground **allspice**
¼ tsp / 1.25 ml ground **cinnamon**
1 tsp / 5 ml **sea salt**
½ tsp / 2.5 ml freshly ground **black pepper**
½ lb / 227 g lean ground **lamb**
½ lb / 227 g extra lean ground **bison**
6 cups / 1.44 L **Clean Marinara Sauce** (see recipe on page 122) or other Clean Marinara

METHOD

1. Preheat oven to 425°F / 220°C.

2. In a food processor, add onion, garlic, basil, mint and parsley, and pulse until finely chopped. Scrape into a large bowl. Place three bread slices in food processor and pulse to make fine breadcrumbs. Add breadcrumbs to large bowl with onion mixture. Add egg white, tomato paste, red pepper flakes, allspice, cinnamon, salt and pepper, and stir to combine all ingredients. Add lamb and bison, and mix together all ingredients until just combined. Roll a bit of meat mixture into a ball to see if it holds its shape easily. If too moist, make more breadcrumbs from one slice of bread and add to lamb mixture.

3. Using a small ice cream scoop or a soup spoon, scoop out meatball mixture into 28 to 30 portions and roll them into golf-ball-sized rounds. Bake in oven for 18 to 20 minutes until lightly browned on outside and cooked through.

4. In a large saucepot, heat marinara sauce until bubbling. Add meatballs and simmer in sauce to marry flavors, about 10 minutes. Some meatballs may break apart a little. This will thicken and add more flavor and texture to sauce.

5. Serve over your favorite whole wheat pasta or other whole grain such as quinoa.

NUTRITIONAL VALUE
PER SERVING
(5 MEATBALLS, ½ CUP
MARINARA SAUCE):
Calories: 254 |
Calories from Fat: 99 |
Protein: 24 g | Carbs: 14 g |
Total Fat: 11 g |
Saturated Fat: 4 g |
Trans Fat: 0 g | Fiber: 3 g |
Sodium: 575 mg |
Cholesterol: 59 mg

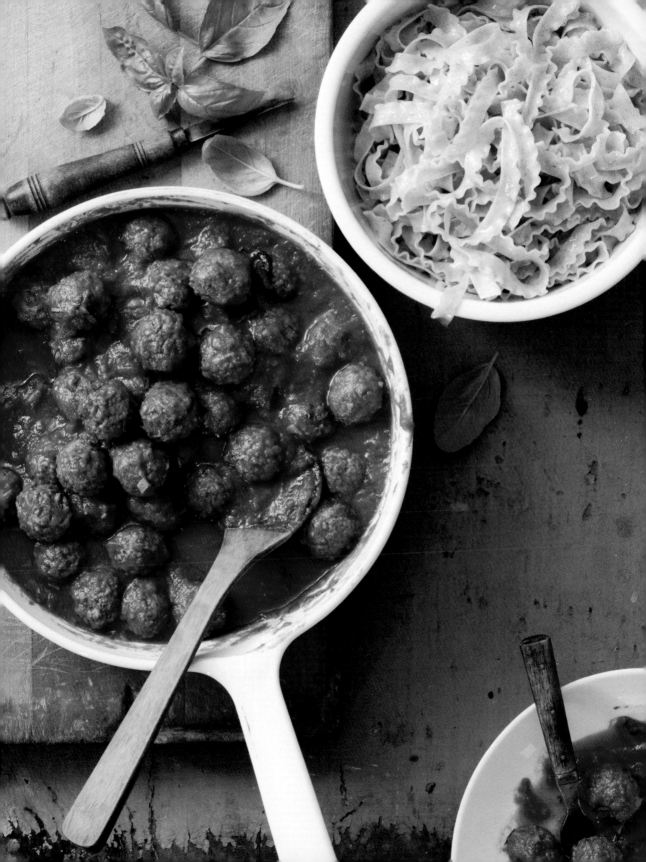

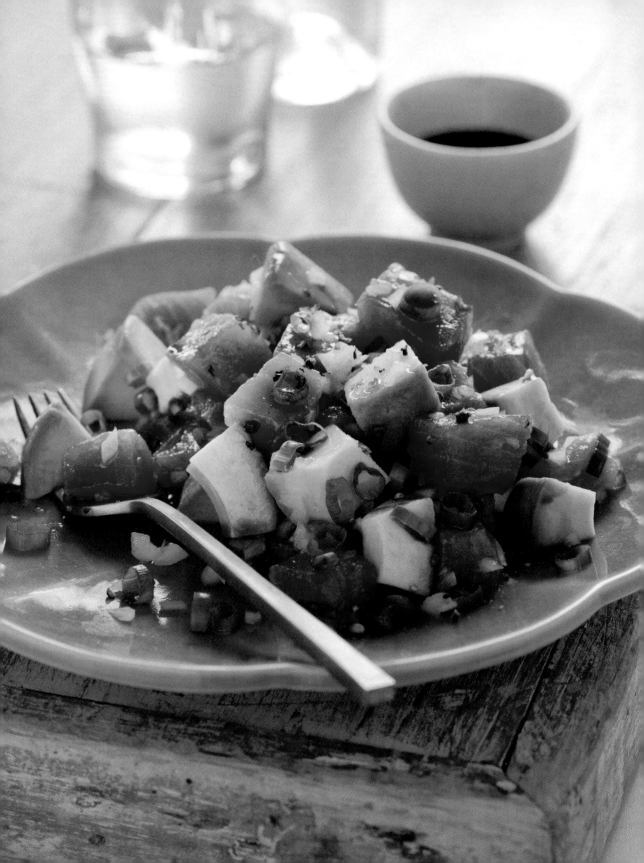

Servings: 4 x ½ cup
Prep time: 10 minutes
Cooking time:
0 minutes

SPICY AHI POKE
with Avocado

Ahi Poke is a raw tuna salad that is easy to make and very fresh. It's popular in Hawaiian cuisine and has started making its way onto American menus, especially in restaurants in California and the rest of the west coast.

INGREDIENTS

½ lb / 227 g sashimi grade raw **ahi tuna**, diced into ½-inch cubes

1 Tbsp / 15 ml minced **onion**

1 **scallion**, green part only, finely chopped

1½ tsp / 7.5 ml low-sodium **soy sauce**

1 tsp / 5 ml **sesame oil**

½ tsp / 2.5 ml ground fresh **chile paste** (found in international section of grocery or Asian grocery stores)

Pinch **sea salt**

Pinch freshly ground **black pepper**

1 **avocado**, pitted and diced into ½-inch cubes

METHOD

1. Mix together all ingredients except avocado. If serving immediately, gently mix in avocado. If not serving immediately, chill, covered, for up to 2 hours. When ready to serve, mix in avocado.

NUTRITIONAL VALUE
PER SERVING:

Calories: 157 |
Calories from Fat: 78 |
Protein: 14 g | Carbs: 5 g |
Total Fat: 9 g |
Saturated Fat: 1 g |
Trans Fat: 0 g | Fiber: 3 g |
Sodium: 112 mg |
Cholesterol: 26 mg

Servings: 4 x 4 oz
Prep time: 5 minutes
Cooking time:
10 minutes

OLIVE TAPENADE STUFFED SOLE

Tapenade is the easiest way to perk up fish filets. Sole is a mild tasting, firm fish, and it's greatly enhanced by this salty olive tapenade.

Note: Olive Tapenade must be made ahead of time.

INGREDIENTS

Eat-Clean Cooking Spray (see page 348)
1 lb / 454 g wild caught **sole filets**, boneless and skinless
8 tsp / 40 ml **Olive Tapenade** (see recipe on page 360) or other Clean tapenade, divided
1 tsp / 5 ml chopped **flat leaf parsley**

METHOD

1. Preheat oven to 400°F / 200°C. Spray a baking sheet lightly with Eat-Clean Cooking Spray and lay sole filets on baking sheet. Divide olive tapenade among filets, about 2 tsp / 10 ml per filet, and spread evenly over top.

2. Roll up filets, starting at thicker end, and secure closed with one or two toothpicks.

3. Bake in oven until fish is opaque and set, about 10 minutes. Using a spatula, carefully remove from baking sheet and divide among four plates. Remove toothpicks and garnish with fresh parsley.

NUTRITIONAL VALUE
PER SERVING:
Calories: 130 |
Calories from Fat: 39 |
Protein: 1 g | Carbs: 0.3 g |
Total Fat: 4 g |
Saturated Fat: 1 g |
Trans Fat: 0 g | Fiber: 0 g |
Sodium: 124 mg |
Cholesterol: 55 mg

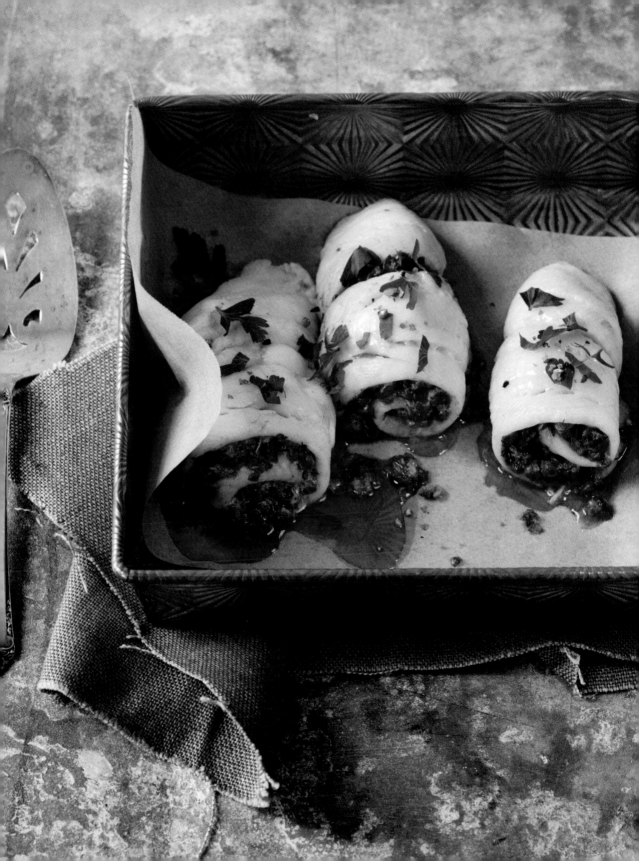

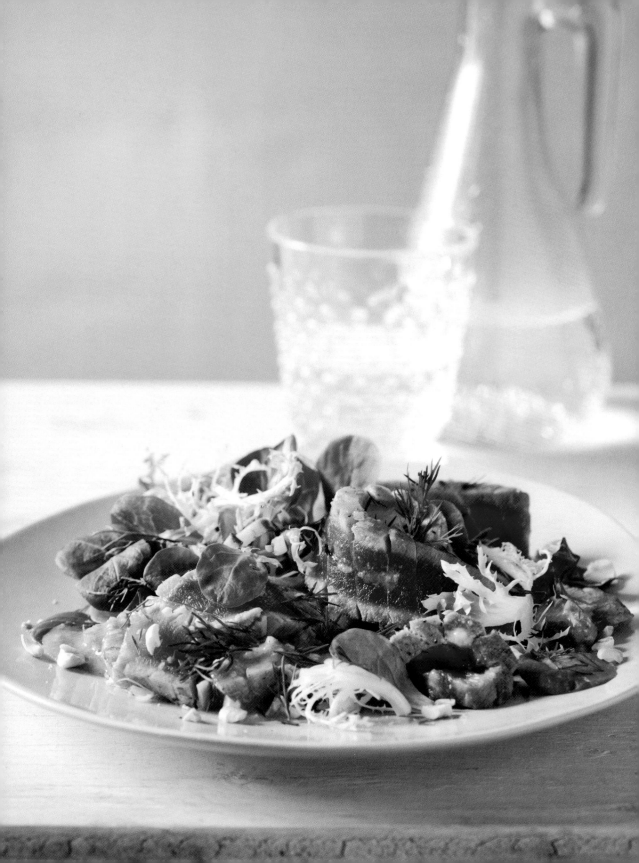

Servings: 4 x 4 oz
Prep time: 10 minutes
Cooking time:
4 minutes

YELLOWFIN TUNA
with Cashew Sauce

Yellowfin tuna, also called "ahi" tuna, is caught in the tropical and subtropical waters of the world. It's best to purchase your yellowfin tuna frozen, as it tends to degrade in quality after it's caught. To make this recipe, simply allow your tuna to thaw before cooking.

INGREDIENTS

CASHEW SAUCE

2 Tbsp / 30 ml unsalted unsweetened natural **cashew butter**

2 Tbsp / 30 ml warm **water**

2 tsp / 10 ml low-sodium **soy sauce**

2 tsp / 10 ml natural unsweetened **rice vinegar**

1 tsp / 5 ml **honey**

½ tsp / 2.5 ml ground fresh **chili paste**

½ tsp / 2.5 ml **Asian fish sauce**

1 clove **garlic**, minced

TUNA

1 lb / 454 g good quality wild **yellowfin tuna**

Eat-Clean Cooking Spray (see page 348)

½ tsp / 2.5 ml **sea salt**

¼ tsp / 1.25 ml freshly ground **black pepper**

4 cups / 960 ml **mixed greens**

1 Tbsp / 15 ml finely chopped toasted **cashews**

2 Tbsp / 30 ml chopped fresh **dill**

METHOD

1. Whisk together all cashew sauce ingredients until well combined.

2. Heat a grill or grill pan to high heat. Spray both sides of tuna with Eat-Clean Cooking Spray, and season with salt and pepper. Grill for 2 minutes on each side until opaque on outside, but still pink on inside. (Overcooked yellowfin will be dry; it is best to serve fish rare.)

3. Remove tuna to a cutting board and thinly slice against grain. Place mixed greens on a serving platter and arrange sliced tuna over greens. Pour cashew sauce over top of tuna and sprinkle with cashews and dill.

NUTRITIONAL VALUE
PER SERVING
(4 OZ TUNA, 2 TBSP /
30 ML SAUCE):
Calories: 297 |
Calories from Fat: 116 |
Protein: 6 g | Carbs: 13 g |
Total Fat: 13 g |
Saturated Fat: 3 g |
Trans Fat: 0 g | Fiber: 3 g |
Sodium: 526 mg |
Cholesterol: 52 mg

Servings: 4 x 4 oz
Prep time: 10 minutes
Cooking time:
3-9 minutes

BLACKENED SOLE

Despite what the name suggests, "blackened" food is not burnt. Blackening is a cooking technique used when preparing proteins, such as chicken, fish and other seafood. The food, in this case, sole, is dredged in a spice mixture and then cooked over high temperature in a cast iron skillet, resulting in a black-brown colored fish that is delightfully spicy.

INGREDIENTS

1 tsp / 5 ml cracked **black peppercorns**
2 tsp / 10 ml **paprika**
1 tsp / 5 ml **garlic powder**
1 tsp / 5 ml **onion powder**
1 tsp / 5 ml dried **basil**
½ tsp / 2.5 ml **sea salt**
¼ tsp / 1.25 ml **white pepper**
¼ tsp / 1.25 ml **cayenne pepper**
1 lb / 454 g wild **Dover sole fillets**, boneless
Eat-Clean Cooking Spray (see page 348)
1 **lemon**, cut into 4 wedges

METHOD

1. In a spice grinder or clean coffee grinder, place all ingredients from peppercorns to cayenne pepper and grind into a fine powder. Transfer to a small bowl and set aside.

2. Heat a large cast iron skillet over medium-high heat. Sprinkle rub evenly over both sides of sole fillets, and gently pat and rub in until completely coated. Spray skillet with Eat-Clean Cooking Spray, and lay sole in skillet in a single layer, working in batches. Cook for 1 to 2 minutes on one side, then, using a perforated or slotted metal spatula, carefully flip sole. Sole is a delicate fish and will fall apart if not handled gently. Cook for 1 more minute and remove to a baking sheet.

3. Using a paper towel, wipe out skillet and return to heat. Spray with more Eat-Clean Cooking Spray and add more sole fillets in a single layer to skillet and cook as before, repeating until all sole is cooked. Divide blackened sole among four plates and serve with lemon wedges for squeezing over top.

NUTRITIONAL VALUE
PER SERVING (4 OZ SOLE):
Calories: 123 |
Calories from Fat: 24 |
Protein: 20 g | Carbs: 3 g |
Total Fat: 1 g |
Saturated Fat: 0 g |
Trans Fat: 0 g | Fiber: 1 g |
Sodium: 327 mg |
Cholesterol: 52 mg

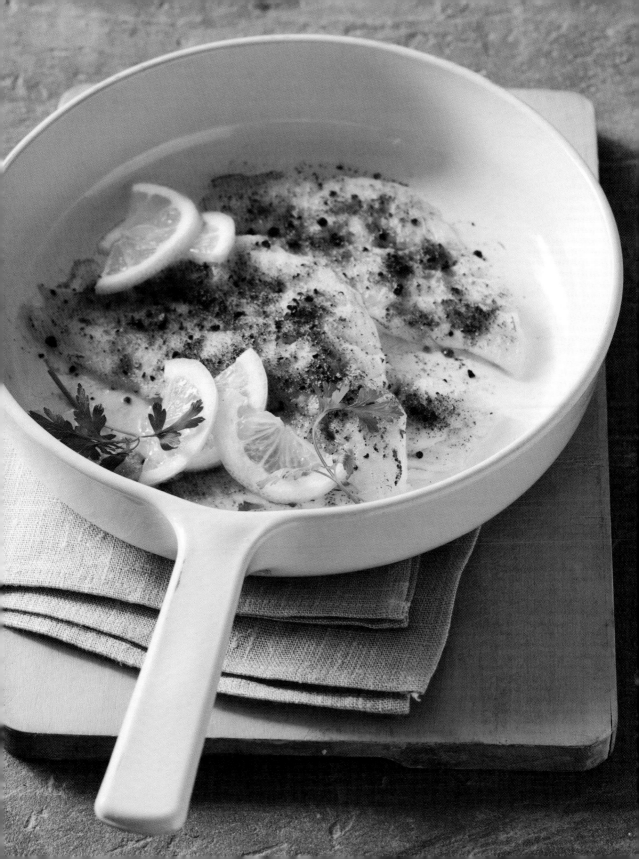

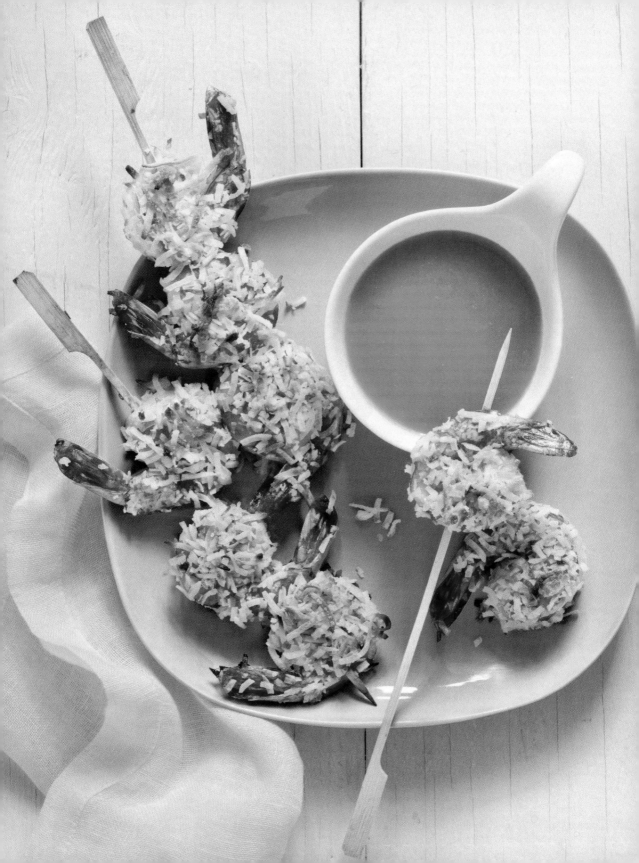

Servings:
4 x 2 skewers
Prep time: 10 minutes
Total time: 18 minutes

COCONUT SHRIMP
with Spicy Orange Dipping Sauce

Coconut shrimp are typically made with whole eggs, white flour, sweetened coconut and lots of oil for frying. I've lightened up this version by using egg whites and unsweetened coconut and skipping the fat fry – baked is the way to go.

INGREDIENTS

1 lb / 454 g wild caught **shrimp**, peeled and deveined (24 shrimp)
1 **egg white**
½ tsp / 2.5 ml toasted **sesame oil**
⅛ tsp / 0.625 ml **sea salt**
Pinch freshly ground **black pepper**
½ cup / 60 ml unsweetened shredded **coconut**
Eat-Clean Cooking Spray (see page 348)
Spicy Orange Dipping Sauce (see recipe on page 360)

METHOD

1. Preheat oven to 450°F / 230°C.

2. Thread shrimp onto eight skewers. In a small bowl, beat egg white with sesame oil. Using a pastry brush, brush sesame-egg wash onto both sides of shrimp and season with salt and pepper.

3. Place shredded coconut into a shallow container that is long enough to fit shrimp skewers. Place one shrimp skewer into coconut and coat both sides. Place on a baking sheet and repeat with remaining skewers. Discard remaining coconut.

4. Spray both sides of coconut shrimp with Eat-Clean Cooking Spray and place in oven. Bake 5 minutes on one side, then turn over and continue baking until shrimp are cooked through and coconut is lightly browned, about 2 to 3 minutes longer. Remove and serve with Spicy Orange Dipping Sauce.

NUTRITIONAL VALUE
PER SERVING
(4 OZ SHRIMP, 1 TBSP /
15 ML SAUCE):
Calories: 276 |
Calories from Fat: 127 |
Protein: 26 g | Carbs: 10 g |
Total Fat: 14 g |
Saturated Fat: 3 g |
Trans Fat: 0 g | Fiber: 1 g |
Sodium: 303 mg |
Cholesterol: 172 mg

NOTE *If using wood or bamboo skewers, you will need to soak in water for 30 minutes before using.*

Servings: 4 x 5 oz
Prep time: 15 minutes
Cooking time:
4 minutes

GRILLED BLUE MARLIN
with Strawberry Nectarine Salsa

The Blue Marlin is a fatty fish with a sharp, pointy nose. Using his bill, he can kill, injure or simply stun his prey and return later to eat at his leisure. Perhaps he's waiting two-and-a-half to three hours to keep his metabolism running on high!

INGREDIENTS

SALSA

1 cup / 240 ml fresh **strawberries**,
   stemmed and quartered
2 **nectarines**, pits removed and
   cut into ½-inch pieces
1 **red chili pepper** (red jalapeño),
   seeded and finely chopped
1 Tbsp / 15 finely chopped **red onion**
2 Tbsp / 30 ml fresh **lime juice**
1 Tbsp / 15 ml chopped fresh **mint**
1 Tbsp / 15 ml chopped fresh **cilantro**
Scant pinch **sea salt**
Scant pinch **black pepper**

MARLIN

4 x 5 oz / 140 g wild caught
   Hawaiian blue marlin steaks
   (can substitute swordfish or tuna)
1 Tbsp / 15 ml fresh **lime juice**
Eat-Clean Cooking Spray (see page 348)
1 tsp / 5 ml **sea salt**, divided
½ tsp / 2.5 ml freshly ground
   black pepper, divided

METHOD

1. In a medium bowl, combine salsa ingredients and place in refrigerator to allow flavors to meld while you prepare marlin.

2. Place marlin steaks in a shallow dish and squeeze lime juice over top, lifting up edges of steaks to allow juice to reach underside. Let marlin marinate in lime juice for 5 minutes.

3. Heat a grill or grill pan to medium-high heat and spray with Eat-Clean Cooking Spray. Spray top of marlin steak and season with half of salt and half of pepper. Place on grill and cook for 2 minutes. Turn, spray with more Eat-Clean Cooking Spray and season with remaining salt and pepper. Cook until desired doneness, about 2 more minutes for medium rare. This fish is better undercooked than overcooked.

4. Remove marlin steaks to a serving plate and spoon salsa over top.

NUTRITIONAL VALUE
PER SERVING (5 OZ
MARLIN, ½ CUP /
120 ML SALSA):

Calories: 262 |
Calories from Fat: 79 |
Protein: 33 g | Carbs: 13 g |
Total Fat: 3 g |
Saturated Fat: 1 g |
Trans Fat: 0 g | Fiber: 2 g |
Sodium: 328 mg |
Cholesterol: 60 mg

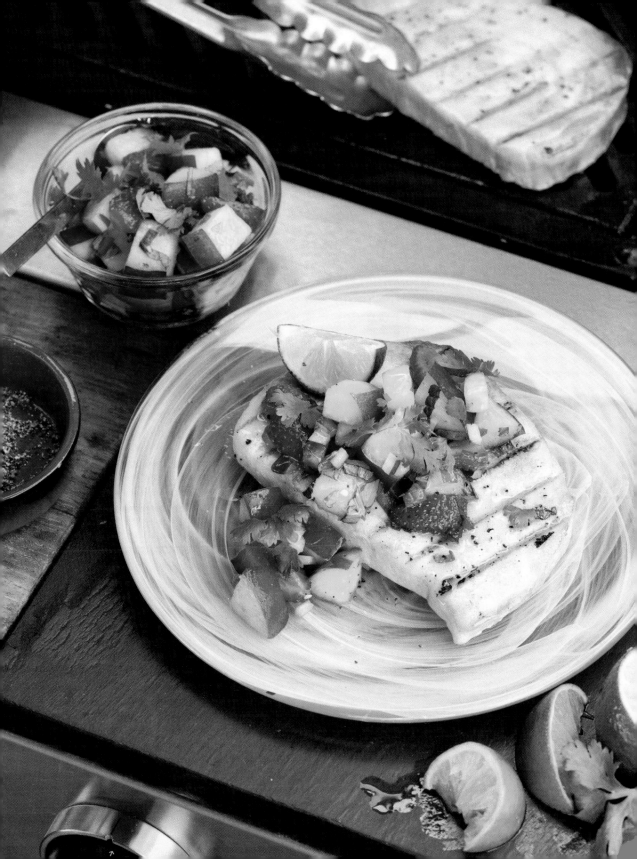

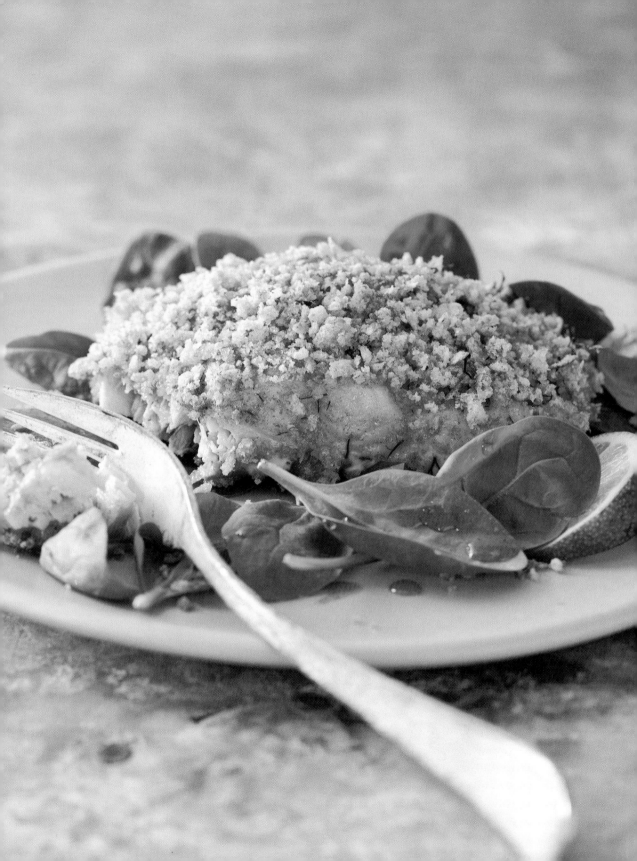

Servings: 4 x 5 oz
Prep time: 10 minutes
Cooking time:
15 minutes

CRUNCHY BAKED GINGER DILL SALMON

Baked salmon is a delicious and healthy meal that can be prepared in a hurry. The tangy lime, used in both the coating mixture and the sauce, really brings this dish to the next level of exciting flavor.

INGREDIENTS

Eat-Clean Cooking Spray (see page 348)
4 x 5 oz / 140 g wild caught **salmon filets**, skin removed
¼ cup / 60 ml **whole wheat flour**
¼ cup / 60 ml fresh **lime juice**
1 Tbsp / 15 ml **agave nectar**
1 Tbsp / 15 ml finely chopped fresh **dill**
1 tsp / 5 ml finely grated fresh **ginger**
¼ tsp / 1.25 ml fresh **chili paste**
¼ tsp / 1.25 ml **sea salt**
⅛ tsp / 0.625 ml freshly ground **black pepper**
¼ cup / 60 ml dried whole wheat **breadcrumbs**
¼ cup / 60 ml low-sodium **chicken** or **vegetable broth**
4 cups / 960 ml **baby spinach**, lightly packed

METHOD

1. Preheat oven to 450°F / 230°C. Spray a baking dish with Eat-Clean Cooking Spray.

2. Have ready three shallow vessels, such as pie tins, baking dishes or plastic storage containers for three-step breading procedure. In first container, place flour. In second container, whisk together lime juice, agave, dill, ginger, chili paste, salt and pepper. In third container, place breadcrumbs.

3. Place a salmon filet in flour and lightly coat both sides, dip both sides in lime juice mixture and coat with breadcrumbs, both sides. Place in baking dish and repeat with remaining filets of salmon. Bake in oven for 8 to 10 minutes until golden brown and salmon is almost firm, but still has a little give when touched.

4. While salmon is cooking, pour lime juice mixture into a small saucepan and place on stove over medium-high heat. If there are any large clumps of flour in mixture, remove them with a spoon. Add chicken broth and bring to a boil, whisking. Cook until mixture thickens, about 1 minute, then remove from heat and set aside.

5. Divide spinach among four plates, and place a filet of salmon on top of each. Drizzle 1 Tbsp / 15 ml of lime ginger sauce on greens around salmon and serve immediately.

NUTRITIONAL VALUE
PER SERVING
(6 OZ SALMON):
Calories: 133 |
Calories from Fat: 33 |
Protein: 3 g | Carbs: 20 g |
Total Fat: 4 g |
Saturated Fat: 1 g |
Trans Fat: 0 g | Fiber: 3 g |
Sodium: 278 mg |
Cholesterol: 11 mg

Servings: 6
Prep time: 20 minutes
Cooking time:
Approximately 3 hours
Chill time: 4-24 hours

PUERCO PIBIL
(Braised Boar in Mexican Achiote Sauce)

Puerco pibil, also known as cochinita pibil, is a slow-roasted pork dish from the Yucatan Peninsula of Mexico. It's traditionally made by marinating the meat in very acidic citrus juice, and then roasting it while it's wrapped in banana leaves. I've skipped that step, but don't worry – it's just as flavorful as the original.

INGREDIENTS

2 lbs / 908 g **boar** or **pork shoulder**, cut into 2-inch cubes and trimmed of any excess fat
3 Tbsp / 45 ml ground **annatto seeds**, or achiote powder (found in Mexican or
    International section of some grocery stores, or in specialty grocery stores)
5 large cloves **garlic**, peeled
Juice of 3 **limes**
Juice of 1 **orange**
¼ cup / 60 ml **cider vinegar**
2 tsp / 10 ml ground **cumin**
1 tsp / 5 ml **allspice**
2 **habañero peppers**, stems removed and halved (for a less spicy sauce,
    remove seeds and ribs; wash hands thoroughly afterward)
2 tsp / 10 ml **sea salt**
1 tsp / 5 ml freshly ground **black pepper**

METHOD

1. Place boar or pork in a Dutch oven or large heatproof ceramic dish. Add rest of ingredients to a blender or food processor and blend until smooth. Pour processed mixture over meat, cover, and refrigerate for at least 4 hours and up to 24 hours.

2. Preheat oven to 350°F / 175°C. Place meat, covered, in oven for 15 minutes to bring to a simmer. At this point, reduce heat to 275°F / 135°C and slowly cook until fork-tender and easily pulls apart, 2½ to 3 hours. Using a slotted spoon, remove meat from sauce and shred using two forks. Pour sauce into a saucepan and bring to a boil over high heat. Reduce heat to medium-low and simmer to reduce by about a third, 5 to 7 minutes.

3. Divide shredded meat among six plates and pour a quarter-cup sauce over top. Serve with Spanish rice or on tortillas, as shown.

NUTRITIONAL VALUE
PER SERVING:

Calories: 381 |
Calories from Fat: 188 |
Protein: 39 g | Carbs: 7 g |
Total Fat: 21 g |
Saturated Fat: 7 g |
Trans Fat: 0 g | Fiber: 1 g |
Sodium: 741 mg |
Cholesterol: 136 mg

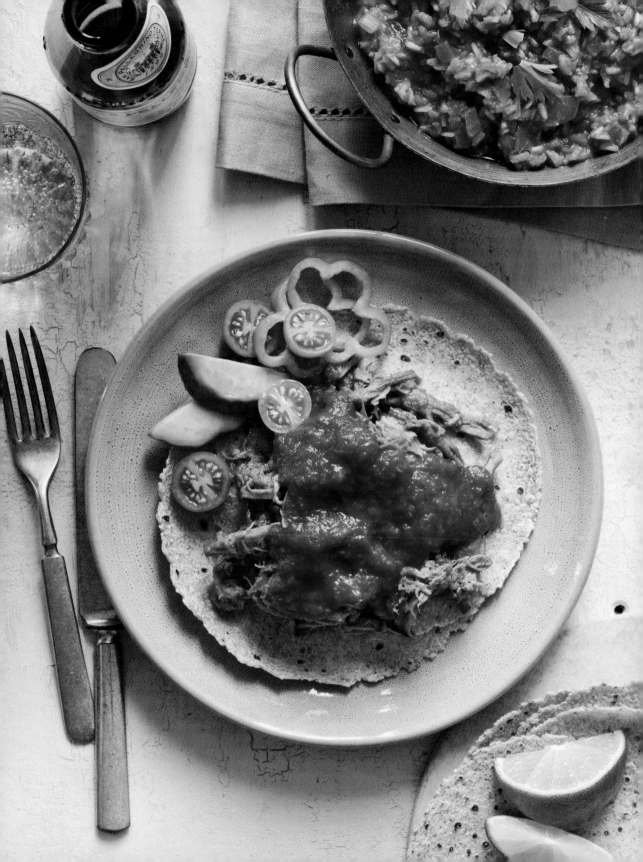

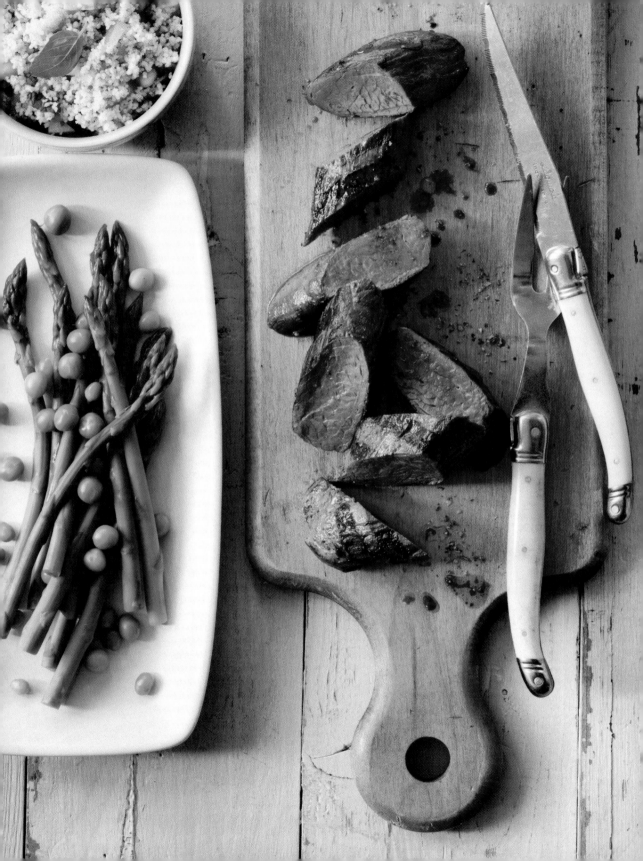

Servings: 6 x 4 oz
Prep time: 10 minutes
Cooking time:
4-7 minutes

CHILI RUBBED GRILLED OSTRICH TENDERLOIN

Ostrich is very lean and actually tastes much like steak. To ensure that it's tender, cook it rare to medium rare. The following chili rub recipe is delicious on almost anything – beef, pork, chicken and even fish, so if you can't find ostrich meat, a beef or pork tenderloin will work just as well. Pick your head up out of the sand and try this tasty dish tonight!

INGREDIENTS

1 tsp / 5 ml ground **cumin**
1 tsp / 5 ml **chili powder**
½ tsp / 2.5 ml smoked **paprika**
½ tsp / 2.5 ml **garlic powder**
½ tsp / 2.5 ml ground **coriander**
⅛ tsp / 0.625 ml **cinnamon**
⅛ tsp / 0.625 ml ground **cloves**
⅛ tsp / 0.625 ml **ginger**
⅛ tsp / 0.625 ml freshly ground **black pepper**
1½ lbs / 681 g **ostrich tenderloin**
1 tsp / 5 ml **sea salt**
Eat-Clean Cooking Spray (see page 348)

METHOD

1. In a small bowl, combine all ingredients from cumin to black pepper and set aside.

2. Heat a grill or grill pan to high heat. Season all sides of tenderloin with sea salt. Coat meat evenly with rub, using your fingers to pat and rub it in. Spray tenderloin with Eat-Clean Cooking Spray and grill 2 minutes on each side, but not more than 6 to 7 minutes total. You want tenderloin rare to medium rare to ensure tenderness. Let rest 5 to 10 minutes. Slice against the grain and serve.

NUTRITIONAL VALUE
PER SERVING
(4 OZ OSTRICH):
Calories: 154 |
Calories from Fat: 46 |
Protein: 24 g | Carbs: 1 g |
Total Fat: 6 g |
Saturated Fat: 0 g |
Trans Fat: 0 g | Fiber: 1 g |
Sodium: 572 mg |
Cholesterol: 88 mg

Servings: 4
Prep time: 15 minutes
Cooking time:
12-14 minutes

SALMON
with Sun-Dried Tomato Tapenade in Parchment

Baking salmon in parchment allows it to steam while it cooks, which results in a moist, flavorful salmon that is perfectly executed every time.

INGREDIENTS

2 cloves **garlic**
1 cup / 240 ml fresh **basil** leaves
¼ cup / 60 ml **sun-dried tomatoes** in olive oil, drained
¼ cup / 60 ml pitted **kalamata olives**
Zest of 1 **lemon**
2 Tbsp / 30 ml fresh **lemon juice**
1 tsp / 5 ml fresh **thyme** leaves
Pinch **sea salt**
4 x 4 oz wild **salmon** filets, skin and pin bones removed
Freshly ground **black pepper**

METHOD

1. Preheat oven to 400°F / 200°C.

2. In a food processor, place garlic, basil, sun-dried tomatoes, olives, lemon zest and juice, thyme, salt and pepper. Pulse until mixture resembles a chunky paste. Scrape tapenade into a bowl and set aside.

3. Cut four 12 x 16-inch pieces of parchment. Season both sides of salmon with pepper. Place one filet on each piece of parchment, and spread 2 Tbsp / 30 ml tapenade on top of each piece of salmon. Bring long sides of parchment together, and fold down toward filet, leaving one inch between parchment and top of salmon. Then fold remaining two sides of parchment under fillet. Packet should be securely closed without being too tight.

4. Place salmon on a baking sheet and bake in oven until fish is opaque and very gently flakes apart, 12 to 14 minutes. Divide packets among four dinner plates and pull packets apart at table.

NUTRITIONAL VALUE
PER SERVING
(4 OZ SALMON, 2 TBSP /
30 ML TAPANADE):
Calories: 142 |
Calories from Fat: 64 |
Protein: 19 g | Carbs: 5 g |
Total Fat: 13 g |
Saturated Fat: 1 g |
Trans Fat: 0 g | Fiber: 1 g |
Sodium: 585 mg |
Cholesterol: 45 mg

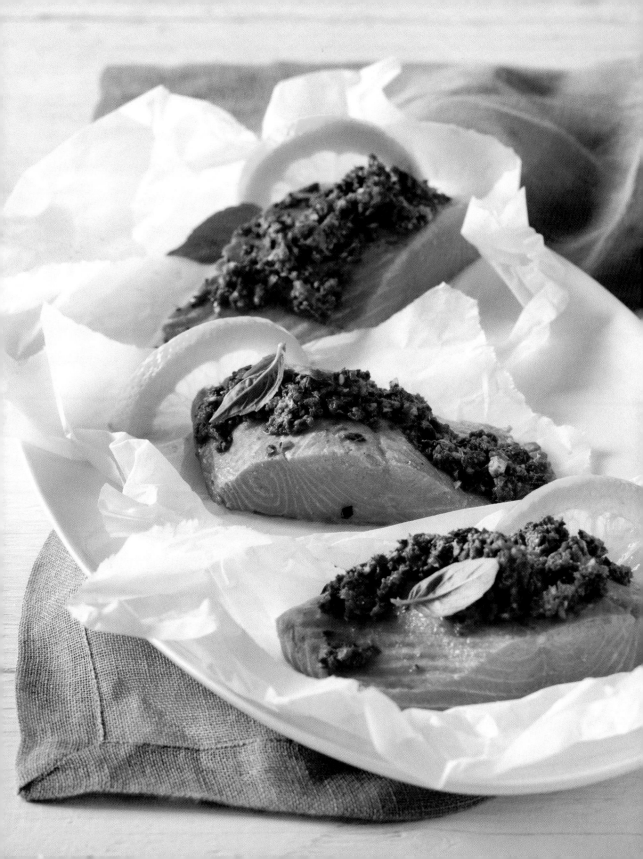

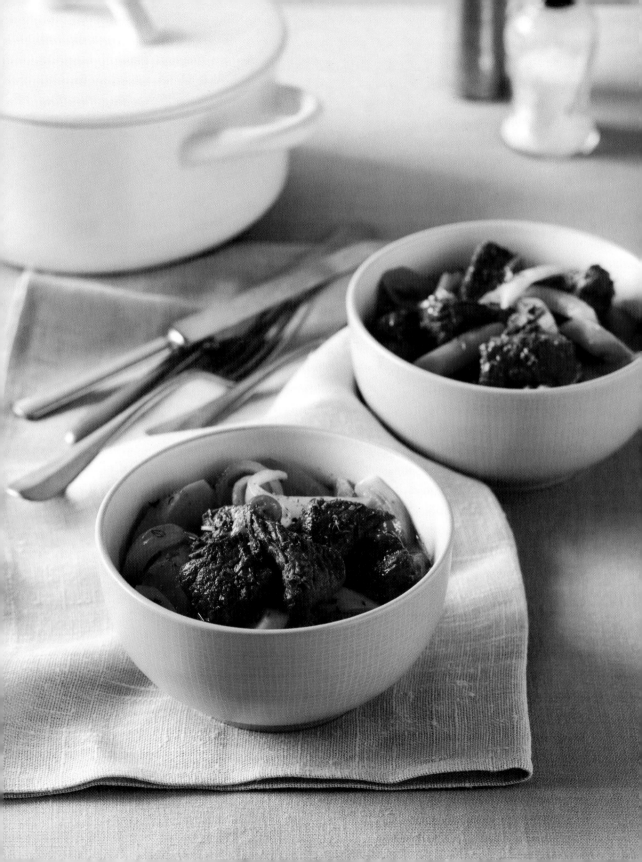

Servings: 4 x 1 cup
Prep time: 10 minutes
Cooking time:
4 hours, 5-7 minutes

VENISON BOURGUIGNON

*Bourguignon is a well-known French recipe typically made with beef. I've used venison –
a more flavorful, less fatty protein – but kept the cooking method the same, resulting in
a healthier dish with the same warm, comforting taste.*

INGREDIENTS

1 Tbsp / 15 ml + 1 tsp / 5 ml **olive oil**, divided

1 lb / 454 g **venison shoulder**, cut into 2-inch chunks

1 large **carrot**, peeled and sliced diagonally

1 **yellow onion**, peeled and sliced

2 cloves **garlic**, chopped

1 tsp / 5 ml **sea salt**

¼ tsp / 1.25 ml freshly ground **black pepper**

1 Tbsp / 15 ml **whole wheat flour**

1 cup / 240 ml **dry red wine** (such as a Bordeaux or a Burgundy)

1 to 2 cups / 240 to 480 ml low-sodium **beef broth**

1 Tbsp / 15 ml **tomato paste**

1 Tbsp / 15 ml chopped fresh **thyme**

1 tsp / 5 ml chopped fresh **rosemary**

1 **bay leaf**

METHOD

1. Preheat oven to 275°F / 135°C.

2. Heat 1 Tbsp / 15 ml olive oil in a large Dutch oven or braising pot over medium-high
heat. Pat venison dry with a paper towel and place in pot in a single layer, being careful
not to overcrowd. Cook without moving until brown on one side, 2 minutes. Turn and
brown on other side, 2 minutes. Remove to a bowl and set aside.

3. Add remaining 1 tsp / 5 ml olive oil to pot. Add carrot, onion and garlic, and sauté
until starting to brown, 1 to 2 minutes. Place venison and any accumulated juices back
in pot. Season with salt and pepper. Sprinkle in flour and stir to coat. Add red wine and
enough beef broth to almost cover venison and vegetables. Stir in tomato paste, thyme,
rosemary and bay leaf. Cover and place in preheated oven until venison is fork-tender
and almost falling apart, about 4 hours.

4. Remove bay leaf and discard. Ladle into bowls and serve.

NUTRITIONAL VALUE
PER SERVING:

Calories: 353 |

Calories from Fat: 86 |

Protein: 43 g | Carbs: 11 g |

Total Fat: 9 g |

Saturated Fat: 5 g |

Trans Fat: 0 g | Fiber: 2 g |

Sodium: 687 mg |

Cholesterol: 128 mg

A "How-to" for Fish

High in protein and low in saturated fat, fish is gaining popularity on dinner tables across North America. I am a big advocate of fish as it's an excellent protein choice for the Eat-Clean Diet lifestyle. Not only is fish tasty, it's also high in omega-3 fatty acids, which makes it a brain food. And according to the Mayo Clinic's *Women's HealthSource Newsletter*, fish is lower in calories, total fat and saturated fat than comparable portions of red meat or poultry. You'd be wise to make these gifts from rivers, lakes and oceans part of your regular diet.

I've heard from many people who are reluctant to try cooking fish because they aren't sure how to purchase the correct type or handle it the right way. They enjoy eating fish in restaurants, but wouldn't attempt to recreate those dishes at home.

The following pages serve as your "how-to" guide when it comes to purchasing and preparing fish. It's easier than you think, and I'm not just saying that for the "halibut!" Don't miss this opportunity to add such a nutritious food to your culinary repertoire.

Shopping for Fish

Fresh fish can be separated into three main categories: lean, moderate fat and high fat. Lean fish contains one to five percent fat, while high-fat fish contain up to 35 percent fat. Fatty fish have a darker flesh and a stronger taste than lean fish. Keep in mind that the fats in these fish are healthy fats your body needs for health and even weight loss, and should definitely be included in your diet – just watch your portions.

The most cost-effective way to purchase fresh fish is to buy it whole, which means either you or the fishmonger will need to gut and scale it before cooking, but you can skip this step by buying filets of fish. Fish is sold at supermarkets and retail fish markets.

LEAN
Black Sea Bass, Brook Trout, Cod, Haddock, Hake, Halibut, Ocean Perch, Red Snapper, Rockfish, Tilapia

MODERATE FAT
Barracuda, Striped Bass, Swordfish, Trout, Tuna, Whiting

HIGH FAT
Herring, Butterfish, Mackerel, Salmon, Smelt, Sturgeon, Yellowtail

Choosing a Fish

Use your senses to pick out a fish. Look at its eyes. If they are dull, hazy or sunken, this fish is not fresh. Take a whiff of your fish. If it smells like the ocean, you're good to go. If it smells sour or "fishy," leave it. If you are purchasing fish filets, look out for discoloration. The flesh should be moist with a skin that shines. When picking out frozen fish, watch for discoloration or visible blood. The package should also be free of ice crystals.

Cooking A Fish

Some of the healthier ways to prepare fish include poaching, baking, grilling and broiling. Overcooking your fish will toughen the meat and ruin the flavor, so it's important to pay attention while it cooks and keep an eye on the clock.

No matter which cooking method you choose, your fish is finished when its flesh is opaque and flakes easily with a fork. Cooking times do vary for different fish, but a standard guide is as follows:

- For each inch of thickness, your fish will need to cook for 10 minutes.
- If your fish is frozen, it will need to cook for 20 minutes per inch.

Using Parchment

One of the simplest ways to cook fish is to cook it in parchment; the fish cooks in its own steam and remains moist throughout the cooking process. Begin by cutting a large piece of parchment and drizzling it with a small amount of oil. Your parchment should be big enough for one or two filets and vegetables/herbs, if you choose to include them. Rinse filets and lay flat on the parchment. Add herbs and vegetables if desired. If adding vegetables such as potatoes and carrots you may need to parboil them first. Fold parchment in half and seal the edges together by folding them over. Place parchment packet on a baking sheet and bake for 20 to 25 minutes or until the fish flakes with a fork.

This dish is perfect to serve at dinner parties. Cut an "X" through the top layer of parchment, folding the points back to reveal the contents. It's a surprise that will have your guests shouting, "Oh my cod!"

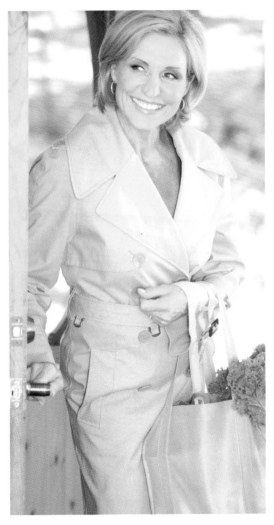

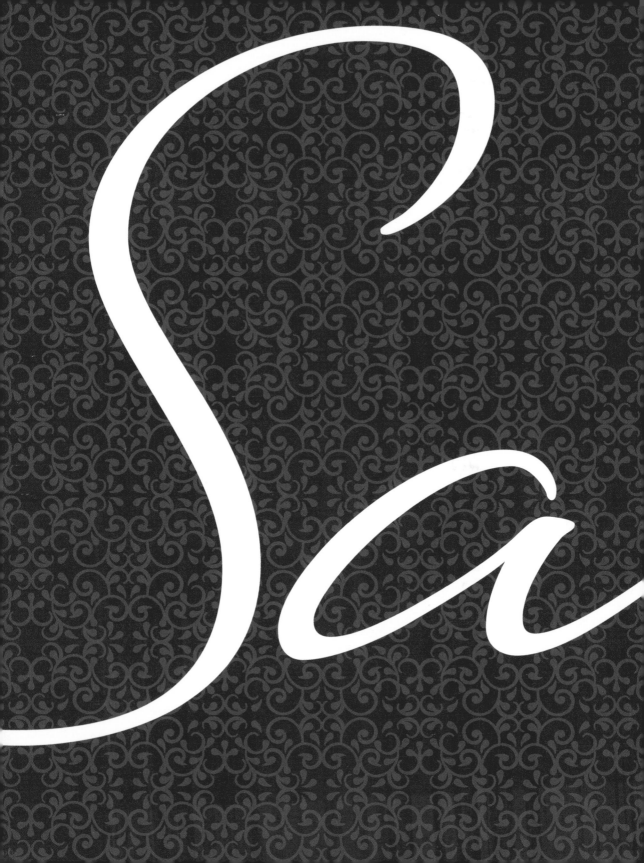

10

Salads

258 PEACH AND HEIRLOOM TOMATO CAPRESE SALAD

261 CELERIAC AND FENNEL SALAD
with Pomegranate Seeds

262 COLD SOBA NOODLE SALAD
with Cashew Miso Dressing

265 SUMMER ROOT VEGETABLE SALAD
with Fresh Cherries

266 ROASTED SWEET POTATO AND SPINACH SALAD

269 GRILLED TREVISO AND ENDIVE
with Cranberries and Pumpkin Seeds

270 WARM BRUSSELS SPROUTS SALAD
with Walnuts and Lemon

273 ASIAN PEAR, WATERCRESS, PEA
SHOOT AND BLUE CHEESE SALAD

274 WINTER GREENS
with Cherries and Walnuts

277 ORZO AND CHICKPEA SALAD
with Roasted Red Peppers and Dill

278 BEETS, BLOOD ORANGES AND ARUGULA
with Feta

Servings: 4 x 1 cup
Prep time: 10 minutes
Cooking time:
0 minutes

PEACH AND HEIRLOOM TOMATO CAPRESE SALAD

This salad is best during summer when peaches and heirloom tomatoes are in season and at their peak. Heirloom tomatoes can be found at farmers' markets and in some finer grocery stores. If you can't find heirloom tomatoes, flavorful vine-ripened tomatoes are a good substitute, and can be found at most grocery stores year round.

INGREDIENTS

1 Tbsp / 15 ml **white balsamic vinegar**
1 Tbsp / 15 ml fresh **lemon juice**
1 Tbsp / 15 ml **extra virgin olive oil**
⅛ tsp / 0.625 ml **sea salt**
Pinch freshly ground **black pepper**
2 large ripe **heirloom tomatoes**, sliced
2 large ripe **peaches**, pits removed and sliced
2 fresh **mozzarella balls**, ovolini-shaped (egg shaped), sliced
Small handful fresh **basil** leaves, thinly sliced

METHOD

1. In a small bowl, whisk together vinegar, lemon juice, olive oil, salt and pepper. Set aside. To assemble salad, layer sliced tomatoes, peaches and mozzarella across a serving platter. Drizzle with dressing and sprinkle with thinly sliced basil.

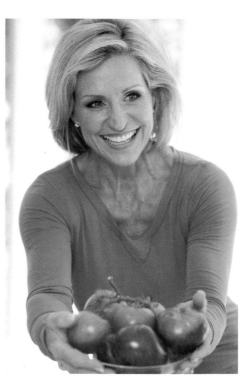

NUTRITIONAL VALUE
PER SERVING:

Calories: 207 |
Calories from Fat: 114 |
Protein: 14 g | Carbs: 13 g |
Total Fat: 13 g |
Saturated Fat: 6 g |
Trans Fat: 0 g | Fiber: 2 g |
Sodium: 125 mg |
Cholesterol: 30 mg

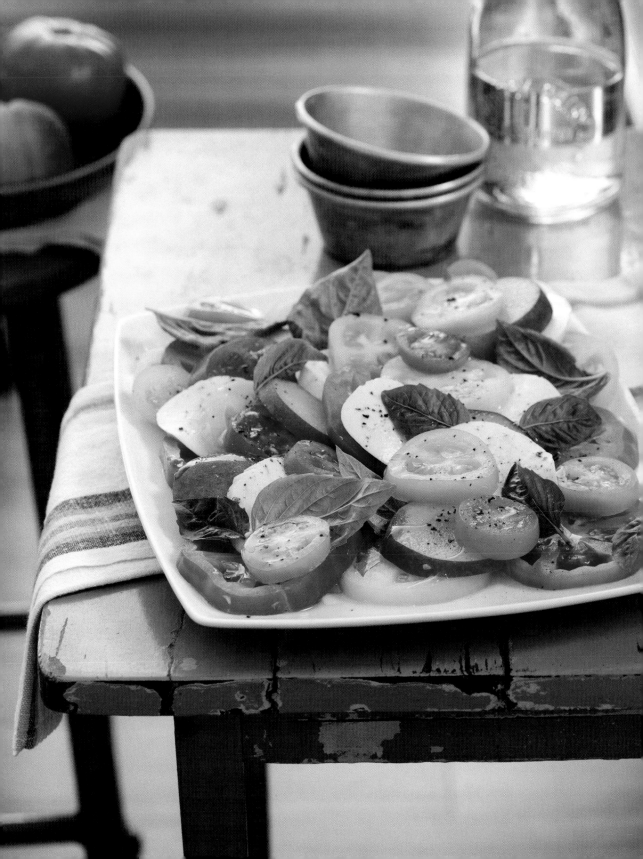

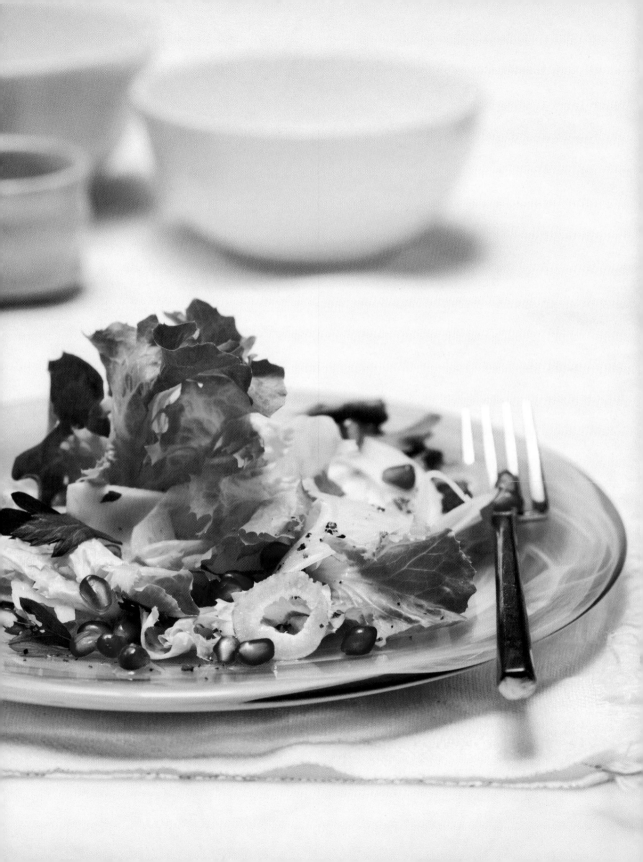

Servings: 4 x 1 cup
Prep time: 15 minutes
Cooking time:
0 minutes

CELERIAC AND FENNEL SALAD
with Pomegranate Seeds

Celeriac, an ingredient common in European cuisine, is a special kind of celery grown for its very large and robust root. This root is also known as celery root, turnip rooted celery or knob celery. It's not a pretty vegetable, but it adds a delicious flavor to every bite.

INGREDIENTS

1 Tbsp / 15 ml **lemon juice**
1 tsp / 5 ml chopped fresh **parsley**
½ tsp / 2.5 ml **honey**
⅛ tsp / 0.625 ml **sea salt**
Pinch freshly ground **black pepper**
1 Tbsp / 15 ml **extra virgin olive oil**
½ small **celeriac**, peeled
½ medium bulb **fennel**, stalks removed and ends trimmed
2 cups / 480 ml **escarole**, stems removed, leaves torn into bite-sized pieces
½ **pomegranate**

METHOD

1. In a large bowl, whisk together lemon juice, parsley, honey, salt and pepper. Whisk in olive oil and set aside.

2. Using a mandolin slicer or sharp chef's knife, thinly slice celeriac and fennel until almost paper-thin. Transfer to large bowl containing vinaigrette and add escarole. Gently toss to combine and transfer to a large serving plate. Hold pomegranate over salad, cut-side-down, and using handle of a long wooden spoon, tap top of pomegranate to release seeds. Any remaining seeds can be removed using your fingers, and sprinkled over top of salad.

NUTRITIONAL VALUE
PER SERVING:

Calories: 89 |
Calories from Fat: 34 |
Protein: 2 g | Carbs: 13 g |
Total Fat: 4 g |
Saturated Fat: 0.5 g |
Trans Fat: 0 g | Fiber: 4 g |
Sodium: 126 mg |
Cholesterol: 0 mg

Servings: 7 x 1 cup
Prep time: 5 minutes
Cooking time:
5 minutes

COLD SOBA NOODLE SALAD
with Cashew Miso Dressing

Popular in Japan, soba noodles are thin noodles that consist of at least 30 percent buckwheat, which is a very healthy grain. Soba noodles are very similar to spaghetti noodles, although they are darker in color. You can eat them hot, but they are also quite delicious cold – just like in this salad!

Note: Cashew Miso Dressing must be made ahead of time.

INGREDIENTS

6 oz / 168 g **buckwheat soba noodles**
½ cup / 120 ml **Cashew Miso Dressing** (recipe on page 361)
½ **red pepper**, seeded and thinly sliced
½ **yellow pepper**, seeded and thinly sliced
1 cup / 240 ml **radishes**, thinly sliced into half moons
½ **English cucumber**, thinly sliced into half moons
2 **scallions**, chopped fine
1 tsp / 5 ml **sesame seeds**, to garnish

METHOD

1. Cook noodles according to package directions. Drain, rinse with cold water and drain again.

2. Transfer noodles to a large bowl. Pour ½ cup / 120 ml Cashew Miso Dressing over noodles and toss to combine. Add all vegetables and toss again to combine. Transfer to a serving bowl and sprinkle sesame seeds over top.

NUTRITIONAL VALUE
PER SERVING (1 CUP SALAD,
1 TBSP DRESSING):
Calories: 87 |
Calories from Fat: 32 |
Protein: 2 g | Carbs: 12 g |
Total Fat: 4 g |
Saturated Fat: 1 g |
Trans Fat: 0 g | Fiber: 1 g |
Sodium: 122 mg |
Cholesterol: 0 mg

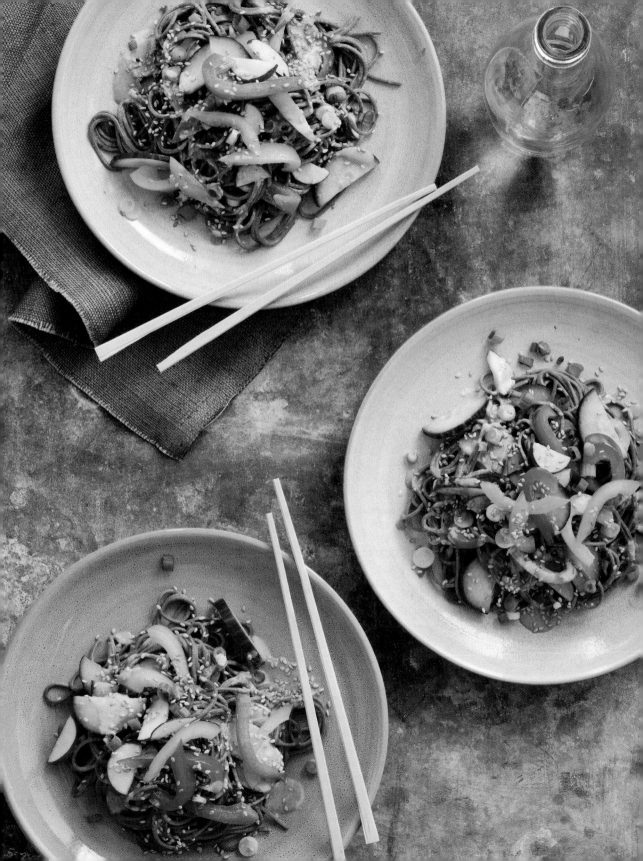

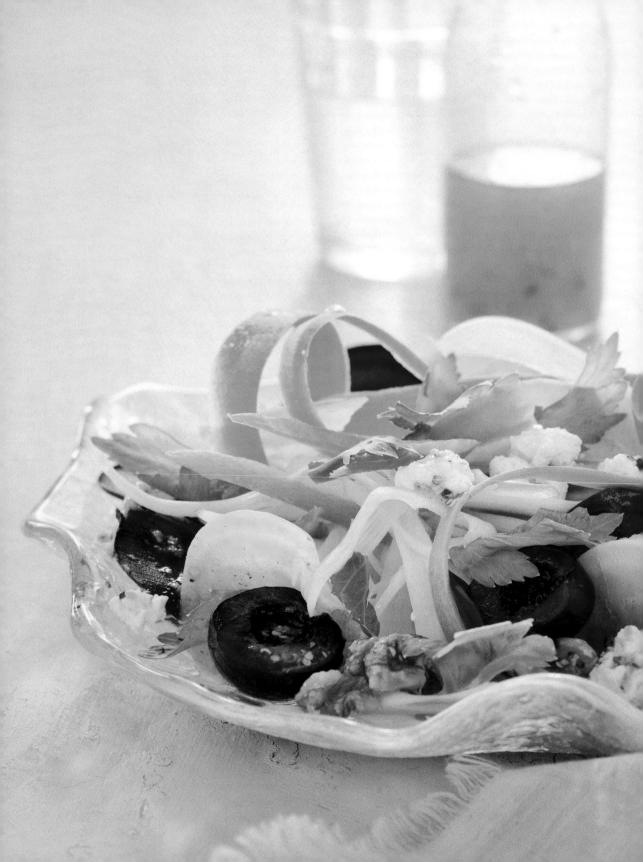

Servings: 6 x 1 cup
Prep time: 15 minutes
Cooking time:
5 minutes

SUMMER ROOT VEGETABLE SALAD
with Fresh Cherries

This salad is light, crunchy and colorful – perfect for an early summer lunch or light late dinner. The cherries bring a subtle sweetness that creates a level of simple sophistication.

Note: Yogurt Cheese must be made ahead of time.

INGREDIENTS

3 Tbsp / 45 ml **walnut** pieces, toasted
½ medium bulb **fennel**
1 medium **carrot**, peeled
2 small raw **beets**, peeled
1 Tbsp / 15 ml **white balsamic vinegar**
½ tsp / 2.5 ml **whole grain mustard**
⅛ tsp / 0.625 ml **sea salt**
Pinch freshly ground **black pepper**, plus more to garnish
1 Tbsp / 15 ml **extra virgin olive oil**
1 stalk **celery**, thinly sliced on diagonal, plus leaves
1 cup / 240 ml fresh **cherries**, bing and/or Ranier, pitted and halved
¼ cup / 60 ml **Yogurt Cheese** (see page 348)

METHOD

1. Preheat oven to 350°F / 175°C. Spread walnuts on a baking sheet and place in oven to toast, about 5 minutes. Remove and set aside.

2. Using a mandolin or sharp chef's knife, very thinly slice fennel, carrot and beets so they are almost paper-thin. Keep beets separate so they don't discolor other ingredients.

3. In a small bowl, whisk together vinegar, mustard, salt and pepper, and then olive oil.

4. On a large serving plate, spread out slices of beets, carrot and fennel. Add sliced celery. Drizzle dressing over top. Sprinkle with celery leaves. Top with cherry halves and toasted walnuts. Place teaspoon-sized dollops of Yogurt Cheese over top. Grind a little black pepper over top, if desired.

NUTRITIONAL VALUE
PER SERVING:
Calories: 93 |
Calories from Fat: 45 |
Protein: 3 g | Carbs: 11 g |
Total Fat: 5 g |
Saturated Fat: 1 g |
Trans Fat: 0 g | Fiber: 2 g |
Sodium: 104 mg |
Cholesterol: 0 mg

Servings: 6 x 1 cup
Prep time: 20 minutes
Cooking time:
20-25 minutes

ROASTED SWEET POTATO AND SPINACH SALAD

Sweet potatoes are big on taste and offer low-glycemic-index healthy carbs to boot. Their sweetness, combined with the heat of the cayenne and the sourness of the vinaigrette makes a perfectly balanced flavor.

SALAD INGREDIENTS

2 **sweet potatoes**, peeled and diced into ½-inch cubes (about 4 cups / 960 ml)
1 **red pepper**, seeded and cut into 1-inch pieces
3 tsp / 15 ml **extra virgin olive oil**, divided
¼ tsp / 1.25 ml ground **cumin**
Pinch **cayenne pepper**
¼ tsp / 1.25 ml **sea salt**
⅛ tsp / 0.625 ml freshly ground **black pepper**
4 cups / 960 ml **baby spinach**, lightly packed

VINAIGRETTE INGREDIENTS

2 tsp / 10 ml **white balsamic vinegar**
1 tsp / 5 ml fresh **lemon juice**
1 small clove **garlic**, finely grated
½ tsp / 2.5 ml **ginger**, finely grated
½ tsp / 2.5 ml **honey**
¼ tsp / 1.25 ml ground **cumin**
¼ tsp / 1.25 ml **sea salt**
⅛ tsp / 0.625 ml freshly ground **black pepper**
1 Tbsp / 15 ml **extra virgin olive oil**

METHOD

1. Preheat oven to 450°F / 230°C.

1. Place sweet potato and red pepper on two baking sheets in a single layer. Drizzle 2 tsp / 10 ml olive oil over potatoes and 1 tsp / 5 ml olive oil over red pepper, and sprinkle salt and pepper over top of both. Sprinkle cumin and cayenne over top of potatoes. Place in oven and roast for 20 to 25 minutes, stirring once or twice, until soft and caramelized.

2. In a small bowl, whisk together all vinaigrette ingredients except olive oil. Drizzle in olive oil while whisking again.

3. Place spinach in a large serving bowl. Add roasted sweet potato and red pepper. Drizzle vinaigrette over top and toss to combine. Divide among six plates and serve.

NUTRITIONAL VALUE
PER SERVING:
Calories: 139 |
Calories from Fat: 22 |
Protein: 2 g | Carbs: 26 g |
Total Fat: 3 g |
Saturated Fat: 0.5 g |
Trans Fat: 0 g | Fiber: 0 g |
Sodium: 78 mg |
Cholesterol: 0 mg

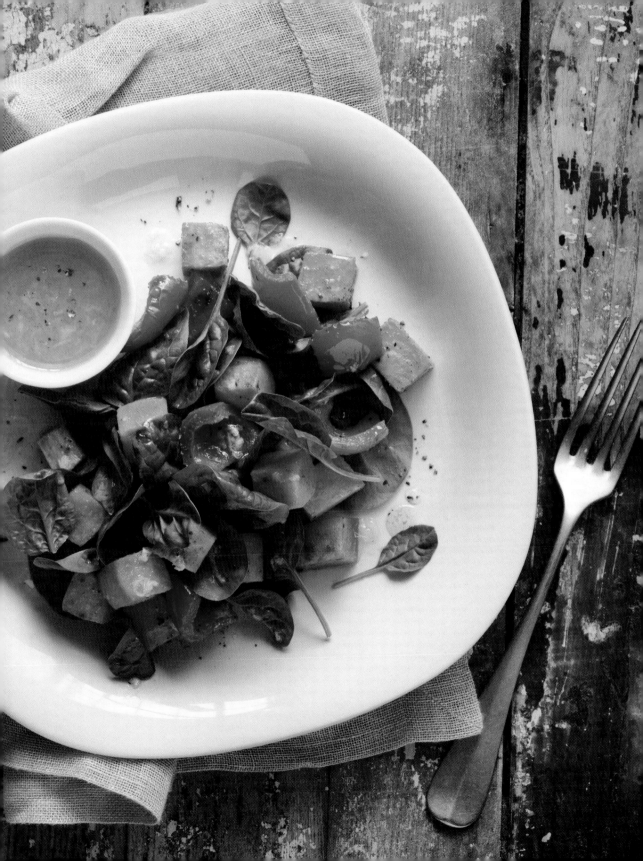

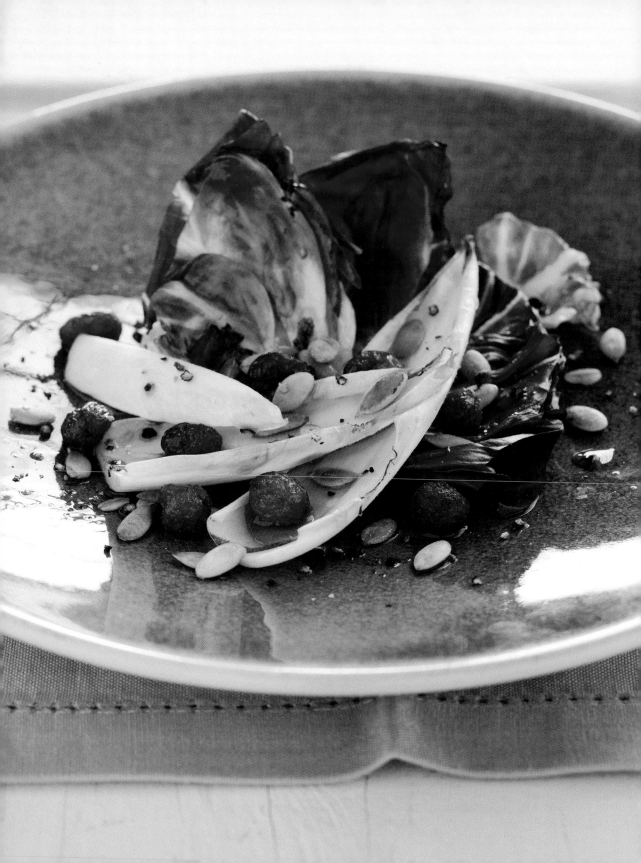

Servings: 8 x 1 cup
Prep time: 5 minutes
Cooking time:
3 minutes

GRILLED TREVISO AND ENDIVE
with Cranberries and Pumpkin Seeds

Gaining popularity on cooking shows and in high-end restaurants, treviso is a flavorful type of radicchio. It's crunchy and bitter, and can be prepared and eaten in many ways, including grilled, braised or used in stuffings. Here I've grilled it and paired it with complementary cranberries.

INGREDIENTS

1 head **treviso** or **radicchio**, halved, core intact
4 to 5 heads **Belgian endive**, halved, core intact
Eat-Clean Cooking Spray (see page 348)
¼ cup / 60 ml dried **cranberries**
¼ cup / 60 ml shelled **pumpkin seeds**, unsalted (pepitas)
1 Tbsp / 15 ml **white balsamic vinegar**
1 Tbsp / 15 ml **extra virgin olive oil**
¼ tsp / 1.25 ml **sea salt**
⅛ tsp / 0.625 ml freshly ground **black pepper**

METHOD

1. Preheat a grill or grill pan to medium-high heat. Spray both sides of treviso/radicchio and endive with Eat-Clean Cooking Spray and place on grill, cut side down. Cook for 1 to 2 minutes, just until marks appear, and turn over. Cook one minute longer and remove to a cutting board. Cut into two-inch strips and place in a large serving bowl.

2. Add cranberries and pumpkin seeds. Drizzle with vinegar and extra virgin olive oil, and season with salt and pepper. Toss to combine and distribute seasoning and serve.

NUTRITIONAL VALUE
PER SERVING:
Calories: 128 |
Calories from Fat: 56 |
Protein: 7 g | Carbs: 14 g |
Total Fat: 7 g |
Saturated Fat: 1 g |
Trans Fat: 0 g | Fiber: 11 g |
Sodium: 150 mg |
Cholesterol: 0 mg

Servings: 4 x 1 cup
Prep time: 10 minutes
Cooking time:
4 minutes

WARM BRUSSELS SPROUTS SALAD
with *Walnuts and Lemon*

Cooking Brussels sprouts is an art. Boiled, they often resemble (and taste like) mushy green balls, but roasted or sautéed, they bring a delightful flavor to the table that is worthy of applause.

INGREDIENTS

1 lb / 454 g **Brussels sprouts**, stalk ends trimmed and dry outer leaves removed
1 Tbsp / 15 ml **extra virgin olive oil**
1 clove **garlic**, minced
½ tsp / 2.5 ml **sea salt**
⅛ tsp / 0.625 ml freshly ground **black pepper**
Juice of 1 **lemon**
½ cup / 120 ml chopped toasted **walnuts**

METHOD

1. Using slicing blade of a food processor or a sharp knife, thinly slice Brussels sprouts an eighth of an inch thick.

2. Heat olive oil in a very large skillet over medium-high heat. Add garlic and cook until fragrant but not brown, 1 minute. Add sliced Brussels sprouts, season with salt and pepper, and toss to coat in oil. Cook 3 minutes until heated through and slightly wilted but not brown, stirring occasionally. Remove from heat and add lemon juice and walnuts. Toss to combine and transfer to a serving plate, or divide among four plates and serve.

NUTRITIONAL VALUE
PER SERVING:
Calories: 180 |
Calories from Fat: 115 |
Protein: 6 g | Carbs: 14 g |
Total Fat: 13 g |
Saturated Fat: 1 g |
Trans Fat: 0 g | Fiber: 5 g |
Sodium: 260 mg |
Cholesterol: 0 mg

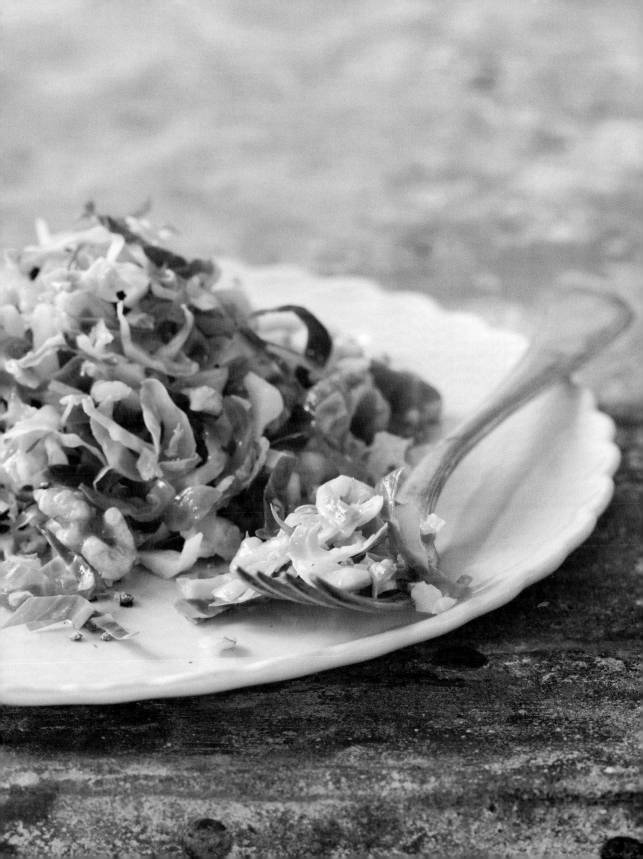

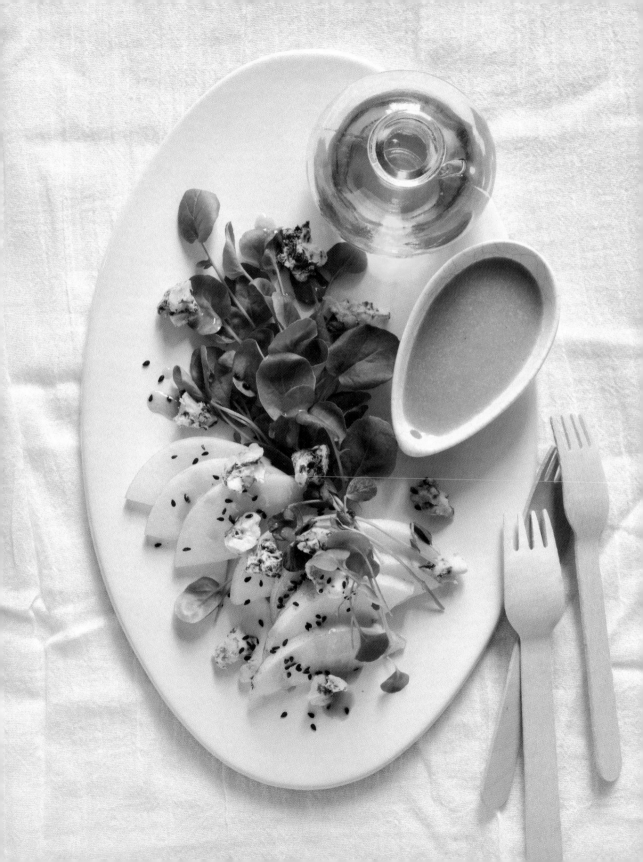

ASIAN PEAR, WATERCRESS, PEA SHOOT AND BLUE CHEESE SALAD

Asian pears may seem to have more in common with apples than typical pears. An Asian pear is round and similar in size to an apple, but has the sweetness and flavor of a pear. Its crunch makes the Asian pear a delightful addition to this summery salad.

Note: Tahini Sauce must be made ahead of time.

INGREDIENTS

DRESSING

1 Tbsp / 15 ml **Tahini Sauce** (see page 354)
1½ tsp / 7.5 ml **white balsamic vinegar**
1 tsp / 5 ml fresh **lemon juice**
½ tsp / 2.5 ml reduced-sodium **soy sauce**
1 tsp / 5 ml **honey**
⅛ tsp / 0.625 ml **sea salt**
⅛ tsp / 0.625 ml freshly ground **black pepper**
1 Tbsp /15 ml **extra virgin olive oil**

SALAD

1 bunch **watercress**, stems trimmed to remove root ball (if there is one attached)
2 **Asian pears**, cored and thinly sliced
¼ cup / 60 ml **pea shoots**
1 oz / 28 g **blue cheese**, crumbled
½ tsp / 2.5 ml **black sesame seeds**

METHOD

1. Whisk together all dressing ingredients.

2. To arrange salad, divide watercress among four large plates, keeping it together in a little bundle. Drizzle dressing over stems of watercress and onto plate. Fan out pear slices on side of watercress. Sprinkle pea shoots, crumbled blue cheese and sesame seeds over top. Serve immediately.

NUTRITIONAL VALUE
PER SERVING:
Calories: 117 |
Calories from Fat: 65 |
Protein: 4 g | Carbs: 9 g |
Total Fat: 8 g |
Saturated Fat: 2 g |
Trans Fat: 0 g | Fiber: 3 g |
Sodium: 207 mg |
Cholesterol: 5 mg

TIP *Pea shoots can be bought in herb section of grocery store in little plastic pots, growing live; just snip with scissors and use.*

Servings: 4 x 1 cup
Prep time: 10 minutes
Cooking time:
5 minutes

WINTER GREENS
with Cherries and Walnuts

There is something about roasted nuts that makes me warm and happy inside. This salad contains toasted walnuts that pair beautifully with sweet cherries and bitter greens. Pair with a protein for a perfect light lunch.

INGREDIENTS

¼ cup / 60 ml **walnut** pieces
1 tsp / 5 ml **white balsamic vinegar**
½ tsp / 2.5 ml **Dijon mustard**
Pinch **sea salt**
Pinch freshly ground **black pepper**
1 Tbsp / 15 ml **walnut oil**
2 cups / 480 ml chopped **escarole**
2 cups / 480 ml chopped **radicchio** (about ½ head)
¼ cup / 60 ml unsweetened dried **bing cherries**

METHOD

1. Preheat oven to 350°F / 175°C. Spread walnut pieces on a baking sheet and place in oven to toast, about 5 minutes. Remove and set aside.

2. In a large bowl, whisk together vinegar and mustard. Season with a pinch of salt and pepper. Whisk in walnut oil. Add escarole, radicchio, cherries and toasted walnuts. Toss to combine.

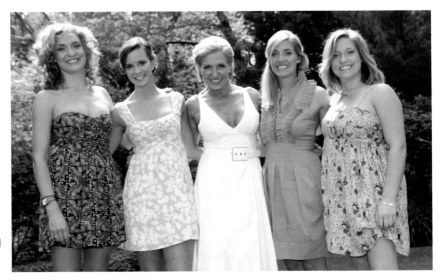

NUTRITIONAL VALUE
PER SERVING:

Calories: 127 |
Calories from Fat: 85 |
Protein: 3 g | Carbs: 11 g |
Total Fat: 9 g |
Saturated Fat: 1 g |
Trans Fat: 0 g | Fiber: 4 g |
Sodium: 78 mg |
Cholesterol: 0 mg

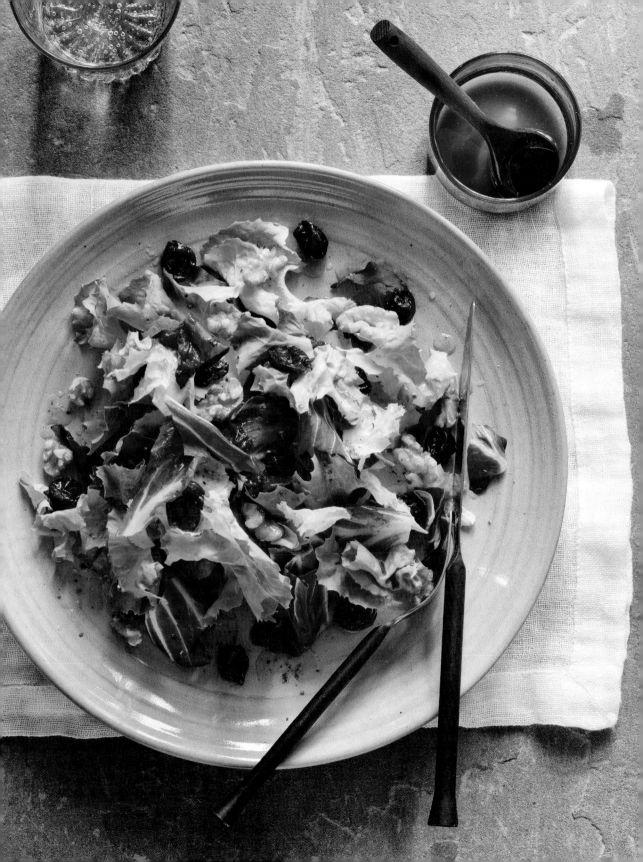

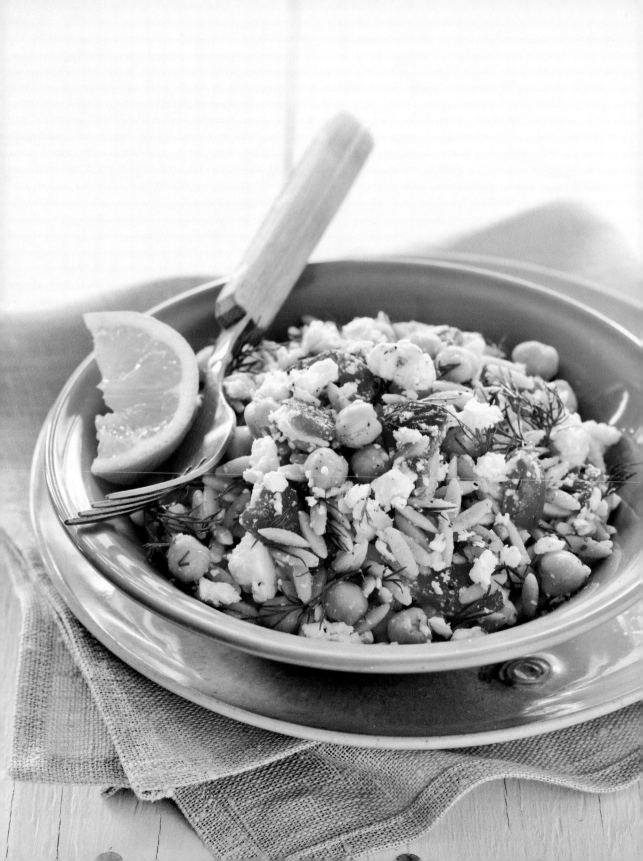

Servings: 5 x 1 cup
Prep time: 5 minutes
Cooking time:
10 minutes

ORZO AND CHICKPEA SALAD
with Roasted Red Peppers and Dill

Orzo may look like grains of rice, but it's actually a tiny pasta. It's often used in soups, stews, casseroles and salads. Look for whole wheat orzo in bulk stores or the organic/healthy section of your supermarket.

INGREDIENTS

¼ tsp / 1.25 ml **sea salt**, plus a pinch, divided
1 cup / 240 ml whole wheat **orzo pasta**
Juice of 1 **lemon**
½ tsp / 2.5 ml **honey**
½ tsp / 2.5 ml **cumin**
Pinch **sea salt** and freshly ground **black pepper**
1 Tbsp / 15 ml **extra virgin olive oil**
1 cup / 240 ml cooked **chickpeas** (if using canned, make sure to purchase BPA-free cans)
½ cup / 120 ml drained and diced roasted **red peppers**
2 Tbsp / 30 ml chopped fresh **dill**
2 oz / 56 g reduced-fat **feta**, crumbled

METHOD

1. Heat a large pot of water over high heat. Season cooking water with a pinch of salt and stir in orzo. Cook according to package directions until tender but firm to bite. Drain and set aside.

2. In a small bowl, whisk together lemon juice, honey, cumin, salt and pepper. Whisk in olive oil.

3. In a large bowl, place cooked orzo, chick peas, roasted red peppers and dill. Pour dressing over top and toss to combine. Add crumbled feta and gently toss together.

NUTRITIONAL VALUE
PER SERVING:

Calories: 220 |
Calories from Fat: 40 |
Protein: 9 g | Carbs: 36 g |
Total Fat: 5 g |
Saturated Fat: 1 g |
Trans Fat: 0 g | Fiber: 8 g |
Sodium: 236 mg |
Cholesterol: 1 mg

Servings: 6 x 1⅓ cups
Prep time: 15 minutes
Cooking time:
1 hour

BEETS, BLOOD ORANGES AND ARUGULA
with Feta

Beets are a very versatile vegetable with a potent, dark red color. They can be boiled, pickled, baked, roasted, grilled and more. When choosing beets, select firm, healthy looking beets with no discoloration, wrinkles or sliminess, and store them in the refrigerator.

INGREDIENTS

SALAD

4 medium **beets**, any kind
   (red, golden, Chioggia)
1 **blood orange**
4 cups / 960 ml **arugula**, loosely packed
2 oz / 56 g low-fat **feta** (about a
   2-inch cube), crumbled

VINAIGRETTE

2 Tbsp / 30 ml **blood orange juice**
   (from reserved membrane,
   see directions below)
1 Tbsp / 15 ml **champagne vinegar**
   or **white wine vinegar**
½ tsp / 2.5 ml **honey**
⅛ tsp / 0.625 ml **sea salt**
Pinch freshly ground **black pepper**
1 Tbsp / 15 ml **extra virgin olive oil**

METHOD

1. Preheat oven to 425°F / 220°C. Place beets in a loaf pan or similar bakeware and add enough water to come half an inch up side of beets. Cover tightly with aluminum foil and cook in oven until tender when pierced with a toothpick, about 1 hour. Remove from oven, uncover, and let sit until cool enough to handle. Peel beets (wear latex or rubber gloves if you don't want to stain your hands and fingernails), cut them into slim wedges and cut wedges into bite-sized pieces.

2. Using a knife, cut away peel and white pith of blood orange. Using a paring knife, segment orange, reserving membrane. Set segments aside.

3. To make vinaigrette, squeeze juice from reserved blood orange membrane into a small bowl. Add vinegar, honey, salt and pepper, and whisk, adding olive oil.

4. Place arugula in a bowl and add half of vinaigrette. Toss to combine. Divide arugula among plates. Add beets and remaining vinaigrette to bowl, and toss to combine. Place beets around arugula. Divide reserved blood orange segments among plates and crumble feta over top. Serve immediately.

NUTRITIONAL VALUE
PER SERVING:
Calories: 81 |
Calories from Fat: 28 |
Protein: 4 g | Carbs: 10 g |
Total Fat: 3 g |
Saturated Fat: 1 g |
Trans Fat: 0 g | Fiber: 2 g |
Sodium: 143 mg |
Cholesterol: 2 mg

NOTE *Save beet tops and use them to make German-Braised Beet Tops and Apples (see recipe page 309) or Bruschetta with Ricotta, Beet Greens and Walnuts (see recipe page 282).*

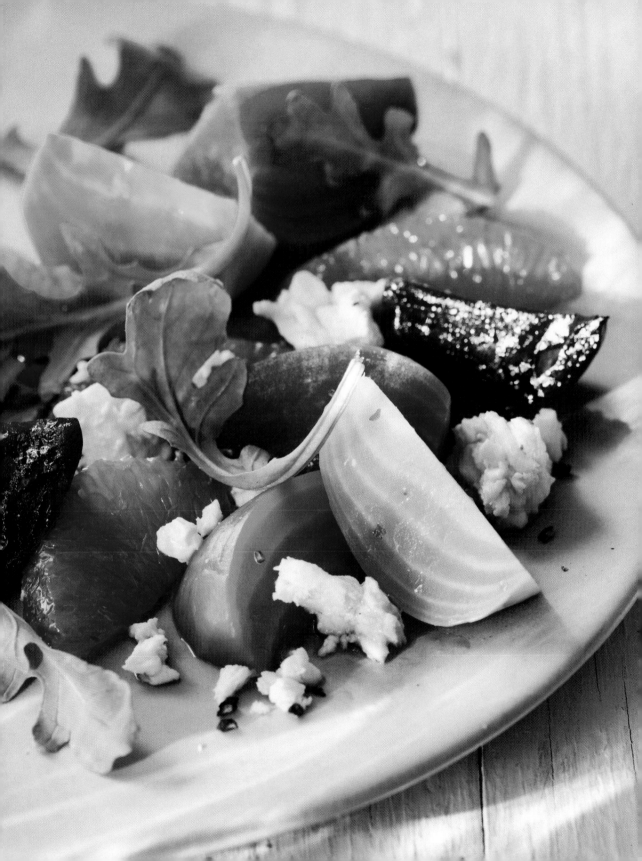

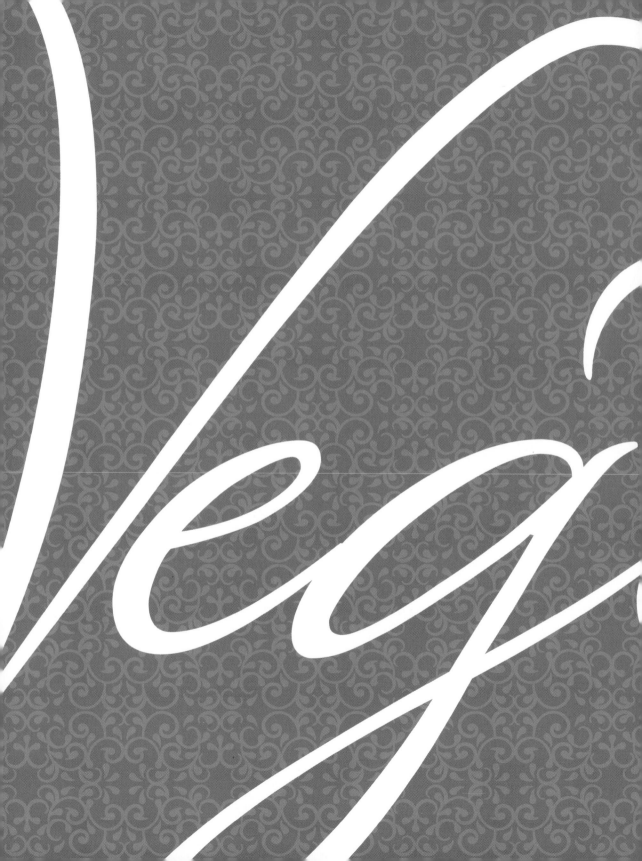

11

Vegetables

282 BRUSCHETTA
with Ricotta, Beet Greens and Walnuts

285 SUGAR SNAP PEAS AND MORELS

286 GRILLED FINGERLING POTATOES

289 PATTY PAN SQUASH

290 SAUTÉED FRESH PEPPERONCINI
with Yogurt Cheese and Baguette

293 BROCCOLI RAAB (RAPINI)
with Sun-Dried Tomatoes

294 CARAMELIZED CREMINI MUSHROOMS
AND PEARL ONIONS

297 BRAISED COLLARD GREENS

298 SMOKY SLATHERED CORN ON THE COB

301 SESAME MANDARIN SLAW

302 COLCANNON
with Kale

305 GRILLED GARLIC SPEARS

306 BABY YELLOW POTATOES
with Parsley

309 GERMAN-BRAISED BEET TOPS AND APPLES

310 ROASTED DELICATA SQUASH

Servings: 4 x 1 cup
Prep time: 5 minutes
Cooking time:
8 minutes

BRUSCHETTA
with Ricotta, Beet Greens and Walnuts

Ricotta is a low-fat whey cheese, typically used in Italian dishes such as lasagna and cannoli. It's soft and mild with a fairly bland flavor, so it works well in combination with stronger tastes, such as the walnuts and greens on this bruschetta.

INGREDIENTS

4 heaping tsp / 20 ml chopped walnuts
4 long diagonally cut ½-inch slices whole wheat French bread
1 whole clove of garlic, peeled
½ cup / 120 ml low-fat ricotta
1 tsp / 5 ml finely grated lemon zest
1¾ tsp / 8.75 ml extra virgin olive oil, divided
1½ cups / 360 ml beet greens, stems removed, and leaves sliced
    into 2-inch pieces (greens from about 3 beets)
Pinch sea salt
Pinch freshly ground black pepper
1 Tbsp / 15 ml fresh lemon juice

METHOD

1. Preheat oven to 350°F / 175°C. Spread walnuts out on a baking sheet and toast in oven for 5 minutes. Remove and set aside.

2. Heat a grill pan or grill to medium-high heat. Place bread slices on grill until marks appear, 30 seconds to 1 minute, then turn and mark other side. Remove and rub garlic on top of each slice.

3. In a small bowl, mix together ricotta and lemon zest. Heat 1 tsp / 5 ml olive oil in a skillet over medium-high heat and spread to coat bottom. Add beet greens and season with salt and pepper. Cook, stirring until wilted, about 2 minutes. Remove from heat and add lemon juice.

4. Spread 2 Tbsp / 30 ml lemon ricotta mixture on each slice of grilled bread. Divide beet greens evenly and place on top of ricotta. Sprinkle 1 heaping tsp / 5 ml toasted walnuts on top of each pile of beet greens, and drizzle ¼ tsp / 1.25 ml oil on top of each bruschetta. Serve immediately.

NUTRITIONAL VALUE
PER SERVING:
Calories: 175 |
Calories from Fat: 50 |
Protein: 8 g | Carbs: 23 g |
Total Fat: 8 g |
Saturated Fat: 2 g |
Trans Fat: 0 g | Fiber: 3 g |
Sodium: 307 mg |
Cholesterol: 10 mg

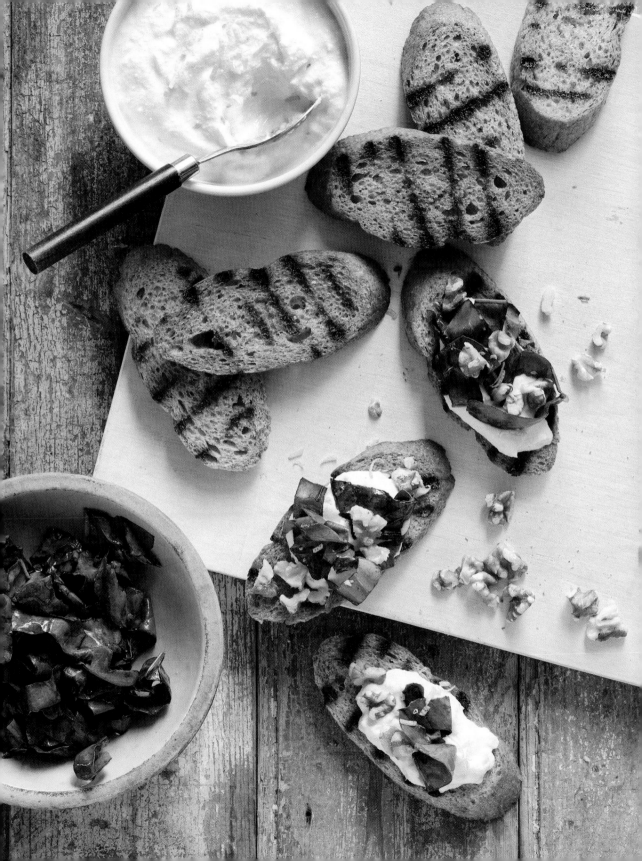

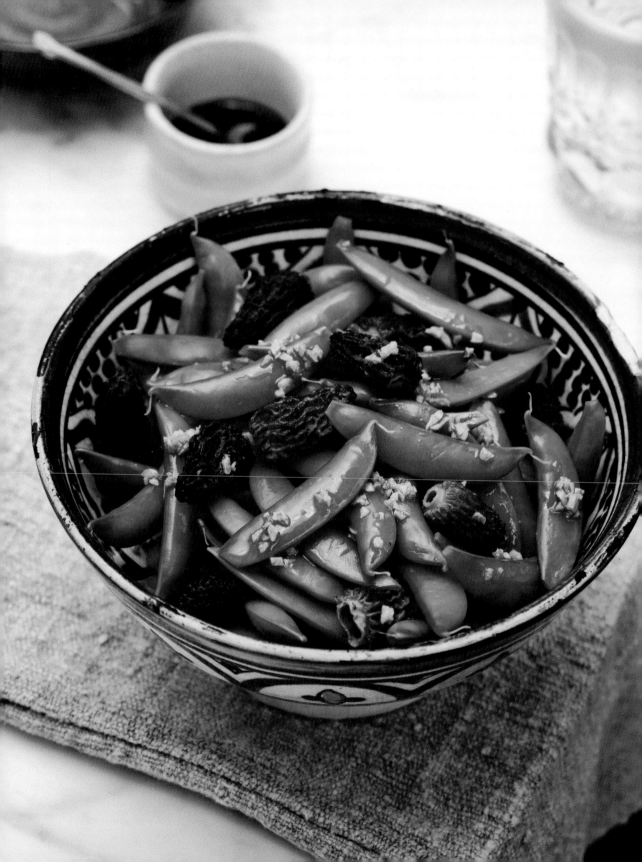

Servings: 4 x 1 cup
Prep time: 10 minutes
Cooking time:
2 minutes

SUGAR SNAP PEAS AND MORELS

This dish is about showcasing the freshest ingredients and allowing them to speak for themselves, rather than covering them up with too many flavors or seasonings. This is just a quick sauté to heat through, retaining the crispness of the fresh peas and the bounce of the morels. In French, sauté literally means "to jump," which is what you want your ingredients to do while they're in the pan!

INGREDIENTS

1 Tbsp / 15 ml extra virgin olive oil
1 lb / 454 g freshest sugar snap peas, stem end and string removed
3 oz / 84 g fresh morel mushrooms, or dried (if using dried morels, be
   sure to rehydrate first according to package directions)
1 clove garlic, minced
1 tsp / 5 ml low-sodium soy sauce
¼ tsp / 1.25 ml sea salt
⅛ tsp / 0.625 ml freshly ground black pepper

METHOD

1. Heat olive oil in a large skillet over medium-high heat. Add snap peas, morels and garlic, and sauté for one minute, stirring or tossing ingredients to combine and ensure that they all get contact with bottom of pan. Add soy sauce, salt and pepper, and stir or toss again to evenly distribute seasoning. Remove from heat and serve immediately.

NUTRITIONAL VALUE
PER SERVING:
Calories: 98 |
Calories from Fat: 30 |
Protein: 3 g | Carbs: 10 g |
Total Fat: 4 g |
Saturated Fat: 0.5 g |
Trans Fat: 0 g | Fiber: 3 g |
Sodium: 203 mg |
Cholesterol: 0 mg

Servings: 6 x ¾ cup
Prep time: 5 minutes
Cooking time:
17 minutes

GRILLED FINGERLING POTATOES

Fingerling potatoes are just like regular potatoes, except, well, they look a little like fingers! They come from a family of heritage potatoes that naturally grow much smaller than regular potatoes, but they can be cooked in the same way. Here I've decided to grill my fingerlings, which gives them a pleasing, slightly charred taste.

INGREDIENTS

1½ lbs / 681 g fingerling potatoes – try different colors!
2 Tbsp / 30 ml extra virgin olive oil
1 large clove garlic, minced
1 Tbsp / 15 ml chopped fresh flat leaf parsley
1 tsp / 5 ml chopped fresh thyme
½ tsp / 2.5 ml sea salt
¼ tsp / 1.25 ml freshly ground black pepper

METHOD

1. Place fingerling potatoes in a pot big enough to allow at least a few inches of room at top. Fill pot with enough cold water to cover potatoes by one inch and place on stove over high heat. Bring to a boil, then reduce heat and simmer until potatoes are tender when pierced with a skewer, about 12 to 15 minutes. Drain, and let sit until cool enough to handle, about 5 minutes.

2. Meanwhile, heat a grill or grill pan to medium-high heat. Cut fingerlings in half lengthwise and gently toss with olive oil, garlic, herbs, salt and pepper. Place potatoes cut side down on grill and let cook until marks develop, about 1 minute. Turn them a quarter-turn to create crosshatch grill marks and cook for 1 minute longer. Remove and serve.

NUTRITIONAL VALUE
PER SERVING:
Calories: 128 |
Calories from Fat: 40 |
Protein: 2 g | Carbs: 19 g |
Total Fat: 5 g |
Saturated Fat: 1 g |
Trans Fat: 0 g | Fiber: 0 g |
Sodium: 194 mg |
Cholesterol: 0 mg

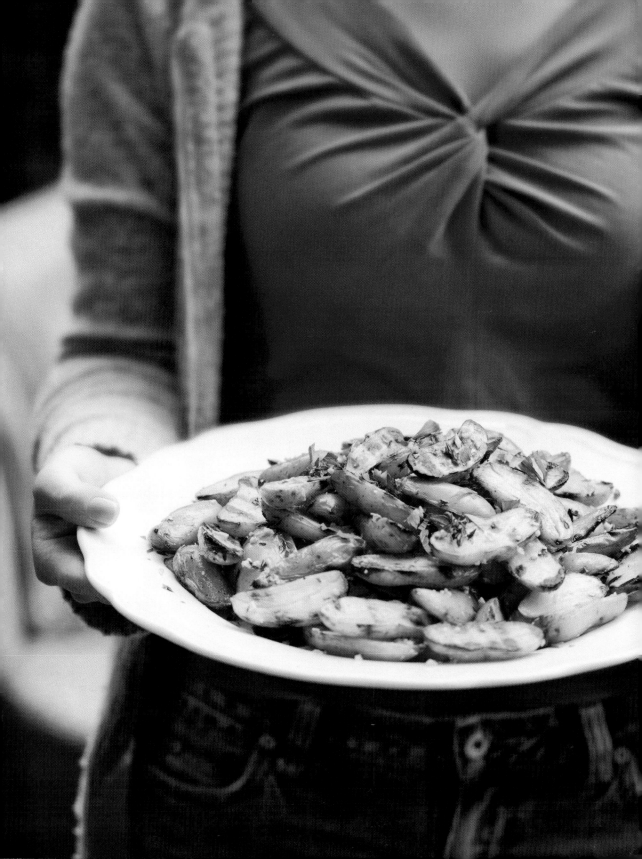

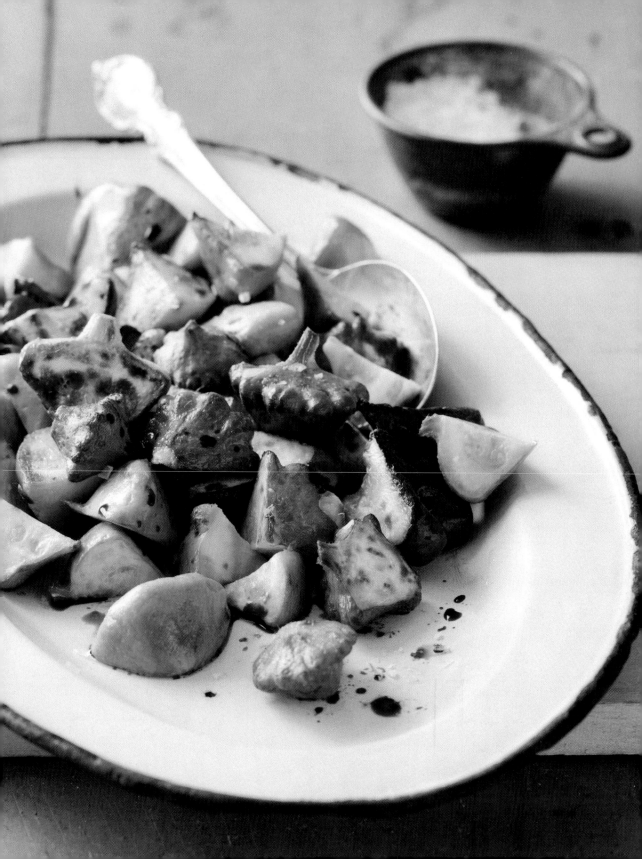

PATTY PAN SQUASH

Servings: 6 x ½ cup
Prep time: 8 minutes
Cooking time: 3-4 minutes

Shaped like a UFO or strange disc, the patty pan squash is a summer squash with a taste similar to that of zucchini. The best patty pan squashes are small, no larger than the width of your palm. They should be uniform in texture, but can be yellow, green or even white in color.

INGREDIENTS

1 lb / 454 g patty pan squash
1 tsp / 5 ml extra virgin olive oil
1 clove garlic, minced
¼ tsp / 1.25 ml sea salt
⅛ tsp / 0.625 ml freshly ground black pepper
1 Tbsp / 15 ml low-sodium soy sauce

METHOD

1. Trim stems from patty pan squash and cut in half top to bottom (the knife will cut through both stem ends). Cut squash into one-inch wedges.

2. Heat olive oil in a large skillet over medium-high heat. Add squash wedges and sauté, stirring or tossing occasionally, until slightly softened and starting to brown, 2 to 3 minutes. (You want squash al dente, so do not overcook.) Stir in garlic and cook for one minute longer. Season with salt and pepper. Add soy sauce, toss to coat, and slide out onto a serving platter. Serve immediately.

NUTRITIONAL VALUE
PER SERVING:
Calories: 22 |
Calories from Fat: 7 |
Protein: 1 g | Carbs: 3 g |
Total Fat: 1 g |
Saturated Fat: 0 g |
Trans Fat: 0 g | Fiber: 1 g |
Sodium: 186 mg |
Cholesterol: 0 mg

Servings: 4 x 2 slices
Prep time: 10 minutes
Cooking time:
3 minutes

SAUTÉED FRESH PEPPERONCINI
with Yogurt Cheese and Baguette

Frequently used in Italian, Greek and Eastern European cuisines, pepperoncini peppers are a type of mild chili pepper that is most commonly pickled and preserved in vinegar. Here I've sautéed them, which helps them retain a satisfying bite without being overpowering.

Note: Yogurt Cheese must be made ahead of time.

INGREDIENTS

2 Tbsp / 30 ml extra virgin olive oil
1½ cups / 360 ml fresh pepperoncini peppers, stemmed and cut into ¼-inch coins
2 cloves garlic, minced
1 tsp / 5 ml fresh lemon juice
¼ cup / 60 ml Yogurt Cheese (see recipe on page 348)
8 x ½-inch slices whole wheat baguette
½ tsp / 2.5 ml coarse sea salt
¼ tsp / 1.25 ml freshly ground black pepper

METHOD

1. Heat olive oil in a large skillet over medium-high heat. Add pepperoncini and sauté until soft, 2 minutes. Add garlic and cook for one minute longer. Remove from heat and stir in lemon juice.

2. Divide Yogurt Cheese evenly among slices of baguette, spreading on top. Place slices on a serving platter. Spoon pepperoncini over top and sprinkle with coarse sea salt and freshly ground black pepper. Serve immediately.

NUTRITIONAL VALUE
PER SERVING:

Calories: 302 |
Calories from Fat: 60 |
Protein: 10 g | Carbs: 48 g |
Total Fat: 7 g |
Saturated Fat: 1 g |
Trans Fat: 0 g | Fiber: 8 g |
Sodium: 420 mg |
Cholesterol: 0 mg

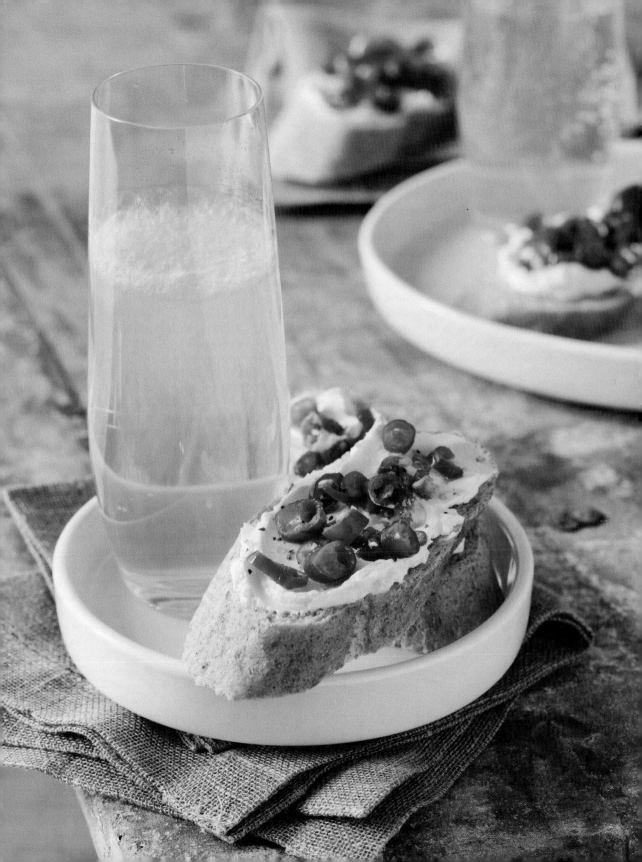

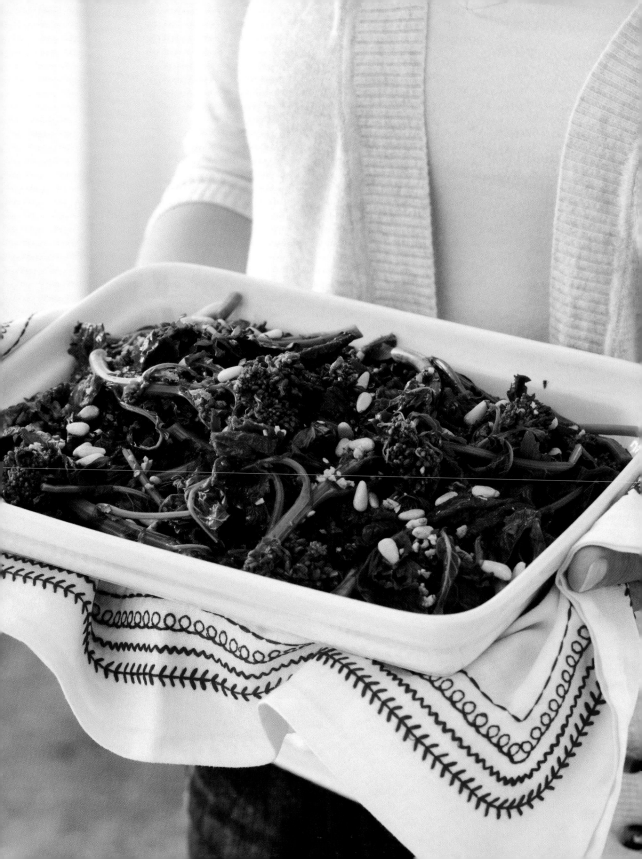

Servings: 4 x ½ cup
Prep time: 5 minutes
Cooking time:
10 minutes

BROCCOLI RAAB (RAPINI)
with Sun-Dried Tomatoes

Rapini is also known as broccoli raab or just raab. Rapini is a leafy mustard green. Its leaves and buds have a mustardy bite much like turnip greens. Serve this vegetable dish alongside your favorite protein such as grilled chicken, lean pork or beef to round out your Clean meal.

INGREDIENTS

1 Tbsp / 15 ml toasted pine nuts
2 heaping Tbsp / 30 ml julienne-cut sun-dried tomatoes in extra virgin olive oil
Pinch red pepper flakes
1 clove garlic, chopped
1 bunch broccoli raab, stalk ends trimmed, and cut into large bite-sized pieces
⅛ tsp / 0.625 ml sea salt
Pinch freshly ground black pepper

METHOD

1. Preheat oven to 350°F / 175°C. Spread pine nuts on a baking sheet and toast in oven until golden brown, 3 to 5 minutes. (Be careful not to burn!)

2. Heat sun-dried tomatoes including oil in a large skillet over medium-high heat. Stir in red pepper flakes and garlic, and cook until fragrant, 1 minute Add broccoli raab and season with salt and pepper. Reduce heat to medium-low and cook until wilted, stirring, about 3 minutes. Add pine nuts and stir to combine. Divide among four plates and serve.

NUTRITIONAL VALUE
PER SERVING:
Calories: 59 |
Calories from Fat: 22 |
Protein: 5 g | Carbs: 5 g |
Total Fat: 2 g |
Saturated Fat: 0 g |
Trans Fat: 0 g | Fiber: 3 g |
Sodium: 139 mg |
Cholesterol: 0 mg

Servings: 4 x ½ cup
Prep time: 10 minutes
Cooking time:
12-15 minutes

CARAMELIZED CREMINI MUSHROOMS AND PEARL ONIONS

The taste of true decadence is in this caramelized mushroom and onion dish. Easy to make, this dish adds so much to a wide variety of meals. I prefer mine spooned over a baked potato or over a crusty whole wheat baguette.

INGREDIENTS

1 tsp / 5 ml olive oil
1 cup / 240 ml pearl onions, thawed
8 oz / 227 g cremini mushrooms, quartered (about 3 cups / 720 ml)
1 clove garlic, minced
½ tsp / 2.5 ml chopped fresh thyme
¼ tsp / 1.25 ml chopped fresh rosemary
⅛ tsp / 0.625 ml sea salt
Pinch freshly ground black pepper
1 cup / 240 ml low-sodium beef broth

METHOD

1. Heat olive oil in a very large nonstick skillet over medium-high heat. Add onions and mushrooms in a single layer, and sauté until browned, stirring occasionally, about 5 minutes. Add garlic, thyme, rosemary, salt and pepper, and cook for 1 minute longer. Add beef broth and simmer until onions are tender and broth has almost completely reduced, stirring once or twice, about 6 to 8 minutes. Remove from heat and serve.

NUTRITIONAL VALUE
PER SERVING:
Calories: 67 |
Calories from Fat: 13 |
Protein: 3 g | Carbs: 10 g |
Total Fat: 2 g |
Saturated Fat: 0 g |
Trans Fat: 0 g | Fiber: 0 g |
Sodium: 104 mg |
Cholesterol: 0 mg

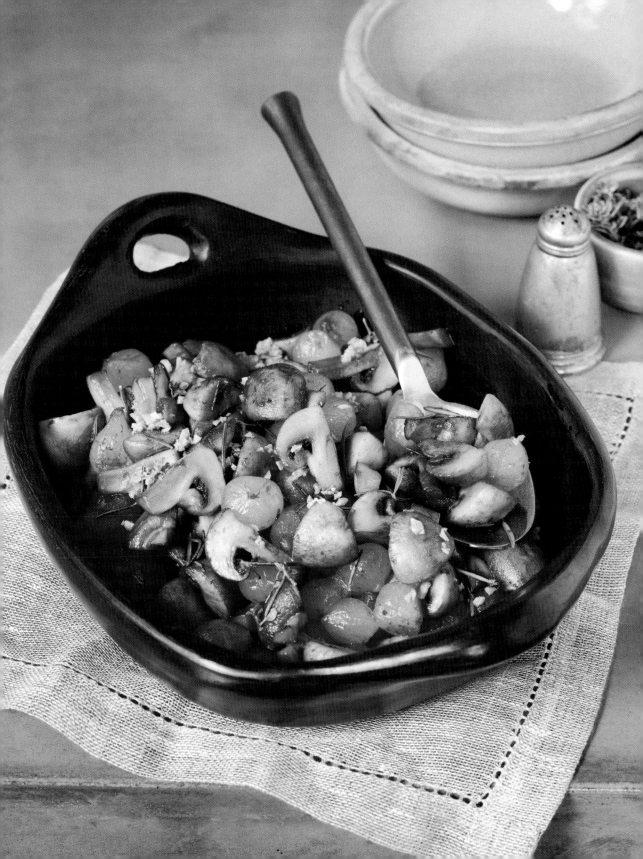

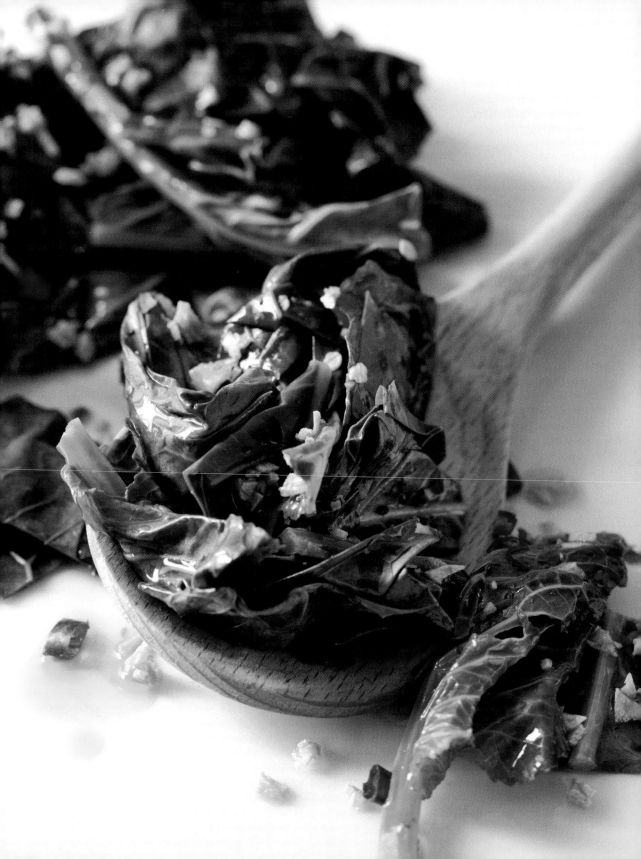

BRAISED COLLARD GREENS

Servings: 4 x ½ cup
Prep time: 10 minutes
Cooking time:
45 minutes

Braising is a method of cooking that combines dry and moist heat. First the food is seared at a high temperature and then it's simmered in a covered pot. Braising your greens is a delicious way to add more vegetables to your diet.

INGREDIENTS

1 Tbsp / 15 ml extra virgin olive oil
2 cloves garlic, chopped
Pinch red pepper flakes
1 bunch collard greens, trimmed and chopped into 2-inch strips (about 12 cups / 3 L)
1 cup / 240 ml low-sodium chicken or vegetable broth
1 Tbsp / 15 ml cider vinegar
2 tsp / 10 ml brown sugar
¼ tsp / 1.25 ml smoked paprika
1 bay leaf
¾ tsp / 3.75 ml sea salt
¼ tsp / 1.25 ml freshly ground black pepper

METHOD

1. Heat olive oil in a large skillet over medium-high heat. Add garlic and red pepper flakes, and cook for 30 seconds. Fold in collards in thirds, stirring, until they start to wilt. Add broth and rest of ingredients. Cover and reduce heat to simmer until tender, about 45 minutes.

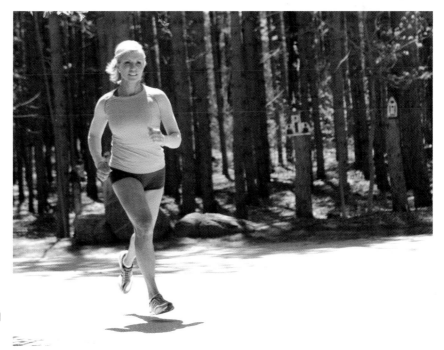

NUTRITIONAL VALUE
PER SERVING:
Calories: 79 |
Calories from Fat: 33 |
Protein: 4 g | Carbs: 9 g |
Total Fat: 4 g |
Saturated Fat: 1 g |
Trans Fat: 0 g | Fiber: 3 g |
Sodium: 470 mg |
Cholesterol: 0 mg

Servings: 4 x ½ cob
Prep time: 8 minutes
Cooking time:
4-5 minutes

SMOKY SLATHERED CORN ON THE COB

Corn on the cob is one of my favorite summer vegetables. It reminds me of the summer fairs and family barbeques I used to attend as a child. This spice-enhanced corn on the cob is sure to impress the guests at your modern-day barbeque or street party – you'll be the talk of the neighborhood!

INGREDIENTS

½ tsp / 2.5 ml smoked paprika
½ tsp / 2.5 ml chili powder
½ tsp / 2.5 ml sea salt
¼ tsp / 1.25 ml freshly ground black pepper
2 ears of corn, husked
1 tsp / 5 ml extra virgin olive oil
2 tsp / 10 ml finely grated Parmigiano Reggiano

METHOD

1. Heat a grill or grill pan to medium-high heat. In a small bowl, mix paprika, chili powder, salt and pepper. Rub ears of corn with olive oil and sprinkle with spice mixture. Place corn on grill and cover. Cook 4 to 5 minutes, turning two or three times, until marked and cooked al dente. Sprinkle corn with Parmigiano Reggiano and serve.

NUTRITIONAL VALUE
PER SERVING
(½ EAR OF CORN):
Calories: 73 |
Calories from Fat: 29 |
Protein: 4 g | Carbs: 9 g |
Total Fat: 2 g |
Saturated Fat: 1 g |
Trans Fat: 0 g | Fiber: 1 g |
Sodium: 337 mg |
Cholesterol: 6 mg

NOTE *One serving is half a cob of corn.*

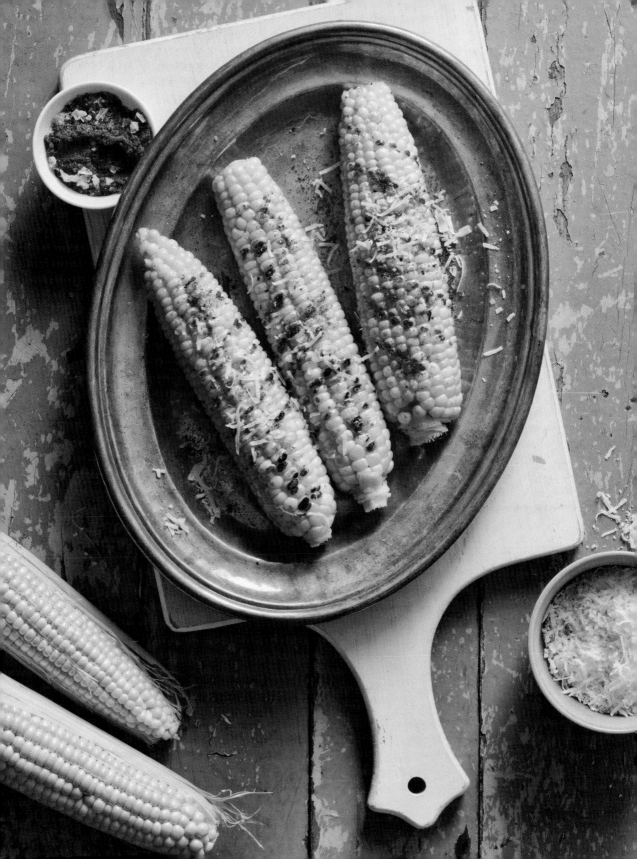

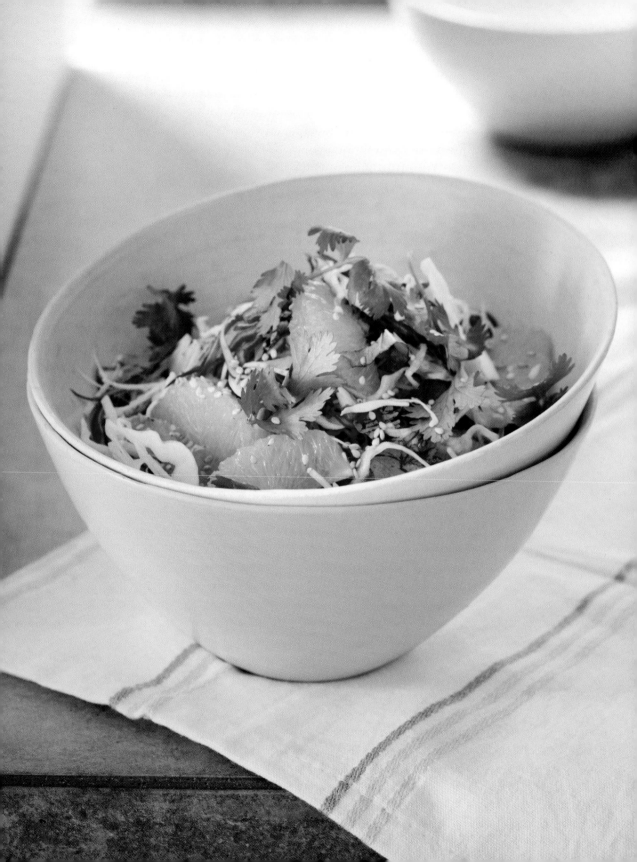

Servings: 6 x 1 cup
Prep time: 15 minutes
Cooking time:
0 minutes

SESAME MANDARIN SLAW

Sesame oil, an oil made from sesame seeds, is known as "the queen of the oils." A potent antioxidant, it's been used as a healing oil for thousands of years, everywhere from India to Holland. Lucky for us, it's also a great oil for cooking, as it lends a pleasant sesame taste to the food it helps cook.

INGREDIENTS

SLAW

⅛ head each purple and green cabbage, thinly sliced
2 mandarin oranges, peeled and chopped
⅛ red onion, thinly sliced
2 Tbsp / 30 ml chopped fresh cilantro
1 Tbsp / 15 ml chopped fresh mint
1 Tbsp / 15 ml toasted sesame seeds

DRESSING

1 Tbsp / 15 ml finely grated fresh ginger
1 Tbsp / 15 ml fresh lime juice
1 Tbsp / 15 ml pure toasted sesame oil
2 tsp / 10 ml agave nectar
1 tsp / 5 ml organic low-sodium tamari
¼ tsp / 1.25 ml fresh chili paste
½ tsp / 2.5 ml sea salt
⅛ tsp / 0.625 ml freshly ground black pepper

METHOD

1. In a large bowl, combine purple and green cabbage, mandarin oranges and red onion.

2. In a small bowl, whisk together all dressing ingredients and pour over slaw in large bowl. Add cilantro, mint and sesame seeds, and toss to combine.

NUTRITIONAL VALUE
PER SERVING:
Calories: 41 |
Calories from Fat: 10 |
Protein: 1 g | Carbs: 7 g |
Total Fat: 1 g |
Saturated Fat: 0 g |
Trans Fat: 0 g | Fiber: 2 g |
Sodium: 10 mg |
Cholesterol: 0 mg

Servings: 6 x 1 cup
Prep time: 15 minutes
Cooking time:
25 minutes

COLCANNON
with Kale

Associated with Halloween, colcannon is a traditional Irish potato dish made with mashed potatoes, kale or cabbage (in this case, both!), milk and butter. I've Cleaned up this version by using olive oil and nutritional yeast, a cheesy-tasting vegan inactive yeast that is high in vitamin B12.

INGREDIENTS

1 lb / 454 g red potatoes, cut into 1-inch chunks
2 Tbsp / 30 ml extra virgin olive oil
1 medium yellow onion, chopped
4 cups / 960 ml thinly sliced green cabbage
4 cups / 960 ml chopped kale, leaves stripped from stems
1½ tsp / 7.5 ml sea salt, divided
2 cloves garlic, finely chopped
½ cup / 120 ml 1% low-fat milk
½ cup / 120 ml low-sodium chicken broth
2 Tbsp / 30 ml nutritional yeast
½ tsp / 2.5 ml freshly ground black pepper
6 tsp / 30 ml shredded low-fat aged cheddar, divided

METHOD

1. Place potatoes in a medium pot filled with cold water and place over high heat. Bring to a boil, and then reduce heat to simmer until potatoes are very tender, 15 to 20 minutes. Drain and place in a large bowl.

2. While potatoes are cooking, heat olive oil in a very large skillet over medium heat. Add onion and cook until soft and translucent, about 5 minutes. Add cabbage, kale and ½ tsp / 2.5 ml sea salt, and stir in with onions. Continue to cook over medium heat until greens are wilted and soft, 10 minutes. Stir in garlic and cook for 1 minute longer. Remove from heat and set aside.

3. Using a potato masher, smash potatoes. Add milk, chicken broth, nutritional yeast, remaining 1 tsp / 5 ml sea salt and black pepper, and mash into potatoes. Add cooked cabbage and kale mixture, and stir to combine. Serve in large bowls, each sprinkled with 1 tsp / 5 ml cheddar. Delicious as a side dish for Irish lamb stew!

NUTRITIONAL VALUE
PER SERVING:
Calories: 409 |
Calories from Fat: 54 |
Protein: 13 g | Carbs: 83 g |
Total Fat: 6 g |
Saturated Fat: 1 g |
Trans Fat: 0 g | Fiber: 8 g |
Sodium: 533 mg |
Cholesterol: 1 mg

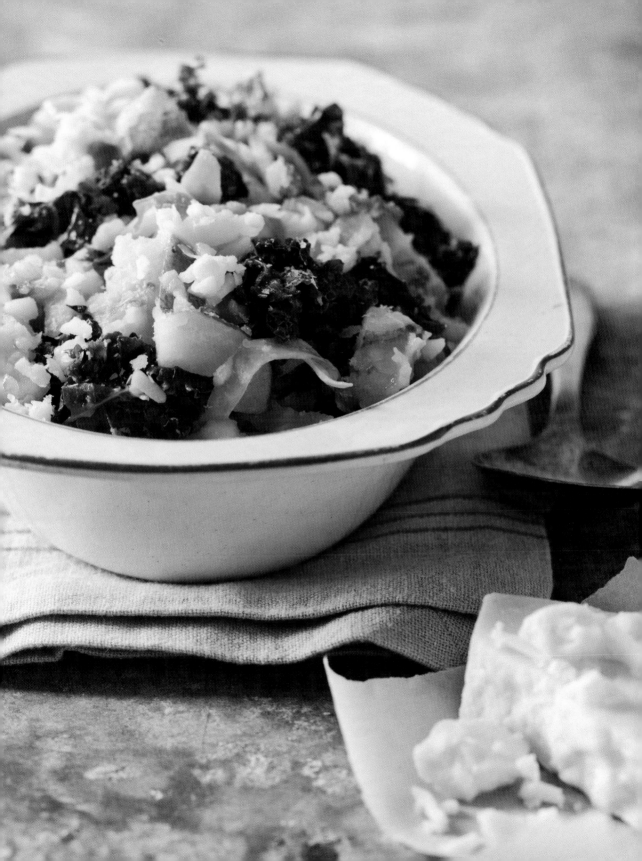

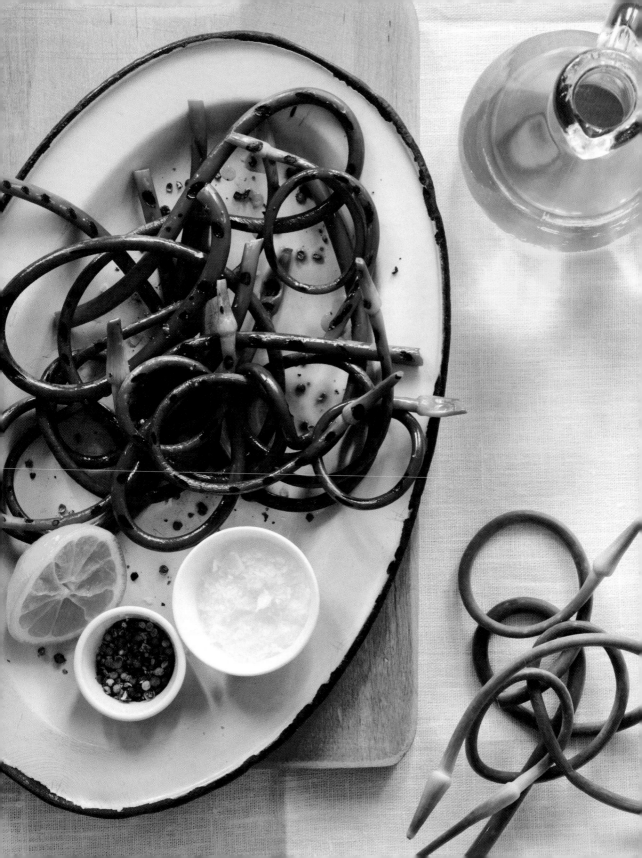

GRILLED GARLIC SPEARS

Servings: 6 x 2²/₃ cups
Prep time: 5 minutes
Cooking time:
4 minutes

When I first started Eating Clean, I made a point to purchase one "new-to-me" vegetable at the supermarket each week. I was delighted to find garlic spears, which are the flowery tops of the elephant garlic plant. Raw, they have a spicy garlic flavor, but they are much more mild when cooked.

INGREDIENTS

1 lb / 454 g garlic spears
1 Tbsp / 15 ml extra virgin olive oil
¼ tsp / 1.25 ml sea salt
⅛ tsp / 0.625 ml freshly ground black pepper
Juice of ½ lemon

METHOD

1. Heat a grill or grill pan to high heat. Trim stalk end of garlic spears half an inch, just enough to remove dry end. Place garlic spears on a baking sheet and drizzle with olive oil. Use your clean hands to gently toss and evenly coat with oil. Sprinkle with salt and pepper.

2. Place garlic spears on grill in an even layer, perpendicular to lines of grate to prevent them from slipping through. Grill until slightly charred and soft, about 2 minutes on each side. Remove to a serving plate and squeeze fresh lemon juice over top. Divide garlic spears among six plates.

NUTRITIONAL VALUE
PER SERVING:

Calories: 89 |
Calories from Fat: 23 |
Protein: 3 g | Carbs: 15 g |
Total Fat: 3 g |
Saturated Fat: 0 g |
Trans Fat: 0 g | Fiber: 1 g |
Sodium: 104 mg |
Cholesterol: 0 mg

Servings: 4 x 1 cup
Prep time: 5 minutes
Cooking time:
15 minutes

BABY YELLOW POTATOES
with Parsley

When choosing vegetables in the supermarket or at your local farmers' market, don't overlook the humble potato. Rich in nutrients and flavor and quick to make, potatoes are the perfect addition to any weeknight dinner. They make excellent lunch leftovers too!

INGREDIENTS

1 tsp / 5 ml sea salt plus a pinch, divided
16 oz / 454 g baby yellow potatoes
½ tsp / 2.5 ml extra virgin olive oil
Pinch freshly ground black pepper
1 tsp / 5 ml chopped fresh parsley

METHOD

1. Bring a medium pot of water to boil over high heat. Add 1 tsp / 5 ml salt and potatoes. Reduce heat to simmer and cook potatoes until tender when pierced with a knife, about 15 minutes. Drain and transfer to a bowl. Toss with olive oil, a pinch of salt and pepper, and parsley.

NUTRITIONAL VALUE
PER SERVING:

Calories: 89 |
Calories from Fat: 5 |
Protein: 2 g | Carbs: 21 g |
Total Fat: 1 g |
Saturated Fat: 0 g |
Trans Fat: 0 g | Fiber: 2 g |
Sodium: 691 mg |
Cholesterol: 0 mg

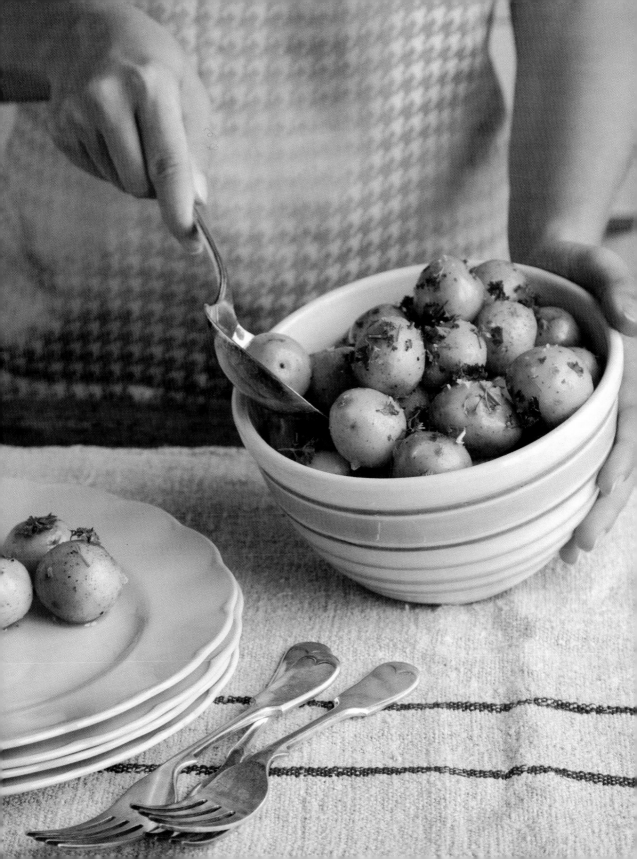

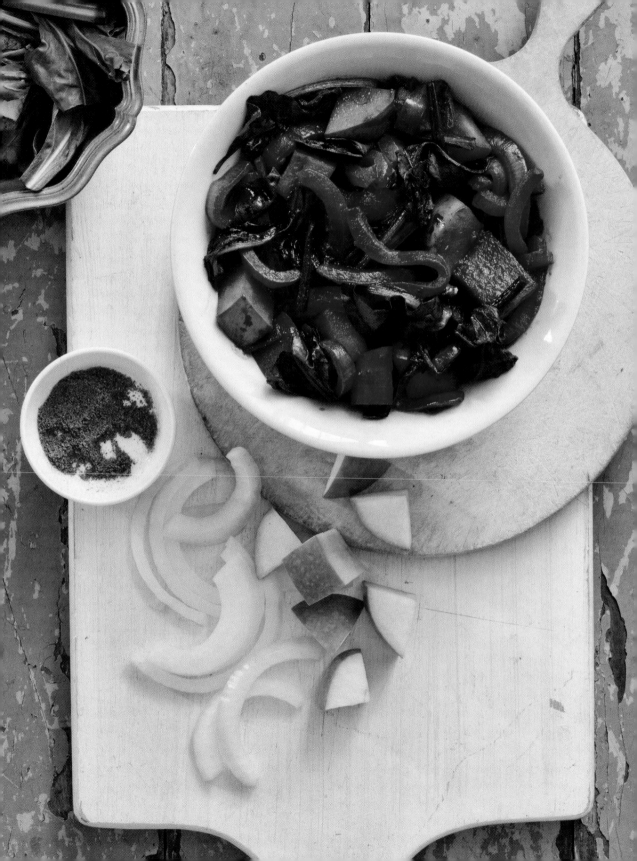

Servings: 4 x ½ cup
Prep time: 10 minutes
Cooking time:
13-15 minutes

GERMAN-BRAISED BEET TOPS AND APPLES

The next time you purchase beets, don't throw anything away. Beet stems and greens are packed with vitamins, minerals and antioxidants, so you can feel good about making this tasty vegetable dish for you and your loved ones.

INGREDIENTS

2 tsp / 10 ml extra virgin olive oil
½ medium yellow onion, thinly sliced
½ apple, such as Granny Smith or Braeburn, cored, thinly sliced and then cut into 1-inch pieces
½ tsp / 2.5 ml sea salt
¼ tsp / 1.25 ml freshly ground black pepper
1 clove garlic, chopped
1 bunch beet tops or Swiss chard, stems and greens divided, each
    cut into 2-inch pieces (about 4 cups / 960 ml)
1 Tbsp / 15 ml unrefined sugar
2 Tbsp / 30 ml red wine vinegar
Pinch ground cloves
½ cup / 120 ml low-sodium chicken or vegetable broth

METHOD

1. Heat olive oil in a large skillet over medium heat. Add onion, apple, salt and pepper and cook until soft, about 3 minutes. Add garlic and cook for 1 minute longer. Add beet stems (reserving greens), sugar, red wine vinegar, ground cloves and broth, and stir to combine. Simmer, partially covered, until stems are al dente, 8 to 10 minutes. Stir in remaining beet greens, cover pan, and cook for 1 minute longer.

NUTRITIONAL VALUE
PER SERVING:
Calories: 74 |
Calories from Fat: 23 |
Protein: 2 g | Carbs: 12 g |
Total Fat: 3 g |
Saturated Fat: 0.5 g |
Trans Fat: 0 g | Fiber: 2 g |
Sodium: 303 mg |
Cholesterol: 0 mg

ROASTED DELICATA SQUASH

Servings: 4 x ½ cup
Prep time: 10 minutes
Cooking time:
15-20 minutes

If you've never tried delicata squash, you're in for a real treat. Yellow in color with a green or green and orange-striped pattern, this oblong vegetable has a creamy texture and sweet taste, which gives it the nickname: "the sweet potato squash."

INGREDIENTS

1 organic delicata squash, washed well, skin on
1 Tbsp / 15 ml extra virgin olive oil
¼ tsp / 1.25 ml Herbes de Provence
½ tsp / 2.5 ml sea salt
¼ tsp / 1.25 ml freshly ground black pepper

METHOD

1. Preheat oven to 425°F / 220°C. Trim ends of squash and halve it lengthwise. Scrape out seeds and discard (or you can clean them and roast them like pumpkin seeds). Place flat side of squash on a cutting board and slice it into half-inch-sized half-rings. Place squash on a baking sheet and drizzle with olive oil. Add Herbes de Provence, salt and pepper. Using your hands, toss to coat squash evenly with seasonings. Spread out in a single layer and roast in oven 15 to 20 minutes, turning once, until golden brown and soft. The entire squash is edible – even the skin!

NUTRITIONAL VALUE
PER SERVING:
Calories: 45 |
Calories from Fat: 34 |
Protein: 1 g | Carbs: 9 g |
Total Fat: 4 g |
Saturated Fat: 0.5 g |
Trans Fat: 0 g | Fiber: 1 g |
Sodium: 306 mg |
Cholesterol: 0 mg

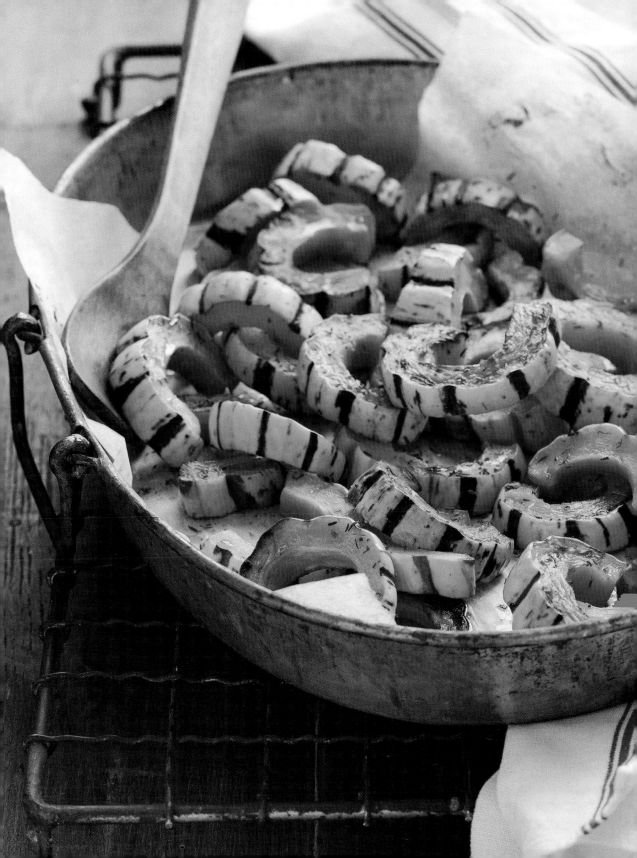

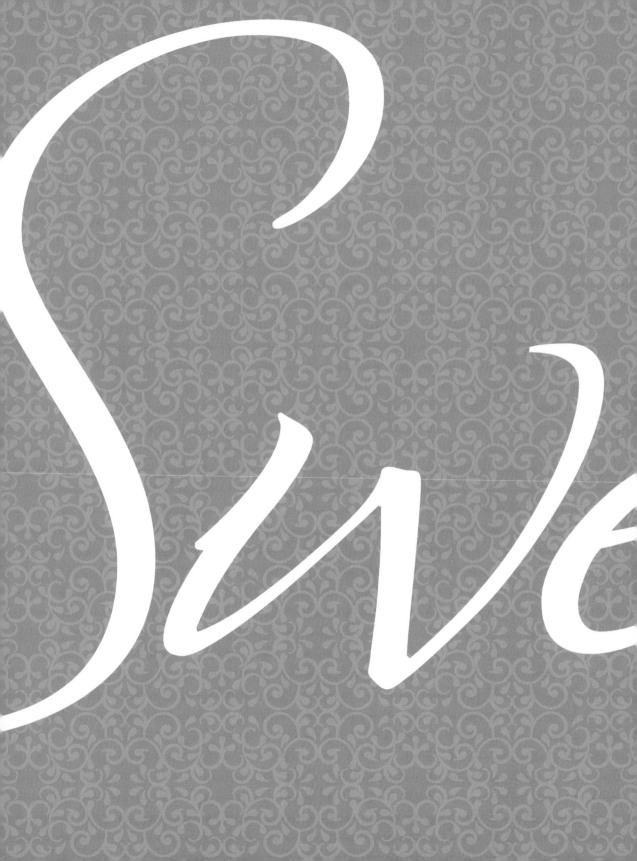

12

Sweets & Breads

314 POACHED PEARS

317 WHITE PEACH SANGRIA

318 MARIONBERRY CRISP
with Walnut Oat Topping

321 WHOLE WHEAT ANGEL FOOD CAKE
with Fresh Strawberries

322 PLUM UPSIDE DOWN CAKE

325 CHOCOLATE ALMOND CAKE

326 HOT SPICED APPLE CIDER

329 CRANBERRY PEAR BELLINI

330 SWEET POTATO CUSTARD
with Spiced Walnut Clusters

333 24 CARROT-TINI

334 RHUBARB WALNUT DESSERT TORTA

337 EFFERVESCENT DESSERT FRUIT SOUP

338 BLUEBERRY BLINTZES

341 BERRY LEMON PARFAIT

342 PAVLOVA
with Fresh Summer Berries

344 *Sweeteners*

Servings: 6
Prep time: 15 minutes
Cooking time:
55-60 minutes

POACHED PEARS

This dish is healthy and simple, yet elegant enough to serve at a fancy dinner party. The pears are "poached," in this case gently simmered, in a bath of red wine, orange juice, vanilla, honey and spices, a brilliant blend of flavors.

INGREDIENTS

6 firm, ripe Bosc pears, peeled, cored, stem intact
1 whole vanilla bean
1 cup / 240 ml red wine
1 cup / 240 ml fresh orange juice
1 Tbsp / 15 ml orange peel, without any white pith
1 cinnamon stick
2 star anise
2 slices fresh ginger
3 Tbsp / 45 ml honey
4 cups / 960 ml water

METHOD

1. Cut a small piece off bottom of each pear so they will stand up straight for serving. Place pears in a medium pot large enough to lay them on their sides in a single layer. Halve vanilla bean lengthwise. Using a small knife, scrape out seeds and add them to pot along with vanilla bean halves. Add rest of ingredients to pot.

2. Bring liquid to a gentle simmer, cover, and poach pears until tender, 15 to 20 minutes. (If there is not enough liquid to completely cover pears, gently turn them over halfway through cooking process.) To test doneness, pierce pears with a skewer, and if there is no resistance, they are done.

3. When done, carefully remove pears using a large plastic slotted strainer and set them aside. Strain poaching liquid into a clean bowl, and then pour it back into poaching pot. Increase heat to a vigorous simmer, and allow liquid to reduce to 1 cup / 240 ml, about 25 to 30 minutes. Liquid will thicken slightly, but will not be as thick as syrup.

4. To serve, spoon liquid into six shallow dessert bowls or plates, and place a pear upright in middle of each. You may wish to add a dollop of honey vanilla Yogurt Cheese on side. Serve immediately. To store, refrigerate and serve cold.

NUTRITIONAL VALUE
PER SERVING
(1 PEAR, 2½ TBSP /
37.5 ML LIQUID):
Calories: 187 |
Calories from Fat: 10 |
Protein: 1 g | Carbs: 39 g |
Total Fat: 1 g |
Saturated Fat: 0 g |
Trans Fat: 0 g | Fiber: 4 g |
Sodium: 9 mg |
Cholesterol: 0 mg

TIP

If you want to make this dish ahead of time, the pears can be poached (and liquid reduced) up to the day before.

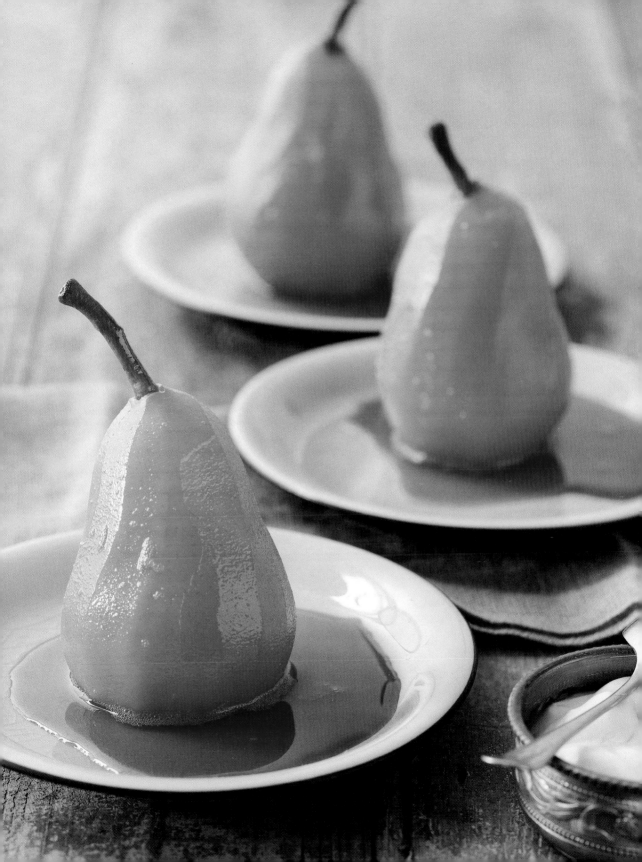

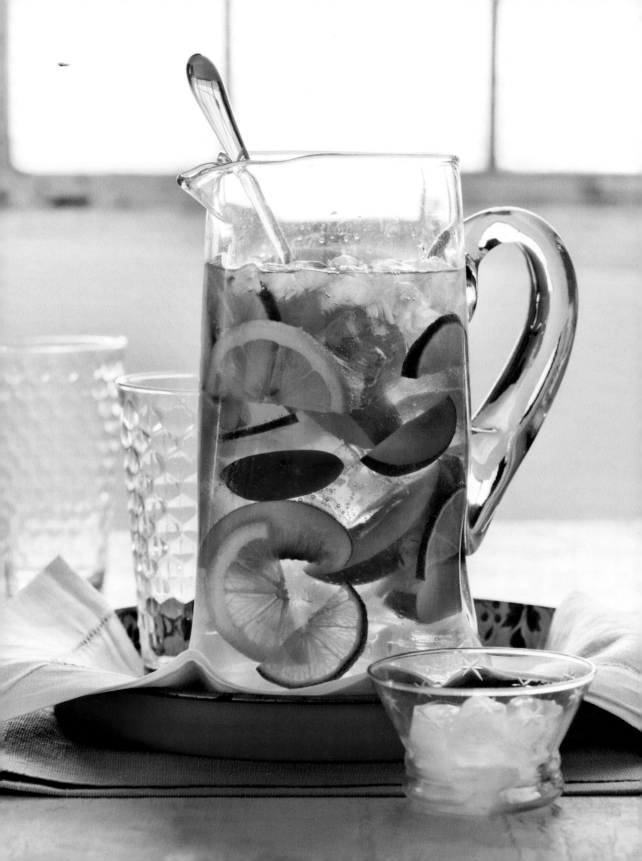

Servings: 4 x 1 cup
Prep time: 10 minutes
Cooking time:
0 minutes

WHITE PEACH SANGRIA

White sangria, or sangria blanca as they say in Spain, is a refreshing wine punch that combines fresh summer fruit with white or sparkling wine. The star of this show is the ripe peach, guaranteed to liven up any summer gathering.

INGREDIENTS

1 ripe peach, pitted and sliced
2 pluots or plums, pitted and sliced
½ orange, washed and thinly sliced into half moons
1 small lemon or ½ large, washed and thinly sliced into half moons
1 small lime or ½ large, washed and thinly sliced into half moons
2 Tbsp / 30 ml cognac
2 Tbsp / 30 ml agave nectar
1 x 750-ml bottle dry white wine, ideally Spanish or Portuguese
Chilled club soda, for topping off sangria

METHOD

1. Add fruit to a large pitcher, then add cognac, agave nectar and white wine. Gently stir to combine. Chill for at least 2 hours to allow flavors to marry (can be made night before). Serve in tall glasses and top with club soda.

NUTRITIONAL VALUE
PER SERVING:
Calories: 248 |
Calories from Fat: 3 |
Protein: 1 g | Carbs: 27 g |
Total Fat: 0 g |
Saturated Fat: 0 g |
Trans Fat: 0 g | Fiber: 4 g |
Sodium: 12 mg |
Cholesterol: 0 mg

Servings: 6 x ½ cup
Prep time: 15 minutes
Cooking time:
40-45 minutes

MARIONBERRY CRISP
with Walnut Oat Topping

Marionberries, also known as marion blackberries, are a cultivated blend of blackberries and raspberries grown in Marion County, Oregon. They are sturdier than blackberries, and have a full, sweet and tart flavor that makes them a perfect filling for crisps and crumbles.

INGREDIENTS

4 cups / 960 ml combination of marionberries and raspberries
Juice of ½ lemon
2 tsp / 10 ml arrowroot powder
2 Tbsp / 30 ml honey
½ cup / 120 ml pitted dates
½ cup / 120 ml old-fashioned rolled oats
½ cup / 120 ml oat flour
¼ cup / 60 ml raw walnut pieces
¼ cup / 60 ml organic raw coconut butter, melted
¼ cup / 60 ml unrefined sugar such as Sucanat
¼ tsp / 1.25 ml nutmeg
¼ tsp / 1.25 ml cinnamon
Pinch sea salt

METHOD

1. Preheat oven to 350°F / 175°C. In a medium bowl combine berries, lemon juice, arrowroot and honey. Stir to combine and scrape into a glass or ceramic baking dish. Place dish on a baking sheet.

2. In a food processor, add dates and pulse until finely chopped. Add rest of ingredients and pulse until walnuts are chopped into smaller pieces and all ingredients are combined. Spread date-walnut topping over berries in an even layer. Place crisp on a rack in middle of oven, and bake until berry filling is bubbling and topping is lightly browned, 40 to 45 minutes. Serve warm.

NUTRITIONAL VALUE
PER SERVING:
Calories: 331 |
Calories from Fat: 103 |
Protein: 7 g | Carbs: 46 g |
Total Fat: 12 g |
Saturated Fat: 6 g |
Trans Fat: 0 g | Fiber: 10 g |
Sodium: 34 mg |
Cholesterol: 0 mg

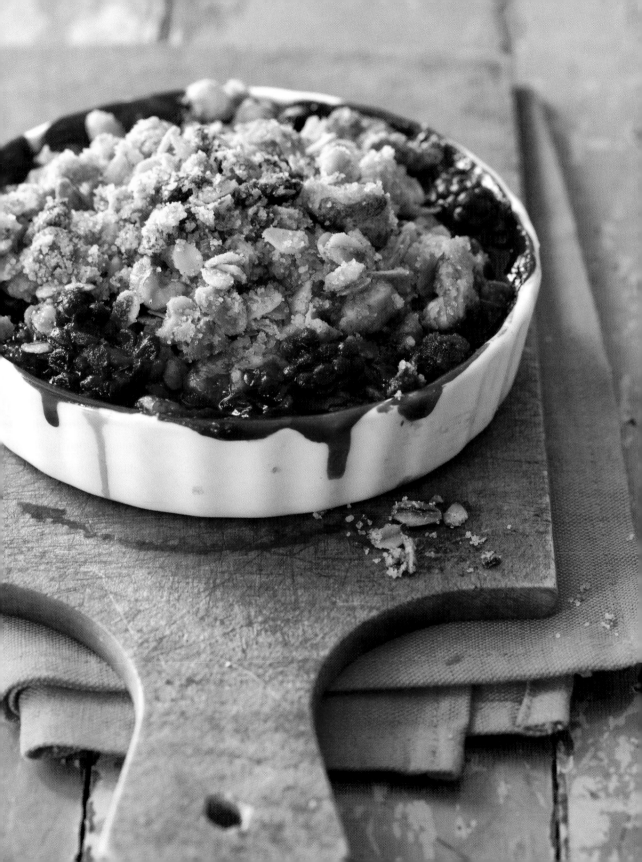

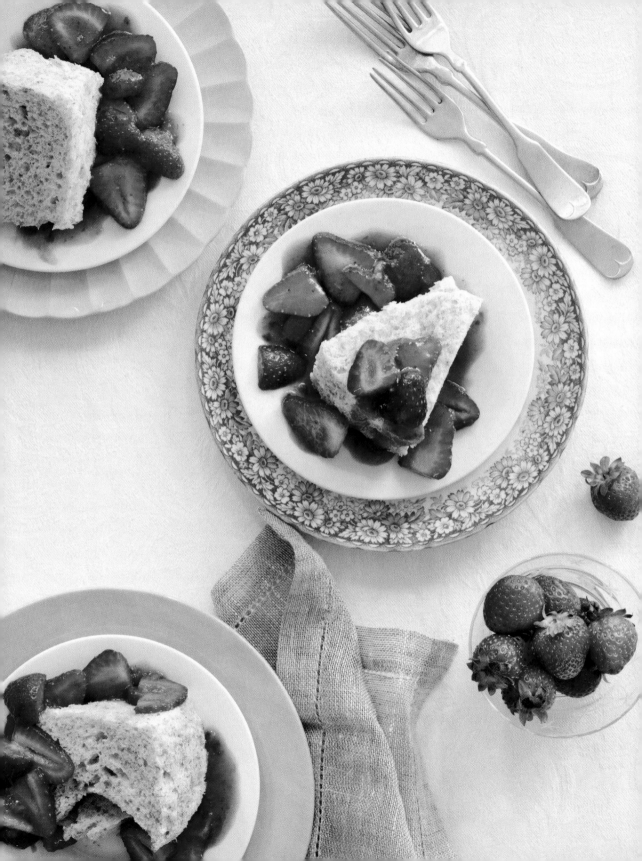

Servings: 12
Prep time: 20 minutes
Cooking time:
35-38 minutes

WHOLE WHEAT ANGEL FOOD CAKE
with Fresh Strawberries

Angel food cake is a delicate, light and foamy, low-fat sponge cake, made by foaming up egg whites and folding them carefully into your dry ingredients. This version is made with whole wheat flour and you'll never know the difference – every bubbly bite will melt in your mouth.

INGREDIENTS

¾ cup / 180 ml whole wheat flour
½ tsp / 2.5 ml sea salt
1½ cups / 360 ml cold egg whites
(about 10 – 12 large egg whites)
1 Tbsp / 15 ml cold water
1 Tbsp / 15 ml fresh lemon juice

1 tsp / 5 ml real vanilla extract
½ cup / 120 ml organic raw turbinado
sugar, ground fine in a spice
grinder or with mortar and pestle
3 cups / 720 ml sliced fresh strawberries
1 tsp / 5 ml agave nectar

METHOD

1. Preheat oven to 350°F / 175°C. Have an ungreased 10-inch tube pan ready.

2. In a small bowl, whisk together flour and salt thoroughly.

3. Using an electric mixer, beat cold egg whites, cold water, lemon juice and vanilla on low speed for 1 minute in a large bowl. Increase mixer speed to medium and beat until egg mixture increases in volume four or five times and looks like small foamy bubbles, about 2 minutes. With mixer on medium speed, gradually beat in finely ground sugar, taking at least 2 minutes. When all sugar is beaten in, foam will be white and hold soft, glossy peaks that bend at the tip. Sift a fine layer of flour mixture (about one-fifth of total) over surface of egg mixture and fold in gently with a rubber spatula, only until flour is almost incorporated. Do not stir. Repeat four more times until all flour is incorporated. Pour batter into tube pan and gently spread it evenly on top.

4. Place pan in oven and bake until a toothpick inserted into middle of cake comes out clean, 35 to 38 minutes. Remove from oven and invert hole in center of tube pan over neck of a bottle to cool. (Alternatively, you can place edges of cake pan over four glasses of even height to cool.)

5. To unmold, slide a thin knife around cake to loosen it from pan, pressing knife against pan so that you won't tear the cake. Repeat cutting method around tube. If bottom of cake pan is removable, lift tube upward, to lift cake from side of pan. Slide knife under cake, pressing edge to bottom of pan to avoid tearing. If bottom is not removable, invert cake and tap pan against counter to detach cake. Let cake drop onto your hand, and let it cool right side up on a rack.

6. Mix together strawberries and agave nectar. To serve, slice cake into 12 slices and top each with ¼ cup / 60 ml strawberries.

NUTRITIONAL VALUE
PER SERVING
(2-INCH SLICE,
¼ CUP BERRIES):
Calories: 85 |
Calories from Fat: 3 |
Protein: 5 g | Carbs: 17 g |
Total Fat: 0 g |
Saturated Fat: 0 g |
Trans Fat: 0 g | Fiber: 2 g |
Sodium: 148 mg |
Cholesterol: 0 mg

Servings: 12
Prep time: 20 minutes
Cooking time:
35-40 minutes

PLUM UPSIDE DOWN CAKE

If you've never cooked with plums, it can be hard to figure out what to do with them, but I'll make it easy for you. Here I've created a delightful twist on pineapple upside down cake by using this sweet and tart fruit, which keeps the cake moist and delicious from top to bottom.

INGREDIENTS

2 Tbsp / 30 ml plus ¼ cup / 60 ml coconut butter, melted
¼ cup / 60 ml turbinado sugar
2 Tbsp / 30 ml unsulfured molasses
8 ripe plums, halved and pitted
1 whole egg
2 egg whites
2 Tbsp / 30 ml plus ¼ cup / 60 ml low-fat buttermilk
½ tsp / 2.5 ml real vanilla extract
1 cup / 240 ml whole wheat pastry flour
¾ tsp / 3.75 ml baking powder
¼ tsp / 1.25 ml baking soda
¼ tsp / 1.25 ml sea salt
¼ cup / 60 ml unsweetened applesauce
¼ cup / 60 ml honey

METHOD

1. Preheat oven to 350°F / 175°C. Place 2 Tbsp / 30 ml coconut butter in a 9-inch cast iron skillet and place in oven until melted (or you can melt it on top of stove). Swirl melted butter around in pan to coat bottom. Sprinkle turbinado sugar evenly over melted coconut butter and drizzle molasses evenly over top. Arrange halved plums, cut side down, in bottom of pan.

2. In a small bowl whisk together egg, egg whites, 2 Tbsp / 30 ml buttermilk and vanilla.

3. In a large bowl, thoroughly blend flour, baking powder, baking soda and salt. Add remaining ¼ cup / 60 ml buttermilk, remaining ¼ cup / 60 ml melted coconut butter, applesauce and honey. Mix together until just combined. Add one-third egg mixture and beat for 1 minute, until combined. Continue adding one-third of egg mixture at a time and beat until just combined, about 30 seconds, scraping down bowl each time to fully incorporate all ingredients. Scrape batter over plums in pan and spread out evenly.

4. Place in oven and bake until a toothpick inserted in center of cake comes out clean, 35 to 40 minutes. Remove and let cool for 5 minutes. To unmold, invert a platter on top of skillet. Turn cake onto platter and lift off skillet. If any fruit or gooey topping is left in pan, scrape it up and spoon it over cake. Best served warm or at room temperature. Refrigerate leftovers after two days.

NUTRITIONAL VALUE
PER SERVING
(2-INCH SLICE):
Calories: 132 |
Calories from Fat: 20 |
Protein: 2 g | Carbs: 27 g |
Total Fat: 2 g |
Saturated Fat: 1 g |
Trans Fat: 0 g | Fiber: 3 g |
Sodium: 96 mg |
Cholesterol: 16 mg

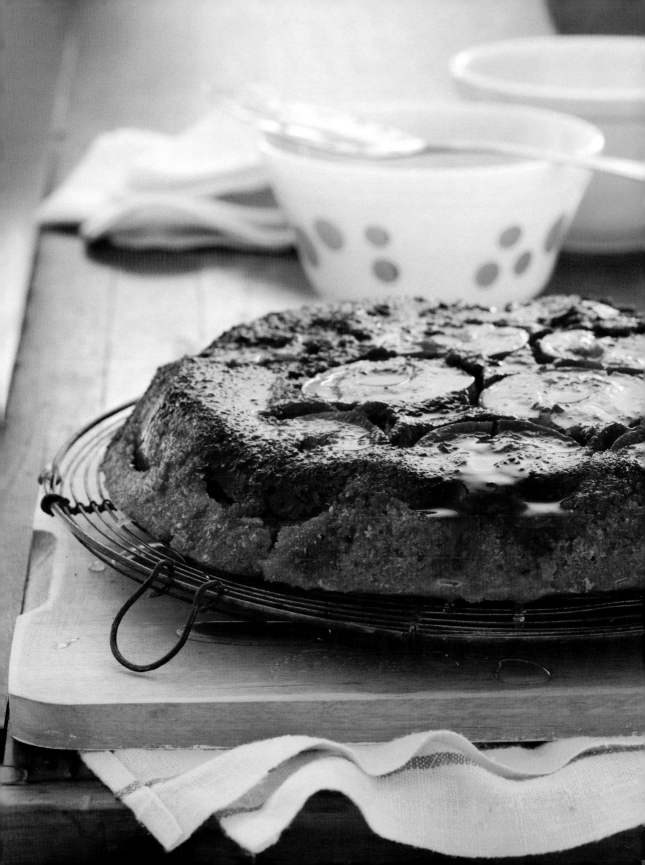

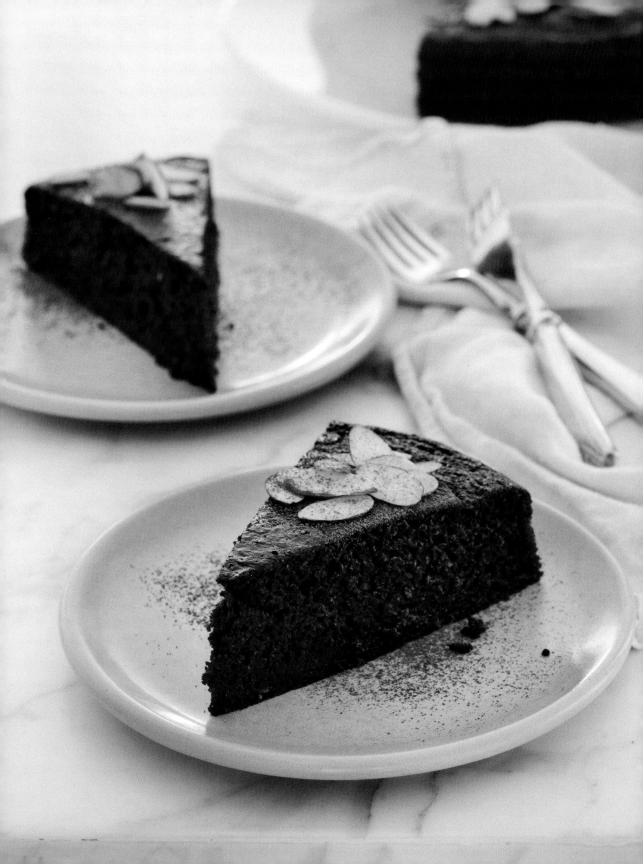

CHOCOLATE ALMOND CAKE

Chocoholics unite! This cake is a slice of heaven. The trick is adding almond butter to the batter, which infuses every bite with a chocolatey-almond flavor that will have your guests begging for seconds.

INGREDIENTS

Eat-Clean Cooking Spray (see page 348)
1 cup / 240 ml plus 1 Tbsp / 15 ml whole wheat flour
½ cup / 120 ml cocoa powder
½ cup / 120 ml unrefined turbinado sugar
2 Tbsp / 30 ml ground golden roasted flaxseed
1 tsp / 5 ml baking powder
1 tsp / 5 ml baking soda
½ tsp / 2.5 ml sea salt
2 egg whites
½ cup / 120 ml unsweetened applesauce
½ cup / 120 ml low-fat buttermilk
¼ cup / 60 ml natural unsalted almond butter
½ tsp / 2.5 ml real almond extract
1 cup / 240 ml freshly brewed very hot coffee
3 Tbsp / 45 ml sliced toasted almonds

METHOD

1. Preheat oven to 350°F / 175°C. Coat a 9-inch round baking pan with Eat-Clean Cooking Spray and 1 Tbsp / 15 ml whole wheat flour, discarding excess flour.

2. Whisk together 1 cup / 240 ml flour, cocoa powder, sugar, flaxseed, baking powder, baking soda and salt in a large bowl. Stir in egg whites, applesauce, buttermilk, almond butter and almond extract. Carefully whisk in hot coffee until thoroughly combined. Batter will be thin.

3. Pour batter into sprayed and floured pan and bake in oven until a toothpick inserted in center comes out almost completely clean, about 40 minutes. Cool 10 minutes and remove from pan to a wire rack. Top with toasted almonds and cut into slices.

NUTRITIONAL VALUE
PER SERVING
(1 SLICE):
Calories: 149 |
Calories from Fat: 47 |
Protein: 5 g | Carbs: 23 g |
Total Fat: 6 g |
Saturated Fat: 1 g |
Trans Fat: 0 g | Fiber: 3 g |
Sodium: 221 mg |
Cholesterol: 1 mg

Servings: 4 x 1 cup
Prep time: 5 minutes
Cooking time:
10 minutes

HOT SPICED APPLE CIDER

It doesn't feel like winter is upon us until I smell the glorious scent of Hot Spiced Apple Cider brewing on the stovetop. Settle down and cozy up by the fire with this festive drink the whole family can enjoy, rum omitted for the little ones of course!

INGREDIENTS

1 quart unfiltered apple cider
1 slice of lemon
1 tsp / 5 ml whole cloves
1 cinnamon stick, plus 3 more to garnish
1 star anise
½ nut of nutmeg (the whole nutmeg, sliced in half; alternatively,
    you can use a pinch of grated or ground nutmeg)
¼ cup / 60 ml dark rum (optional)

METHOD

1. Place apple cider, slice of lemon, cloves, 1 cinnamon stick, star anise, and piece of nutmeg in a medium pot. Bring cider to a gentle simmer and allow lemon and spices to infuse their flavor for 10 minutes, keeping heat very low.

2. Using a hand-held perforated strainer with holes small enough to catch cloves, strain all of spices and lemon slice out of cider. Save cinnamon stick, which can be used again to garnish one mug of cider, but discard other ingredients. Stir dark rum into cider, if desired. Ladle into mugs and garnish each with a cinnamon stick. Serve hot.

NUTRITIONAL VALUE
PER SERVING
(WITH ALCOHOL):
Calories: 160 |
Calories from Fat: 1 |
Protein: 0 g | Carbs: 30 g |
Total Fat: 0 g |
Saturated Fat: 0 g |
Trans Fat: 0 g | Fiber: 0.5 g |
Sodium: 9 mg |
Cholesterol: 0 mg

NUTRITIONAL VALUE
PER SERVING
(WITHOUT ALCOHOL):
Calories: 128 |
Calories from Fat: 1 |
Protein: 0 g | Carbs: 30 g |
Total Fat: 0 g |
Saturated Fat: 0 g |
Trans Fat: 0 g | Fiber: 0.5 g |
Sodium: 9 mg |
Cholesterol: 0 mg

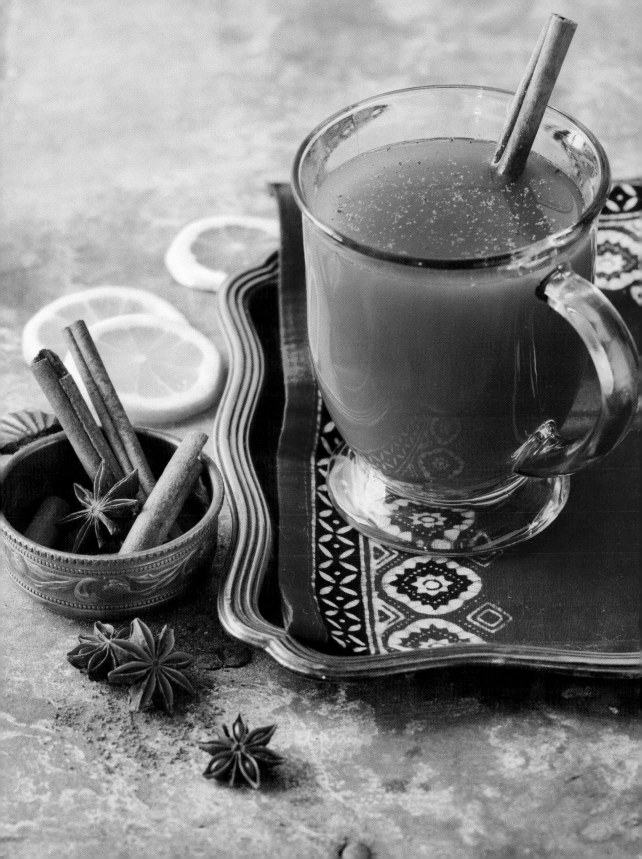

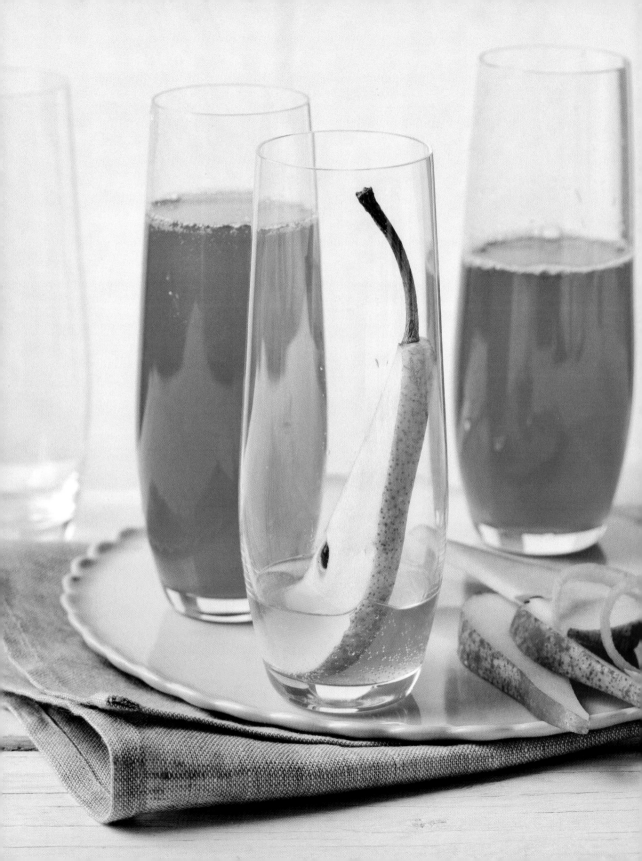

Servings: 12 x ¾ cup
Prep time: 10 minutes
Cooking time:
0 minutes

CRANBERRY PEAR BELLINI

Invented (by a genius) in the 1940s, the bellini is a summery cocktail that typically combines peach juice and prosecco, a dry sparkling wine. I've created a more festive bellini that includes cranberry and pear juice – perfect for holiday parties all year round.

INGREDIENTS

1½ cups / 360 ml organic unsweetened pear purée or juice, chilled
1½ cups / 360 ml organic unsweetened cranberry juice, chilled
1 x 750 L bottle prosecco, cava, brut champagne, or dry
    sparkling wine, chilled (about 3 cups / 720 ml)
2 x 12-oz cans club soda, chilled
Pear slices, to garnish
Lemon zest, to garnish

METHOD

1. In a large pourable measuring cup or small pitcher, combine pear purée and cranberry juice. Pour ¼ cup / 60 ml juice mixture into 12 champagne flutes.

2. Add ¼ cup / 60 ml prosecco (or other sparkling wine), and top with ¼ cup / 60 ml of club soda. Garnish with a slice of pear and a twist of lemon zest, if desired.

NUTRITIONAL VALUE
PER SERVING:
Calories: 71 |
Calories from Fat: 1 |
Protein: 0 g | Carbs: 10 g |
Total Fat: 0 g |
Saturated Fat: 0 g |
Trans Fat: 0 g | Fiber: 1 g |
Sodium: 15 mg |
Cholesterol: 0 mg

Servings: 7 x ½ cup
Prep time: 15 minutes
Cooking time:
6 minutes

SWEET POTATO CUSTARD
with Spiced Walnut Clusters

Custard is a traditional dessert from Europe that is made with milk, using eggs as a thickening agent. This version uses tofu and sweet potato purée, which makes it deliciously vegan. It's the perfect dessert for Thanksgiving or anytime!

Note: Sweet potato purée must be made ahead of time.

INGREDIENTS

SWEET POTATO CUSTARD

2 cups / 480 ml sweet potato purée
1 x 12-oz / 375 g package silken soft tofu, drained well
2 Tbsp / 30 ml honey
1 tsp / 5 ml real vanilla
1 tsp / 5 ml freshly squeezed lemon juice
1 tsp / 5 ml finely grated lemon zest
¼ tsp / 1.25 ml ground cinnamon
⅛ tsp / 0.625 ml each ground cloves, nutmeg and ginger
⅛ tsp / 0.625 ml sea salt

SPICED WALNUT CLUSTERS

½ cup / 120 ml chopped walnuts
2 Tbsp / 30 ml unrefined sugar
½ tsp / 2.5 ml finely chopped fresh rosemary
⅛ tsp / 0.625 ml cayenne pepper
¼ tsp / 1.25 ml sea salt
1 tsp / 5 ml unsulfured blackstrap molasses

METHOD

1. Place all custard ingredients into a blender or food processor and blend until smooth. Stop blender to scrape down sides with a rubber spatula. Blend for an additional 30 seconds until all ingredients are fully incorporated. Scrape into a container, cover, and refrigerate for at least 2 hours to set custard.

2. Preheat oven to 350°F / 175°C. Place walnuts on a baking sheet and toast in oven until fragrant, being careful not to burn, about 5 minutes. Meanwhile, mix sugar, rosemary, cayenne and salt together in a small bowl. When nuts are done, transfer them to small bowl containing sugar mixture and stir to combine. Add molasses and stir to coat nuts well. Scrape nuts back onto baking sheet and pat them out in a single layer, keeping nuts clumped together. Place back in oven for 1 minute. Remove, and let cool and harden into clusters.

3. To serve, scoop ½ cup / 120 ml custard into a dish and top with 1 heaping Tbsp / 15 ml of spiced walnut clusters.

NUTRITIONAL VALUE
PER SERVING:
Calories: 184 |
Calories from Fat: 54 |
Protein: 6 g | Carbs: 26 g |
Total Fat: 6 g |
Saturated Fat: 1 g |
Trans Fat: 0 g | Fiber: 2 g |
Sodium: 181 mg |
Cholesterol: 0 mg

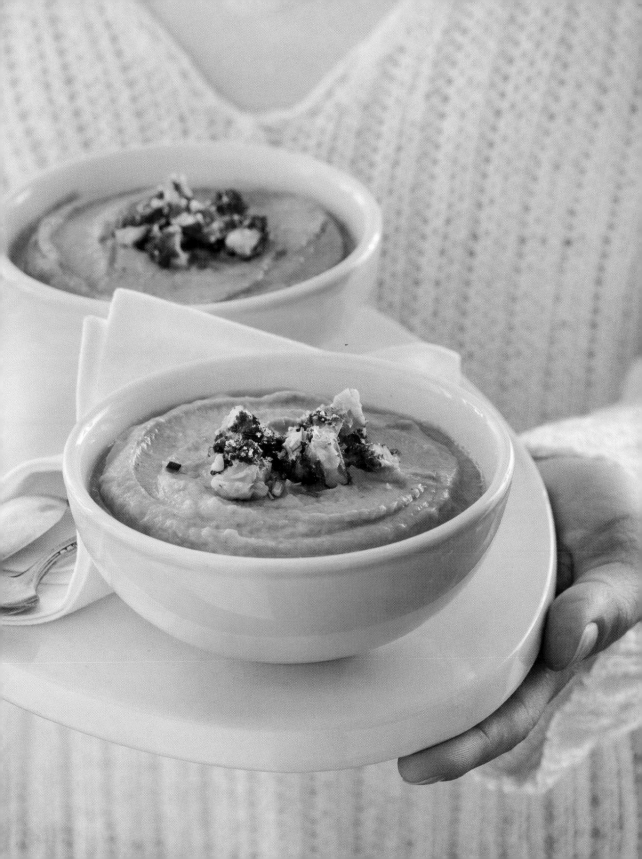

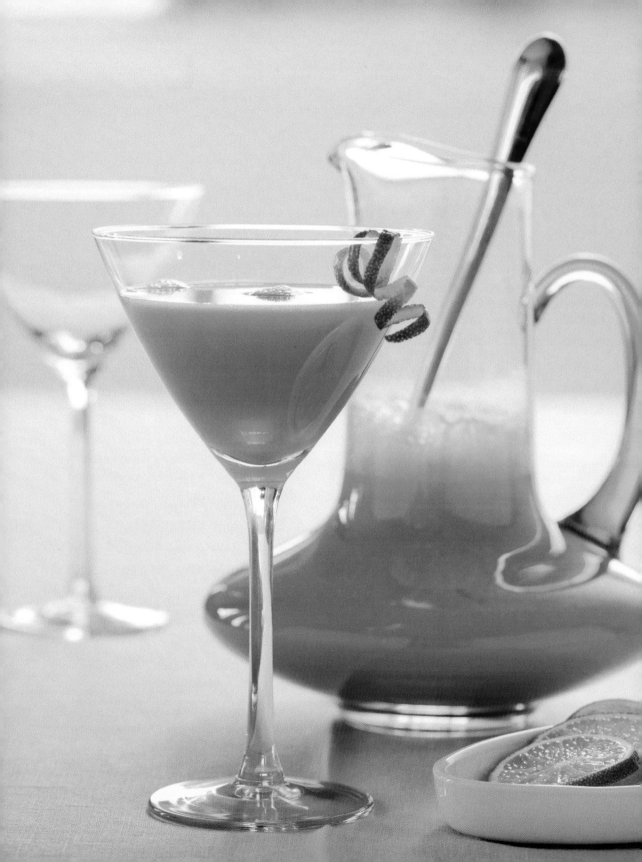

Servings: 2 x ½ cup
Prep time: 5 minutes
Cooking time:
0 minutes

24 CARROT-TINI

Every now and then you just want to get dressed up and enjoy a cocktail. This one contains carrot juice, which is chock full of beta carotene, known for its cancer-preventing and antioxidant properties. Relaxing and healthy ... what a treat!

INGREDIENTS

1 oz / 28 g gin or vodka (optional)
¼ cup / 60 ml 100% carrot juice
¼ cup / 60 ml blend of any of the following: 100% pineapple, apple,
    orange, peach, papaya, pear and white grape juice
1 Tbsp / 15 ml fresh lime juice
1 tsp / 5 ml agave nectar
Dash orange bitters
¼ cup / 60 ml chilled club soda

METHOD

1. Place two martini glasses in freezer. Fill a shaker with ice. Add all ingredients except club soda to shaker. Shake vigorously for 5 to 10 seconds. Transfer chilled martini glasses to counter. Strain carrot-tini into two glasses. Top each with club soda and garnish with a strip of lime zest.

NUTRITIONAL VALUE
PER SERVING
(WITH ALCOHOL):
Calories: 78 |
Calories from Fat: 1 |
Protein: 0 g |
Carbs: 9 g | Total Fat: 0 g |
Saturated Fat: 0 g |
Trans Fat: 0 g | Fiber: 0 g |
Sodium: 13 mg |
Cholesterol: 0 mg

NUTRITIONAL VALUE
PER SERVING
(WITHOUT ALCOHOL):
Calories: 37 |
Calories from Fat: 0.5 |
Protein: 0.4 g |
Carbs: 9 g | Total Fat: 0 g |
Saturated Fat: 0 g |
Trans Fat: 0 g | Fiber: 0 g |
Sodium: 13 mg |
Cholesterol: 0 mg

Servings: 9
Prep time: 15 minutes
Cooking time:
30 minutes

RHUBARB WALNUT DESSERT TORTA

The word "torta" means different things to different cultures. In Mexico, a torta is a sandwich; in Italy, it's a meat and cheese pie. In most South American countries, it's a sweet cake or bread, which is how torta is defined for this recipe.

INGREDIENTS

½ cup / 120 ml chopped walnuts
Zest and juice of ½ organic orange
¼ cup / 60 ml dried cranberries
1 cup / 240 ml whole wheat flour
1½ tsp / 7.5 ml baking powder
1 tsp / 5 ml ground cinnamon
¼ tsp / 1.25 ml sea salt
1 whole egg
4 egg whites
⅓ cup / 80 ml turbinado sugar
¼ cup / 60 ml coconut oil, melted
1 tsp / 5 ml pure vanilla extract
2 cups / 480 ml diced rhubarb (½-inch pieces)
Eat-Clean Cooking Spray (see page 348)

METHOD

1. Preheat oven to 350°F / 175°C. Spread walnuts on a baking sheet and toast in oven until golden brown, about 5 minutes. Remove and set aside.

2. In a small saucepan, combine orange juice and cranberries. Bring to a simmer over medium-high heat. Remove from heat and set aside while cranberries plump up.

3. In a small bowl, whisk together orange zest, flour, baking powder, cinnamon and salt.

4. In a large bowl, whisk together egg and egg whites, sugar, melted coconut oil and vanilla. Add dry ingredients to wet ingredients and stir to combine.

5. Drain cranberries, discarding juice. Using a rubber spatula, fold in cranberries, toasted walnuts and rhubarb just enough to combine. Batter will be thick and chunky.

6. Spray a 9 x 9-inch cake pan lightly with Eat-Clean Cooking Spray. Scrape batter into cake pan and spread evenly. Bake until a toothpick inserted in center comes out clean, about 30 minutes. Serve warm.

NUTRITIONAL VALUE
PER SERVING
(3 X 3-INCH SQUARE):
Calories: 208 |
Calories from Fat: 108 |
Protein: 6 g | Carbs: 15 g |
Total Fat: 12 g |
Saturated Fat: 6 g |
Trans Fat: 0 g | Fiber: 3 g |
Sodium: 99 mg |
Cholesterol: 21 mg

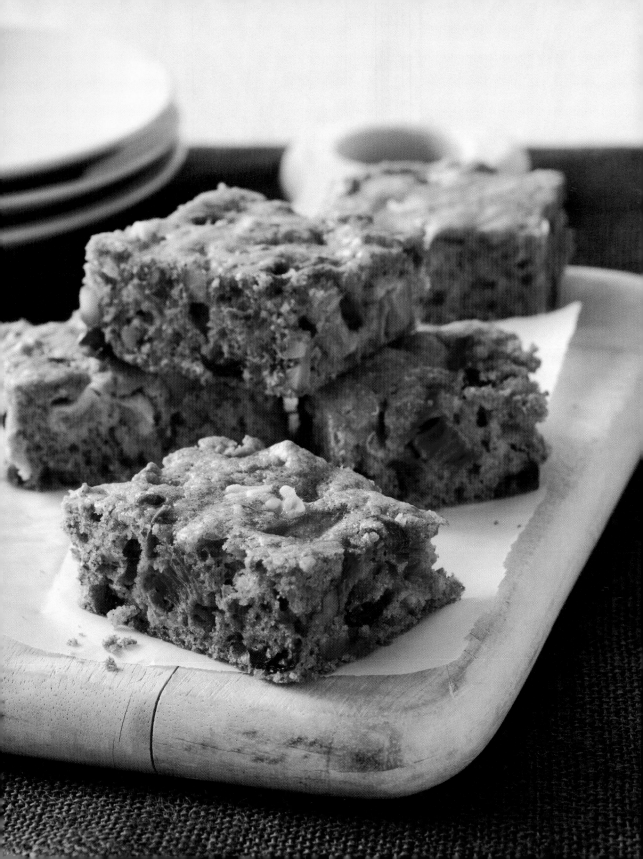

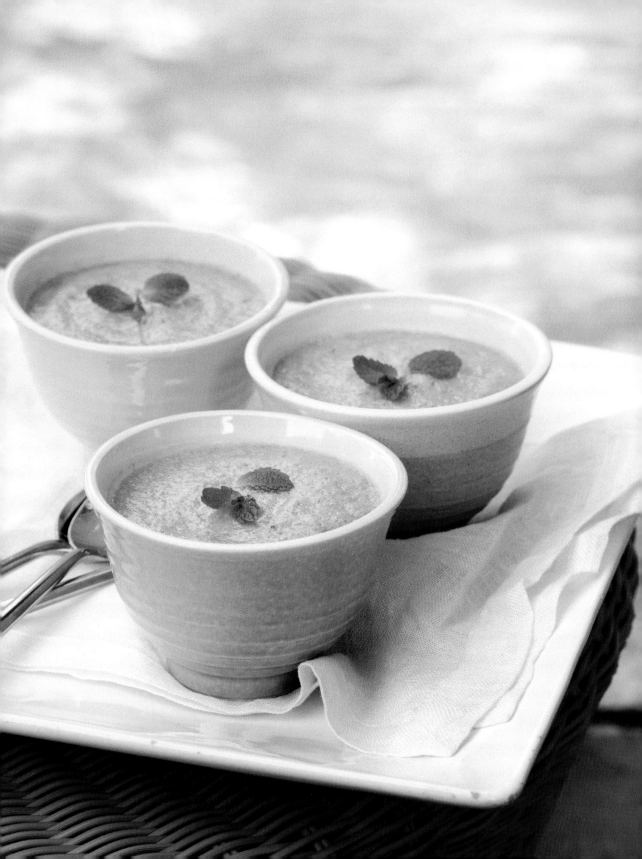

Servings: 6 x 1 cup
Prep time: 10 minutes
Cooking time:
0 minutes
Chill time: 1-2 hours

EFFERVESCENT DESSERT FRUIT SOUP

This fruit soup is light, refreshing and the perfect way to keep an Eat-Clean dieter satisfied and on track with his or her goals at the same time. It's especially refreshing on warm summer nights!

INGREDIENTS

4 cups / 960 ml chopped very ripe Tuscan-style cantaloupe
2 cups / 480 ml chopped very ripe fresh pineapple, core removed
1 cup / 240 ml fresh strawberries, hulled and halved
Juice of 1 lime
2 cups / 480 ml raw organic unsweetened kombucha tea
Fresh mint, to garnish

METHOD

1. Add cantaloupe, pineapple, strawberries and lime juice to a blender or food processor and blend for several minutes until very smooth.

2. Place in refrigerator, covered, until chilled, 1 to 2 hours. When ready to serve, stir in kombucha tea, but do not blend any further. Ladle into bowls and garnish with mint, if desired.

NUTRITIONAL VALUE
PER SERVING:
Calories: 83 |
Calories from Fat: 3 |
Protein: 1 g | Carbs: 22 g |
Total Fat: 0 g |
Saturated Fat: 0 g |
Trans Fat: 0 g | Fiber: 2 g |
Sodium: 22 mg |
Cholesterol: 0 mg

BLUEBERRY BLINTZES

Servings: 4
Prep time: 15 minutes
Cooking time:
25-30 minutes

A blintz is a very thin pancake or crepe that is folded around a delicious filling, which usually contains cheese. Blintzes can be made sweet or savory. Here I've chosen blueberries – a colorful, sweet filling bursting with flavor that makes this treat perfect for dessert or a special Sunday brunch.

Note: Yogurt Cheese must be made ahead of time.

INGREDIENTS

CREPE BATTER
¼ cup / 60 ml 1% low-fat milk
¼ cup / 60 ml water
1 whole egg
1 egg white
½ tsp / 2.5 ml agave nectar
1 tsp / 5 ml virgin coconut oil, melted
½ cup / 120 ml whole wheat flour
Pinch sea salt
Eat-Clean Cooking Spray (see page 348)

CHEESE FILLING
½ cup / 120 ml Yogurt Cheese
   (see recipe on page 348)
½ cup / 120 ml reduced-fat ricotta cheese
Zest of ½ lemon
1 tsp / 5 ml agave nectar
½ tsp / 2.5 ml real vanilla extract

BLUEBERRY SAUCE
2 cups / 480 ml fresh or
   frozen blueberries
Juice of ½ lemon
1 tsp / 5 ml agave nectar
½ tsp / 2.5 ml arrowroot powder

METHOD

1. Combine all crepe batter ingredients in a blender. Blend until smooth and free of lumps, about 15 seconds. Stop blender and scrape down sides, and then blend for a few seconds more. Refrigerate batter for 15 minutes, to give crepes a more tender texture.

2. In a small bowl, whisk together cheese filling ingredients until thoroughly combined. Place in refrigerator until ready to use.

3. In a small saucepan, stir together all blueberry sauce ingredients. Turn heat to medium-high and bring to a gentle boil, stirring, until blueberries are partially broken down, 3 to 5 minutes. Set aside to cool slightly and thicken.

4. Heat an 8-inch nonstick skillet over medium heat and lightly coat with Eat-Clean Cooking Spray. Pour ¼ cup / 60 ml crepe batter into pan and swirl to coat bottom. Let cook until batter is set, about 30 seconds. Using a heatproof rubber spatula, loosen edges of crepe and carefully flip. Cook for 10 more seconds, and then remove from pan to a plate or baking sheet. Crepes should be lightly browned, but still tender and pliable, not crispy. Repeat until all batter is used. There should be enough crepe batter to make five to six crepes, in case you need a practice run.

5. To assemble, place a crepe on a plate, spoon ¼ cup / 60 ml cheese filling in center, fold over edges and carefully turn over so seams are facing down. Top with ¼ cup / 60 ml blueberry sauce. Repeat with remaining three crepes. Serve immediately.

NUTRITIONAL VALUE
PER SERVING
(1 CREPE WITH ¼ CUP /
60 ML FILLING AND
¼ CUP / 60 ML SAUCE):
Calories: 178 |
Calories from Fat: 43 |
Protein: 9 g | Carbs: 26 g |
Total Fat: 5 g |
Saturated Fat: 2 g |
Trans Fat: 0 g | Fiber: 4 g |
Sodium: 91 mg |
Cholesterol: 8 mg

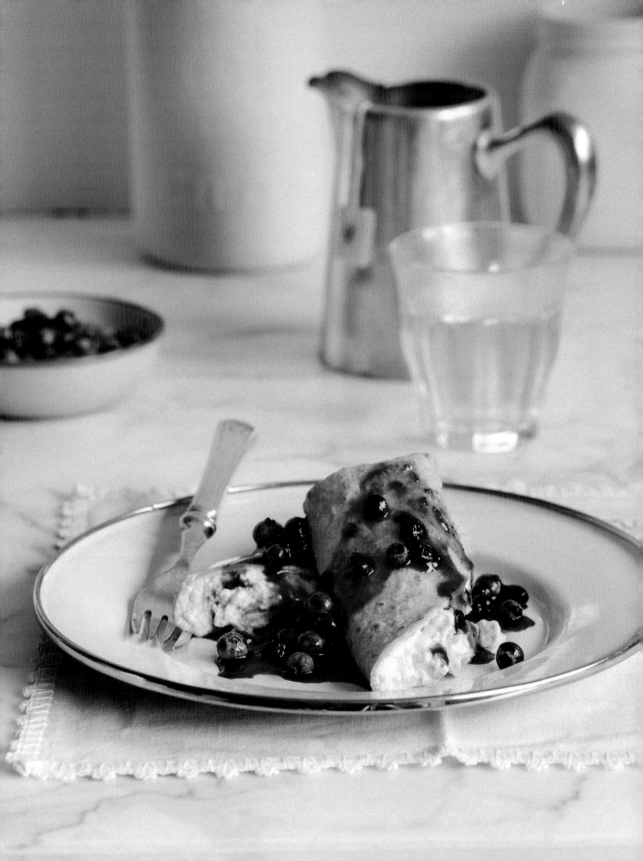

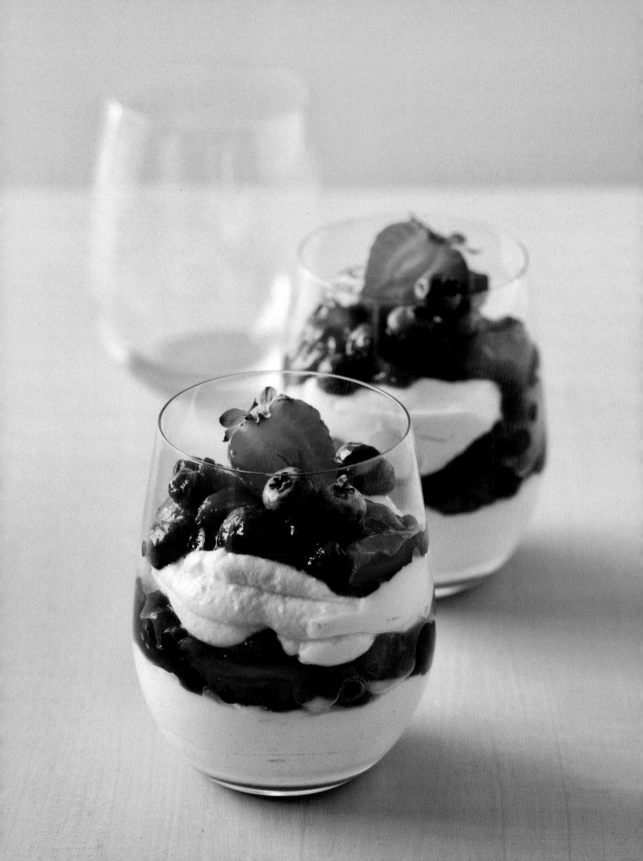

Servings: 6 parfaits
Prep time: 15 minutes
Cooking time:
2-3 minutes

BERRY LEMON PARFAIT

You don't need to add tons of sugar or sweetener to enjoy a sweet dessert. Foods such as fresh berries offer the sweet taste found in nature. Natural sugars are good for you, so you can feel good about your decision to make this slightly sweet and temptingly tart parfait.

Note: Yogurt Cheese must be made ahead of time.

INGREDIENTS

CREAMY LEMON MIXTURE

1 cup / 240 low-fat Yogurt Cheese (see recipe on page 348), drained well
1 x 12-oz / 375 g package silken soft tofu, drained well (must be silken)
2 Tbsp / 30 ml honey
1 tsp / 5 ml freshly squeezed lemon juice
1 tsp / 5 ml finely grated lemon zest
½ tsp / 2.5 ml real vanilla
Scant pinch sea salt

BERRY MIXTURE

1 cup / 240 ml fresh or frozen blueberries
1 cup / 240 ml sliced fresh or frozen strawberries, stems removed
1 Tbsp / 15 ml freshly squeezed lemon juice
½ tsp / 2.5 ml finely grated lemon zest
1 tsp / 5 ml honey
½ tsp / 2.5 ml arrowroot powder

GARNISH INGREDIENTS

Fresh blueberries and strawberry slices, optional
Fresh mint sprigs, optional

METHOD

1. Place all creamy lemon mixture ingredients in a blender and blend until very smooth. Scrape down sides of blender, and blend for another 30 seconds. Scrape into a container, cover, and place in refrigerator for at least 2 hours to chill and set.

2. Place all berry mixture ingredients in a small saucepan over medium high-heat. Bring to a simmer, and let cook, stirring, until liquid thickens but berries still retain their shape, about 2 to 3 minutes. Transfer to a container and refrigerate until ready to use.

3. Serve in decorative glasses, such as martini or parfait glasses. In each glass, layer ⅛ cup / 30 ml berry mixture, then ¼ cup / 60 ml creamy lemon mixture, then ⅛ cup / 30 ml berry mixture again, and finally ¼ cup / 60 ml creamy lemon mixture. Repeat with remaining five glasses. If desired, garnish with fresh berries and/or fresh mint. Serve immediately.

NUTRITIONAL VALUE
PER SERVING:
Calories: 104 |
Calories from Fat: 15 |
Protein: 6 g | Carbs: 16 g |
Total Fat: 2 g |
Saturated Fat: 0 g |
Trans Fat: 0 g | Fiber: 1 g |
Sodium: 37 mg |
Cholesterol: 0 mg

Servings: 8
Prep time: 15 minutes
Cooking time:
1 hour 30 minutes
Cooling time: 1 hour

PAVLOVA
with Fresh Summer Berries

Pavlova is a crusty, fat-free baked meringue named after Russian ballet dancer, Anna Pavlova.

Note: Yogurt Cheese must be made ahead of time.

INGREDIENTS

4 large egg whites, at room temperature
⅛ tsp / 0.625 ml cream of tartar
Pinch sea salt
½ cup / 120 ml unrefined sugar, ground
    superfine in a clean spice grinder
1 tsp / 5 ml arrowroot powder
1 tsp / 5 ml white vinegar
1 cup / 240 ml Yogurt Cheese
    (see recipe on page 348)

1 Tbsp / 15 ml agave nectar
½ tsp / 2.5 ml real vanilla extract
Zest of ½ lemon
2 cups / 480 ml fresh berries, such
    as raspberries, blueberries,
    blackberries and strawberries (if using
    strawberries, quarter or slice)
1 to 2 kiwis, peeled, quartered lengthwise and
    sliced ¼-inch thick crosswise into triangles

METHOD

1. Preheat oven to 250°F / 120°C. Place rack in center of oven.

2. Place a sheet of parchment paper on a baking sheet. Using a pencil, trace a 9-inch round pie pan. Turn parchment over so that pencil is on underside of paper.

3. Place egg whites, cream of tartar and salt in bowl of an electric mixer. Using whisk attachment, beat egg whites on high speed until firm peaks form, about 2 minutes. Add sugar one tablespoon at a time, beating egg whites on medium-high speed until they form shiny peaks and all sugar is incorporated, about 2 minutes.

4. Remove bowl from mixer, sprinkle arrowroot and vinegar onto beaten egg whites, and fold in with a rubber spatula. Do not mix. Scrape meringue into middle of parchment paper and smooth it into shape of drawn circle, creating a well in center of meringue.

5. Bake meringue for 1 hour and 30 minutes. Turn off oven, and with door propped slightly open, allow meringue to cool for 1 hour in oven. Meringue can also be left in oven overnight to cool.

6. In a small bowl, whisk together Yogurt Cheese, agave nectar, vanilla extract and lemon zest.

7. Peel parchment off meringue and place meringue on a plate. Spread yogurt mixture over top, and arrange berries and pieces of kiwi decoratively over top. Serve immediately.

NUTRITIONAL VALUE
PER SERVING:
Calories: 106 |
Calories from Fat: 1 |
Protein: 5 g | Carbs: 23 g |
Total Fat: 0 g |
Saturated Fat: 0 g |
Trans Fat: 0 g | Fiber: 2 g |
Sodium: 57 mg |
Cholesterol: 0 mg

TIP *When making meringue, egg whites should be room temperature, all equipment must be clean and don't let a drop of yolk in!*

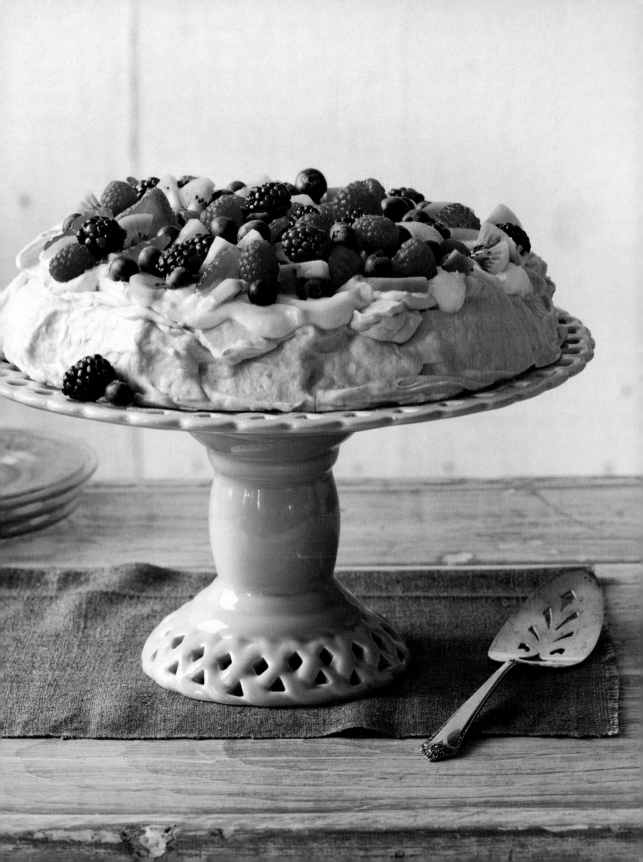

Sweeteners

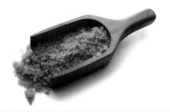

Few of us go through life without a little something sweet now and then. Some of us sweeten everything from our morning coffee to our already-sweetened cereal. Before indulging in sweet treats, have a look at these pages to find out about the many names for sugar along with the chemically made imposters. And remember that just because a sugar is natural doesn't mean you can consume as much as you want. Sugar, by any other name, is a treat. As for the fake stuff, I personally won't touch it, whether the risks are proven or not. Why take the chance? I stick to the real goods – just not too often.

NATURAL SWEETENERS

AGAVE NECTAR:
AKA: Agave syrup
SOURCE: Agave plant (which also gives us tequila)
PRODUCTS: Agave nectar in bottles
RISKS: It doesn't spike blood glucose as quickly as table sugar, but it should still be used in moderation.

STEVIA:
AKA: Truvia
SOURCE: Stevia plant
PRODUCTS: Liquid or powder
RISKS: An all-natural, low-calorie sweetener so far proven to be safe.
EXTRAS: Use sparingly because it has a slightly bitter aftertaste.

UNREFINED SUGARS:
AKA: Barbados sugar, barley malt or sugar, black-strap molasses, cane crystal, cane juice crystals, cane sugar, Demerara sugar, evaporated cane juice, Florida crystals, maple syrup, molasses, muscovado sugar, panocha, raw sugar, sucanat and turbinado sugar
SOURCE: Fruit, sap, or plants
PRODUCTS: Normally sold on its own, but sometimes found in packaged natural foods.

RISKS: While less processed, these sugar products will have the same effect on the blood stream as sugar. However, they contain more micronutrients than pure sucrose.

FRUCTOSE:
AKA: Buttered syrup, carob syrup, corn syrup, crystalline fructose, date sugar, fruit juice, fruit juice concentrate and honey
SOURCE: Honey, fruit or plants
PRODUCTS: Maple syrup, agave nectar (see above), honey, molasses, fruit, fruit juices and fruit juice concentrates.
RISKS: Too much fructose may lead to diabetes.

SUCROSE:
AKA: Beet sugar, brown sugar, caramel, caster sugar, confectioner's sugar, dextran, dextrin, golden sugar or syrup, granulated sugar, icing sugar, powdered sugar, sorghum syrup, sugar, treacle and yellow sugar
SOURCE: Sugarcane or sugar beets
PRODUCTS: Table sugar, baked goods, cereals, desserts, sauces, and just about everywhere
RISKS: Too much sucrose can lead to cellular damage, tooth decay and diabetes.
EXTRAS: If you must, eat it on a full stomach to reduce the incredible load it places on your blood sugar.

HIGH FRUCTOSE CORN SYRUP (HFCS):

SOURCE: Cornstarch

PRODUCTS: Soft drinks, baked goods, condiments and most other processed foods

RISKS: Well documented that this product spikes blood sugar, blocks release of leptin (the hormone that tells you you're full) and is closely linked to diabetes and obesity.

Natural Extras:

Watch out for these sneaky sugar names: dextrose, d-mannose, galactose, glucose, solids, grape sugar, invert sugar, lactose, malt, maltodextrin, maltose and rice syrup

ARTIFICIAL SWEETENERS

SACCHARIN:

AKA: Sweet n' Low, Tab soda and Sugar Twin

SOURCE: Chemically derived

PRODUCTS: Table-top sweeteners and toothpaste

RISKS: An attempt was made to ban this product, but instead for many years products containing it were required to carry a warning label. That has since been repealed.

ASPARTAME:

AKA: Equal and Nutrasweet

SOURCE: Chemically derived

PRODUCTS: 6000+ products (gum, diet products, fillings, desserts, yogurt, and vitamins)

RISKS: The jury is still out on a gamut of rumors linking aspartame's breakdown products to cancer, Alzheimer's and more. It should not be consumed by those with phenylketonuria.

EXTRAS: Don't bake with aspartame because it breaks down when heated.

SUCRALOSE:

AKA: Splenda

SOURCE: Chemically derived from table sugar

PRODUCTS: Splenda, candy, jams, jellies, soft drinks and packaged foods

RISKS: Currently, sucralose is considered safe for all users, but may cause some digestive upset because it suppresses important digestive bacteria.

EXTRAS: It can be used in baking since it is not destroyed at high temperatures.

CYCLAMATE:

AKA: Sweet n' Low and Sugar Twin (Canada)

SOURCE: Chemically derived

PRODUCTS: Table-top sweeteners

RISKS: Banned in U.S. and 55 other countries, but still viable for use in Canada as a tabletop sweetener. Do not use cyclamate when pregnant.

ACESULFAME POTASSIUM:

AKA: Ace-K, Sunett and Sweet One

SOURCE: Chemically derived

PRODUCTS: Gum, candies, baked goods, soft drinks, dairy products, canned food and alcohol

RISKS: Safety is under debate.

EXTRAS: It works synergistically with other sweeteners to enhance their flavor because it tastes awful on its own.

ALCOHOL SWEETENERS:

AKA: Maltitol, Xylitol, Sorbitol, Ethyl Maltol, Erythritol and Mannitol

SOURCE: Chemically derived

PRODUCTS: Toothpaste, mouthwash, candies and gum

RISKS: May cause gastric distress leading to diarrhea.

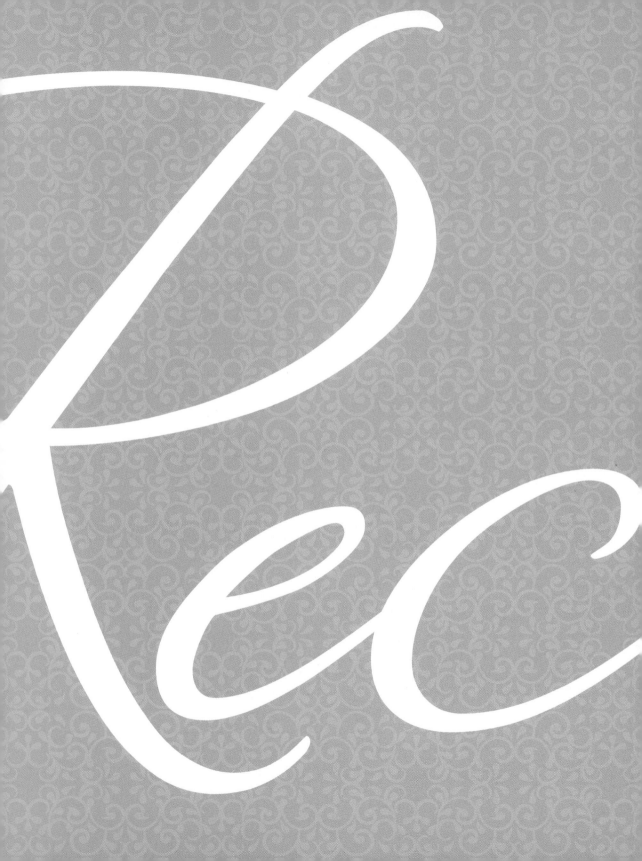

Supportive Recipes

348   YOGURT CHEESE

348   EAT-CLEAN COOKING SPRAY

350   CHIPOTLE RANCHERO SAUCE

350   RASPBERRY SAUCE

351   HERBED YOGURT CHEESE

351   CLEAN COCKTAIL SAUCE

352   SCALLION PISTOU

352   TAHINI SAUCE

353   DASHI *(Ichiban Dashi)*

353   PARMESAN CROUTONS

354   CUCUMBER MIGNONETTE

354   CRISPY HERB AND GARLIC CROUTONS

355   GRILLED PINEAPPLE SALSA

357   CHIMICHURRI

357   ZESTY HUMMUS

358   JERK SEASONING

358   DIJON BLANC SAUCE

359   FIG DEMI-GLACE

360   SPICY ORANGE DIPPING SAUCE

360   OLIVE TAPENADE

361   CASHEW MISO DRESSING

Yogurt Cheese

Servings: 8 x ½ cup
Prep time: 5 minutes
Draining time:
12-24 hours
Makes: 4 cups

The yogurt you use for this recipe must be all natural and free from gelatin or other binding agents.

INGREDIENTS

2 quarts / 1.9 L low-fat plain yogurt, dairy or soy based

METHOD

1. Place four layers of damp cheesecloth in a fine mesh sieve or colander. Place the colander over a bowl.

2. Add yogurt and let it drain overnight in the refrigerator.

3. Discard the water from the bowl.

NUTRITIONAL VALUE
PER SERVING:
Calories: 80 |
Calories from Fat: 14 |
Protein: 12 g | Carbs: 5 g |
Total Fat: 2 g |
Saturated Fat: 2 g |
Trans Fat: 0 g | Fiber: 0 g |
Sodium: 43 mg |
Cholesterol: 5 mg

Eat-Clean Cooking Spray

Yield: 1 cup
Prep time: 2 minutes
Cooking time:
0 minutes

INGREDIENTS

Extra virgin olive oil or other Clean cooking oil

METHOD

1. Place in food-grade spray bottle to spritz over pans, vegetables, or wherever you need a small amount of oil.

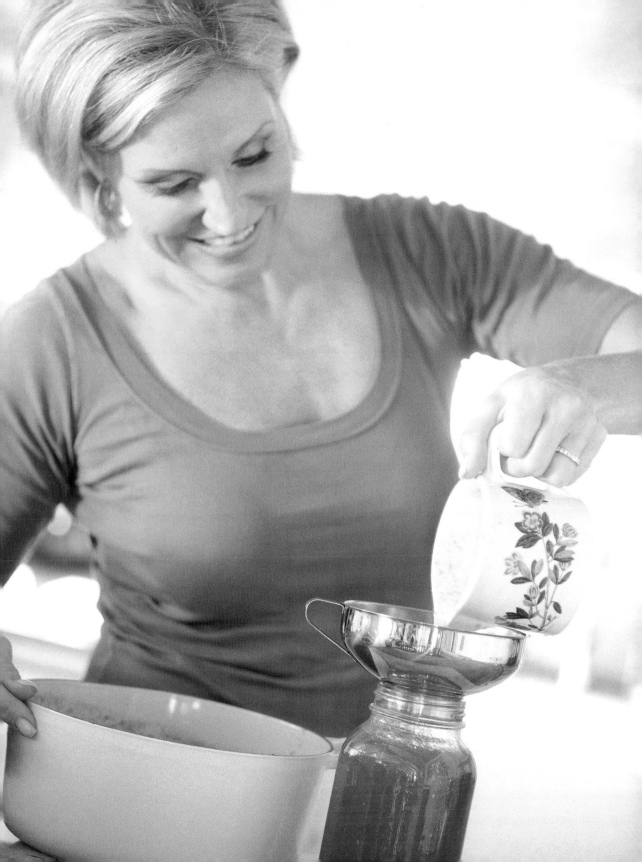

Chipotle Ranchero Sauce:

Use with Huevos Rancheros on page 15.

This sauce can be made in advance and stored for up to one week in the fridge, so when you want to make Huevos Rancheros, it's all ready to go! It's also delicious on burritos, tacos, fajitas – even as a salad dressing!

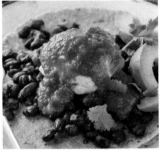

Servings: 10 x ¼ cup
Prep time: 10 minutes
Cooking time: 25-30 minutes
Makes: 2½ cups

INGREDIENTS

1 tsp/ 5 ml extra virgin olive oil
1 cup / 240 ml chopped red onion
3 cloves garlic, chopped
½ red bell pepper, seeded and chopped
2 chipotle peppers in adobo sauce
1 tsp / 5 ml ground cumin
2 cups / 480 ml Clean tomato sauce
½ cup / 60 ml low-sodium chicken or vegetable broth
½ tsp / 2.5 ml sea salt
¼ tsp / 1.25 ml freshly ground black pepper

NUTRITIONAL VALUE
PER SERVING (¼ CUP /
60 ML RANCHERO SAUCE):
Calories: 47 |
Calories from Fat: 6 |
Protein: 1 g | Carbs: 9 g |
Total Fat: 0.5 g |
Saturated Fat: 0 g | Trans
Fat: 0 g | Fiber: 2 g |
Sodium: 132 mg |
Cholesterol: 0 mg

METHOD

1. Heat olive oil in a medium saucepan over medium heat. Add onion, garlic and bell pepper, and cook for 5 minutes. Add remaining ingredients and simmer for 20 to 25 minutes, until onions and peppers are very soft and flavors have combined. Pour into a blender, or use a hand-held immersion blender to blend until very smooth. Use immediately or store, covered, in the fridge for up to one week.

Raspberry Sauce

Use with Multigrain Waffles on page 43.

Servings: 6 x ¼ cup
Prep time: 5 minutes
Cooking time: 3-5 minutes
Makes: 1½ cups

INGREDIENTS

2 cups / 480 ml frozen or fresh raspberries
Juice of ½ lemon
1 tsp / 5 ml arrowroot powder
3 Tbsp / 45 ml honey
Pinch sea salt

NUTRITIONAL VALUE
PER SERVING
(¼ CUP / 60ML):
Calories: 56 |
Calories from Fat: 2 |
Protein: 0 g | Carbs: 14 g |
Total Fat: 0.3 g |
Saturated Fat: 0 g | Trans
Fat: 0 g | Fiber: 3 g |
Sodium: 40 mg |
Cholesterol: 0 mg

METHOD

1. Add raspberries to a small heavy-bottomed saucepan and set burner to medium high. In a small bowl, whisk together lemon juice and arrowroot, and add to raspberries. Add honey and sea salt. Bring to a simmer, whisking, until raspberries break down and sauce thickens, 3 to 5 minutes. Remove from heat and serve.

Herbed Yogurt Cheese

Servings: 16 x 2 Tbsp
Prep time: 10 minutes
Resting time:
120 minutes
Makes: 2 cups

Can be used on sandwiches, in wraps or with pasta as a creamy sauce, or add a little vinegar to make a creamy vinaigrette salad dressing!

Use with Prawn and Herbed Yogurt Cheese Canapés on page 65.

INGREDIENTS

2 cups / 480 ml Yogurt Cheese (see recipe on page. 348), drained well
½ tsp / 2.5 ml minced shallot
½ tsp / 2.5 ml minced garlic
2 tsp / 10 ml fresh chopped chives
2 tsp / 10 ml fresh chopped basil
1 tsp / 5 ml fresh chopped dill
1 tsp / 5 ml fresh lemon juice
¼ tsp / 1.25 ml sea salt
⅛ tsp / 0.625 ml freshly ground black pepper

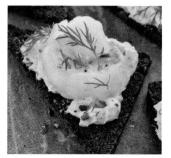

NUTRITIONAL VALUE
PER SERVING
(2 TBSP / 30 ML):
Calories: 15 |
Calories from Fat: 0 |
Protein: 3 g | Carbs: 1 g |
Total Fat: 0 g |
Saturated Fat: 0 g | Trans
Fat: 0 g | Fiber: 0 g |
Sodium: 40 mg |
Cholesterol: 0 mg

METHOD

1. Add all ingredients to a food processor or blender. Process until ingredients are combined and yogurt is smooth, about 15 seconds. Scrape into a container, and if possible, refrigerate for 2 hours to let set. You'll use only 1/2 cup of this spread for the Prawn and Herbed Yogurt Cheese Canapés; store leftovers in the refrigerator for up to three days.

Clean Cocktail Sauce

Servings: 8 x 2 Tbsp
Prep time: 10 minutes
Cooking time:
0 minutes
Makes: 1 cup

Use with Seafood Platter on page 70.

INGREDIENTS

½ medium tomato, cored and finely chopped
½ cup / 120 ml no-salt-added tomato sauce
2 tsp / 10 ml horseradish
2 tsp / 10 ml fresh lemon juice
1 tsp / 5 ml honey
½ tsp / 2.5 ml Worcestershire sauce
¼ tsp / 1.25 ml hot sauce, such as Tobasco
½ tsp / 2.5 ml sea salt

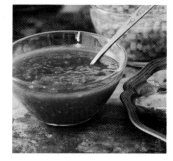

NUTRITIONAL VALUE
PER SERVING
(ABOUT 2 TBSP / 30 ML):
Calories: 11 |
Calories from Fat: 0 |
Protein: 0 g | Carbs: 3 g |
Total Fat: 0 g |
Saturated Fat: 0 g | Trans
Fat: 0 g | Fiber: 0 g |
Sodium: 134 mg |
Cholesterol: 0 mg

METHOD

1. Mix all ingredients together well in a small bowl and refrigerate until ready to serve.

Scallion Pistou

Servings: 24 x 2 tsp
Prep time: 10 minutes
Cooking time:
0 minutes
Makes: 1 cup

Pistou is French for pesto, but made without the addition of cheese. It's delicious added to soups, pasta, whole grains, or spooned over grilled or steamed vegetables.

Use with Summer Vegetable Platter on page 48.

INGREDIENTS

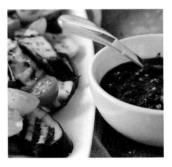

3 scallions, cut into 4-inch sections
1 cup / 240 ml packed basil leaves
1 cup / 240 ml packed mint leaves
2 cloves garlic, smashed
Juice and zest of 1 lemon
2 Tbsp / 30 ml red wine vinegar
¼ cup / 60 ml walnut pieces
½ tsp / 2.5 ml sea salt
¼ tsp / 1.25 ml freshly ground black pepper
½ cup / 120 ml extra virgin olive oil

NUTRITIONAL VALUE
PER SERVING
(2 TSP / 10 ML):
Calories: 34 |
Calories from Fat: 27 |
Protein: 1 g | Carbs: 1 g |
Total Fat: 3 g |
Saturated Fat: 0 g |
Trans Fat: 0 g | Fiber: 1 g |
Sodium: 41 mg |
Cholesterol: 0 mg

METHOD

1. Place the scallions, basil, mint and garlic in a food processor and pulse until roughly chopped. Add lemon zest and juice, red wine vinegar, walnut pieces, salt and pepper, and pulse to combine. While processor is running, slowly stream olive oil in and blend until well combined. You'll only use 1/4 cup of pistou with the Summer Vegetable Platter. To store leftover pistou, lay plastic wrap over surface to prevent it from coming into contact with air. Refrigerate for up to one week, or freeze for up to three months.

Tahini Sauce

Servings: 8 x 2 Tbsp
Prep time: 5 minutes
Cooking time:
0 minutes
Makes: 1 cup

Tahini is a paste made from ground sesame seeds. It is a common Middle-Eastern base for sauces used to dress meat, vegetables and salads.

Use with Curry Spiced Lentil Falafel on page 176.

INGREDIENTS

1 clove garlic, smashed
½ cup / 120 ml tahini, well-stirred
⅓ cup / 80 ml fresh lemon juice
¼ cup / 60 ml water
¼ tsp / 1.25 ml ground cumin
¾ tsp / 3.75 ml sea salt
3 Tbsp / 45 ml extra virgin olive oil

NUTRITIONAL VALUE
PER SERVING
(2 TBSP / 30 ML):
Calories: 144 |
Calories from Fat: 120 |
Protein: 3 g | Carbs: 6 g |
Total Fat: 13 g |
Saturated Fat: 2 g |
Trans Fat: 0 g | Fiber: 1 g |
Sodium: 150 mg |
Cholesterol: 0 mg

METHOD

1. Add all ingredients except olive oil to a blender or food processor, and blend until smooth. While machine is running, slowly stream in olive oil. Stop machine to scrape down sides, and process again to ensure that all ingredients are well blended.

Dashi (Ichiban Dashi)

Servings: 8 x 1 cup
Prep time: 5 minutes
Cooking time:
15 minutes
Makes: 8 cups

"Ichiban Dashi" or "First Dashi" is the base for many Japanese soups and dishes. It is essentially the Japanese version of soup stock.

Use with Japanese Vegetable and Tofu Soup on page 86, and with Egg Drop Soup on page 90.

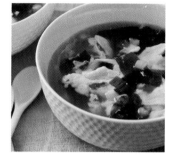

INGREDIENTS

2 x (8 x 4-inch) pieces of dried kelp (kombu)
10 cups / 2.4 L water
¾ oz / 21 g or about 2 cups / 480 ml bonito flakes
  or katsuobushi

NUTRITIONAL VALUE
PER SERVING
(1 CUP / 240 ML):
Calories: 11 |
Calories from Fat: 0 |
Protein: 2 g | Carbs: 1 g |
Total Fat: 0 g |
Saturated Fat: 0 g | Trans
Fat: 0 g | Fiber: 1 g |
Sodium: 52 mg |
Cholesterol: 2 mg

METHOD

1. Add dried kelp and water to a medium soup pot and soak for 10 minutes. Turn heat to high and bring water to a boil. Just as the water is about to boil, remove kelp and discard. Stir in bonito and let water come to a complete boil. Remove any foam that appears on top. Turn off heat and let bonito flakes sink to bottom. Strain through a fine mesh sieve lined with two layers of cheesecloth into a large bowl or soup pot to catch liquid.

Parmesan Croutons

Servings: 4 x
2 croutons
Prep time: 2 minutes
Cooking time:
10 minutes

Have you ever made your own croutons? If not, what are you waiting for? It's simple and they'll taste better than anything store bought, guaranteed.

Use with French Onion Soup on page 82.

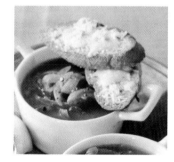

INGREDIENTS

8 x ¼-inch-thick slices whole grain French bread
Eat-Clean Cooking Spray (see page 348)
Pinch sea salt
Pinch freshly ground black pepper
8 tsp / 40 ml freshly grated real Parmesan
  (Parmigiano Reggiano)

METHOD

1. Preheat oven to 350°F / 175°C. Place bread slices on a baking sheet. Spray with Eat-Clean Cooking Spray and sprinkle with salt and pepper. Top each slice with 1 tsp / 5 ml Parmesan. Bake in oven until golden brown, about 10 minutes.

NUTRITIONAL VALUE
PER SERVING
(2 CROUTONS):
Calories: 128 |
Calories from Fat: 24 |
Protein: 6 g | Carbs: 20 g |
Total Fat: 3 g |
Saturated Fat: 1 g |
Trans Fat: 0 g | Fiber: 2 g |
Sodium: 322 mg |
Cholesterol: 4 mg

Cucumber Mignonette

Use with Seafood Platter on page 70.

Servings: 8 x 1 Tbsp
Prep time: 5 minutes
Cooking time:
0 minutes
Makes: ½ cup

INGREDIENTS

¼ cup / 60 ml finely chopped peeled and
    seeded cucumber
1 Tbsp / 15 ml chopped shallot
    (same size pieces as cucumber)
¼ cup / 60 ml champagne vinegar
¼ tsp / 1.25 ml freshly ground black pepper
⅛ tsp / 0.625 sea salt

METHOD

1. In a small bowl, place cucumber and shallot. Add rest of ingredients and stir to combine. Refrigerate until ready to use.

NUTRITIONAL VALUE
PER SERVING
(ABOUT 1 TBSP / 15 ML):
Calories: 4 |
Calories from Fat: 0 |
Protein: 0 g | Carbs: 1 g |
Total Fat: 0 g |
Saturated Fat: 0 g |
Trans Fat: 0 g | Fiber: 0 g |
Sodium: 34 mg |
Cholesterol: 0 mg

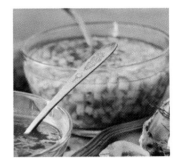

Crispy Herb and Garlic Croutons

It's so easy – and so much healthier – to make your own croutons. Best of all, you can cater the flavors to your own personal tastes. These croutons are subtly seasoned with thyme and rosemary.

Use with Roasted Red Potatoes, Asparagus and Frisée on page 187.

Servings: 16 x 2 Tbsp
Prep time: 5 minutes
Cooking time:
17-20 minutes
Makes: 2 cups

INGREDIENTS

4 cups / 960 ml day-old whole grain bread,
    cut into ¼-inch cubes
Eat-Clean Cooking Spray (see pg 348)
1 clove garlic, minced
1 tsp / 5 ml finely chopped fresh thyme,
    or ¼ tsp / 1.25 ml dried
½ tsp / 2.5 ml finely chopped fresh rosemary
¼ tsp / 1.25 ml sea salt
⅛ tsp / 0.625 ml freshly ground black pepper

NUTRITIONAL VALUE
PER SERVING
(2 TBSP / 30 ML):
Calories: 36 |
Calories from Fat: 5 |
Protein: 1 g | Carbs: 6 g |
Total Fat: 1 g |
Saturated Fat: 0 g |
Trans Fat: 0 g | Fiber: 1 g |
Sodium: 61 mg |
Cholesterol: 0 mg

METHOD

1. Preheat oven to 325°F / 165°C. Place cut bread on a baking sheet and spray thoroughly with Eat-Clean Cooking Spray. Toss with garlic, thyme, rosemary, salt and pepper. Spread out in a single layer and bake in oven, stirring once, until golden brown and crispy, 17 to 20 minutes. Can be stored in an airtight container for up to two weeks.

TIP *Need Eat-Clean breadcrumbs? Put Crispy Croutons in a food processor and process until broken up into crumbs.*

Grilled Pineapple Salsa

This spicy, sweet salsa is perfect with fish, chicken and pork.
Use with Shrimp Tacos on page 144.

Servings: 8 x ¼ cup
Prep time: 15 minutes
Cooking time:
0 minutes
Makes: 2 cups

INGREDIENTS

1 fresh pineapple
½ cup / 120 ml diced jicama
¼ cup / 60 ml diced red onion
1 jalapeño pepper, seeds and ribs removed, diced
1 Anaheim pepper, seeds and ribs removed, diced
Juice of ½ lime
¼ tsp / 1.25 ml sea salt
⅛ tsp / 0.625 ml freshly ground black pepper
1 heaping Tbsp / 17-18 ml finely chopped cilantro
1 heaping Tbsp / 17-18 ml finely chopped fresh mint

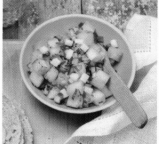

METHOD

1. To prepare pineapple, twist off leafy stalk and discard. Using a sharp chef's knife, cut off top and bottom. Set pineapple on flat bottom, and cut skin away from exterior. If any sharp or fibrous pieces of peel remain, cut them out. Cut pineapple in half lengthwise, and set each half, flat side down, on cutting board. Cut each half into ¼-inch-thick half moons.

2. Heat a grill or grill pan to high. Grill pineapple halves 30 seconds on each side, just long enough to create grill marks, but not cook pineapple. Work in batches, if necessary. Remove to cutting board and dice into ¼-inch cubes. (You need 1 cup / 240 ml of diced grilled pineapple for salsa.) If you don't have enough at this point, grill more pineapple and dice until you have enough. Refrigerate any unused pineapple.

3. Add 1 cup / 240 ml diced grilled pineapple to a medium bowl. Add rest of salsa ingredients and stir to combine. Any unused salsa can be refrigerated, covered, for up to three days.

NUTRITIONAL VALUE
PER SERVING
(¼ CUP / 60 ML):
Calories: 65 |
Calories from Fat: 2 |
Protein: 1 g | Carbs: 17 g |
Total Fat: 0.1 g |
Saturated Fat: 0 g | Trans
Fat: 0 g | Fiber: 2 g |
Sodium: 52 mg |
Cholesterol: 0 mg

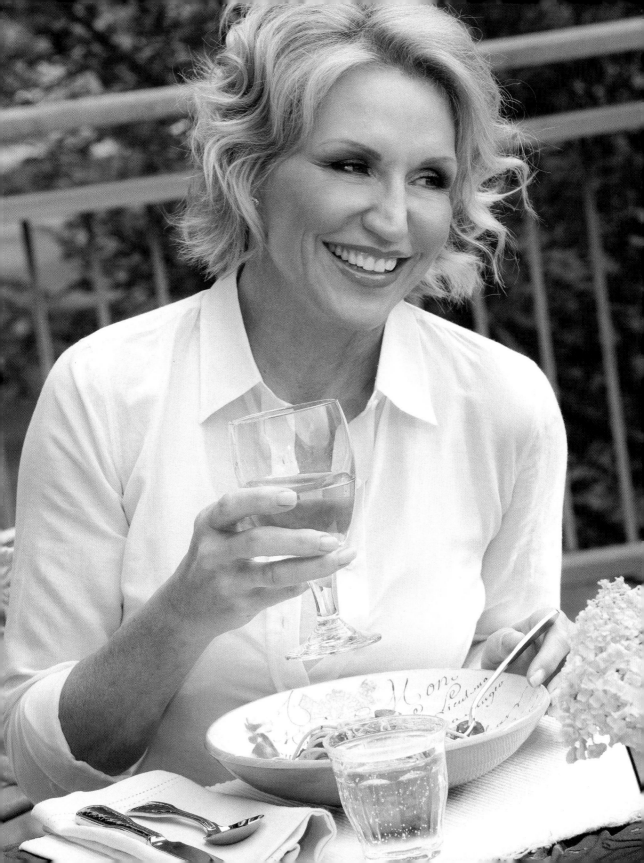

Chimichurri

Servings: 8 x 2 Tbsp
Prep time: 10 minutes
Cooking time:
0 minutes
Makes: 1 cup

Agentine chimichurri is a green sauce used on roast meat and sausages. It also works well as a marinade.

Use with Argentine Cowboy Steak on page 155.

INGREDIENTS

1 bunch cilantro, finely chopped
½ bunch parsley, finely chopped
3 cloves garlic, minced
2 Tbsp / 30 ml aged sherry vinegar
¼ cup / 60 ml + 2 Tbsp / 30 ml extra virgin olive oil
1 tsp / 5 ml sea salt
½ tsp / 2.5 ml freshly ground black pepper

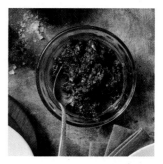

METHOD

1. In a small bowl, stir together all ingredients until combined well.

NUTRITIONAL VALUE
PER SERVING
(2 TBSP / 30 ML):
Calories: 70 |
Calories from Fat: 61 |
Protein: 1 g | Carbs: 2 g |
Total Fat: 7 g |
Saturated Fat: 1 g |
Trans Fat: 0 g | Fiber: 1 g |
Sodium: 207 mg |
Cholesterol: 0 mg

Zesty Hummus

Servings: 14 x 2 Tbsp
Prep time: 10 minutes
Cooking time:
0 minutes
Makes: 1¾ cups

This is not your typical hummus. Cumin and cayenne give it a zip that's sure to please your palate.

Use with Garden Veggie Stuffed Pita Pockets on page 196, and with Quinoa and Black Bean Lunchbowl on page 199.

INGREDIENTS

2 cups / 480 ml cooked chickpeas or
   1 x 15-oz can organic unsalted chickpeas
1 clove garlic
2 Tbsp / 30 ml tahini (sesame seed paste)
Juice of 1 lemon
½ tsp / 2.5 ml ground cumin
⅛ tsp / 0.625 ml cayenne pepper
1 tsp / 5 ml sea salt
⅛ tsp / 0.625 ml freshly ground black pepper
¼ cup / 60 ml extra virgin olive oil

METHOD

1. Add all ingredients up to but not including extra virgin olive oil, to a food processor and pulse blend until combined, but still chunky. While processor is running, slowly stream in olive oil until combined and very smooth. If there are chunky bits stuck to sides of bowl, scrape down sides and blend for another 15 seconds.

NUTRITIONAL VALUE
PER SERVING
(2 TBSP / 30 ML):
Calories: 90 |
Calories from Fat: 51 |
Protein: 3 g | Carbs: 7 g |
Total Fat: 2 g |
Saturated Fat: 1 g |
Trans Fat: 0 g | Fiber: 2 g |
Sodium: 114 mg |
Cholesterol: 0 mg

Jerk Seasoning

Servings: 24 x ½ tsp
Prep time: 10 minutes
Cooking time:
0 minutes
Makes: ¼ cup

Jerk seasoning is a spicy spice rub native to Jamaica. Jerk is also a style of cooking in which meats are dry-rubbed or wet marinated in Jamaican jerk spice.

Use with Jamaican Jerk Steak on page 212.

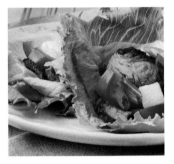

INGREDIENTS

2 tsp / 10 ml ground allspice
2 tsp / 10 ml chopped fresh thyme, or 1 tsp / 5 ml dried
2 tsp / 10 ml unrefined sugar
2 tsp / 10 ml sea salt
2 tsp / 10 ml freshly ground black pepper
1 tsp / 5 ml garlic powder
1 tsp / 5 ml onion powder
½ tsp / 2.5 ml cinnamon
½ tsp / 2.5 ml nutmeg
1 Scotch bonnet pepper, similar to a habañero pepper, destemmed and
   quartered (for a less spicy seasoning, remove ribs and seeds)

NUTRITIONAL VALUE
PER SERVING
(½ TSP / 2.5 ML):
Calories: 4 |
Calories from Fat: 0 |
Protein: 0.1 g | Carbs: 1 g |
Total Fat: 0 g |
Saturated Fat: 0 g |
Trans Fat: 0 g | Fiber: 0.1 g |
Sodium: 131 mg |
Cholesterol: 0 mg

METHOD

1. In a food processor, add all spices up to but not including Scotch bonnet pepper, and pulse to combine. Add Scotch bonnet pepper and process until pepper is ground fine and all ingredients are blended. Can be refrigerated, covered, for up to one week until ready to use.

Dijon Blanc Sauce:

Servings: 8 x 1½ tsp
Prep time: 5 minutes
Cooking time:
2-4 minutes
Makes: ¼ cup

This is a Clean version of classic French Beurre Blanc, or white wine butter sauce, but lighter, and actually contains no butter or white wine! The key is to have all ingredients pre-measured and ready to go because the sauce is very quick to make.

Use with Dover Sole Wrapped Asparagus on page 221.

INGREDIENTS

1 tsp / 5 ml extra virgin olive oil
1 tsp / 5 ml minced shallot
1 Tbsp / 15 ml white wine vinegar
¼ cup / 60 ml low-sodium chicken broth
1 tsp / 5 ml Dijon mustard
2 Tbsp / 30 ml freshly squeezed orange juice
Pinch sea salt
Pinch freshly ground black pepper

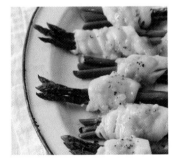

NUTRITIONAL VALUE
PER SERVING:
Calories: 22 |
Calories from Fat: 12 |
Protein: 0 g | Carbs: 3 g |
Total Fat: 1 g |
Saturated Fat: 0 g |
Trans Fat: 0 g | Fiber: 0 g |
Sodium: 114 mg |
Cholesterol: 0 mg

METHOD

1. Heat olive oil in a small skillet or low-sided saucepan over medium-high heat. Add shallot and cook for 1 to 2 minutes or until soft. Add white wine vinegar and chicken broth, and cook until reduced by half, 1 to 2 minutes. Whisk in mustard and orange juice, and season with salt and pepper. Serve immediately.

Servings: 8 x ¼ cup
Prep time: 15 minutes
Cooking time:
22 minutes
Makes: 2 cups

Fig Demi-Glace

Demi-glace means a glaze that has been reduced by half. It is a classic type of French sauce that pairs well with filet mignon.

Use with Filet Mignon on page 229.

INGREDIENTS

1 Tbsp / 15 ml safflower oil
½ medium yellow onion, diced
1 carrot, peeled and diced
1 stalk celery, diced
1 clove garlic, chopped
1 large sprig fresh thyme, leaves stripped from stem
8 parsley stems, each 2 to 4 inches long
1 bay leaf
¼ tsp / 1.25 ml whole black peppercorns
1 tsp / 5 ml tomato paste
¼ cup / 60 ml dry red wine
2 cups / 480 ml plus 1 Tbsp / 15 ml unsalted beef stock, or very low-sodium beef broth, divided
1 tsp / 5 ml arrowroot powder
4 fresh figs, quartered (if fresh figs aren't available, substitute dried)
½ tsp / 2.5 ml sea salt
¼ tsp / 1.25 ml freshly ground black pepper

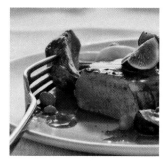

METHOD

1. Heat safflower oil in a shallow, straight-sided pan over medium-high heat. Add onion, carrot and celery, and cook until soft and starting to brown, stirring occasionally, about 5 minutes. Add garlic, thyme leaves, parsley stems, bay leaf and peppercorns, and cook until garlic is fragrant, about 1 minute. Stir in tomato paste. Add red wine and, using a wooden spoon, scrape crusty brown bits off bottom of pan. Allow alcohol from wine to cook off, about 1 minute. Add 2 cups / 480 ml beef stock, bring to a boil, reduce heat and simmer until reduced by half, about 15 minutes. Strain through a fine mesh sieve into a clean pan, and place on stove over medium-low heat.

2. In a small bowl, mix together arrowroot with remaining 1 Tbsp / 15 ml beef stock until there are no lumps, and stir into demi-glace. Add fresh figs and simmer until sauce thickens, about 1 minute. Season with salt and pepper, taste, and make any final adjustments to seasoning. Serve overtop filet mignon (recipe page 229).

NUTRITIONAL VALUE
PER SERVING (¼ CUP /
60 ML DEMI-GLACE):
Calories: 121 |
Calories from Fat: 38 |
Protein: 3 g | Carbs: 17 g |
Total Fat: 1 g |
Saturated Fat: 0 g |
Trans Fat: 0 g | Fiber: 2 g |
Sodium: 294 mg |
Cholesterol: 0 mg

Spicy Orange Dipping Sauce

Use with Coconut Shrimp on page 241.

Use with Coconut Shrimp on page 241.

Servings: 4 x 1 Tbsp
Prep time: 2 minutes
Cooking time: 5 minutes
Makes: ¼ cup

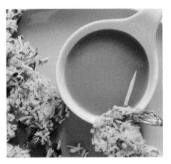

INGREDIENTS

Juice of 1 orange
½ tsp / 2.5 ml agave nectar
½ tsp / 2.5 ml arrowroot powder
¼ tsp / 1.25 ml sambal oelek or other chili sauce
⅛ tsp / 0.625 ml sea salt

METHOD

1. In a small saucepan, combine all ingredients and bring to a boil over high heat. Reduce heat to simmer until thickened, about 3 minutes.

NUTRITIONAL VALUE
PER SERVING
(1 TBSP / 30 ML):
Calories: 37 |
Calories from Fat: 0 |
Protein: 0 g | Carbs: 9 g |
Total Fat: 0 g |
Saturated Fat: 0 g |
Trans Fat: 0 g | Fiber: 0 g |
Sodium: 66 mg |
Cholesterol: 0 mg

Olive Tapenade:

Servings: 12 x 1 Tbsp
Prep time: 10 minutes
Cooking time: 0 minutes
Makes: ¾ cup

Popular in the south of France, tapenade is a spread or dip made with olives, capers, anchovies and olive oil. This tapenade can be used as a dip for vegetables or crusty whole grain bread, as a sandwich spread, as a seasoning for baked fish or chicken, or tossed with whole grains or pasta as a chunky and flavorful sauce.

Use with Olive Tapenade Stuffed Sole on page 234.

Use with Olive Tapenade Stuffed Sole on page 234.

INGREDIENTS

1 cup / 240 ml pitted olives, such as kalamata or nicoise
1 clove garlic, minced
1 Tbsp / 15 ml capers, drained
1 fresh bay leaf, finely chopped
Zest of 1 lemon
2 tsp / 10 ml fresh lemon juice
½ cup / 120 ml chopped parsley
1 Tbsp / 15 ml fresh thyme leaves
1 tsp / 5 ml Dijon mustard
¼ tsp / 1.25 ml anchovy paste
¼ tsp / 1.25 ml red pepper flakes

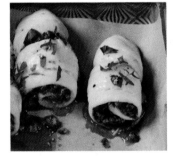

NUTRITIONAL VALUE
PER SERVING
(1 TBSP / 30 ML):
Calories: 45 |
Calories from Fat: 31 |
Protein: 1 g | Carbs: 4 g |
Total Fat: 0.3 g |
Saturated Fat: 0.4 g |
Trans Fat: 0 g | Fiber: 2 g |
Sodium: 382 mg |
Cholesterol: 0 mg

METHOD

1. Add all ingredients to a food processor and pulse until well combined. Use a rubber spatula to scrape down sides of bowl, and then blend until mixture resembles a coarse paste. Scrape into a bowl.

Cashew Miso Dressing

Servings: 1 Tbsp
Prep time: 5 minutes
Cooking time:
0 minutes
Makes: 1¼ cups

You will need only half a cup of this dressing for the Cold Soba Noodle Salad, so use the rest on a tossed green salad, in a lunch wrap to give it a zesty Asian flair, or over steamed vegetables, rice, even grilled chicken or fish!

Use with Cold Soba Noodle Salad on page 262.

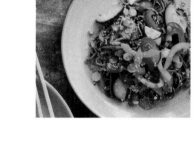

INGREDIENTS

⅓ cup / 80 ml rice wine vinegar
2 Tbsp / 30 ml red miso
1 clove garlic
2 tsp / 10 ml chopped ginger
2 Tbsp / 30 ml honey or agave nectar
3 Tbsp / 45 ml cashew nut butter
1 tsp / 5 ml sesame oil
2 Tbsp / 30 ml extra virgin olive oil

NUTRITIONAL VALUE
PER SERVING
(1 TBSP / 30 ML):

Calories: 41 |
Calories from Fat: 25 |
Protein: 1 g | Carbs: 3 g |
Total Fat: 3 g |
Saturated Fat: 0.5 g |
Trans Fat: 0 g | Fiber: 0 g |
Sodium: 87 mg |
Cholesterol: 0 mg

METHOD

1. Place all ingredients except for extra virgin olive oil in a blender or food processor and blend well. Stop machine and scrape down sides. Start machine again and slowly stream in olive oil until dressing is smooth and all ingredients are thoroughly incorporated.

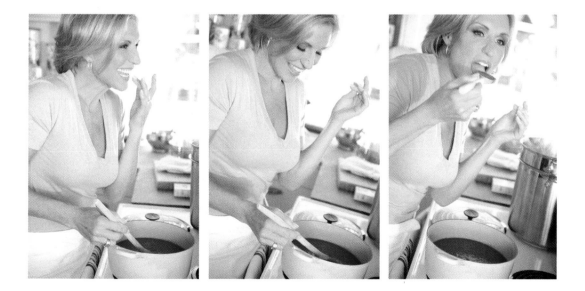

Index

10 Common Culinary Herbs, Their Nutritional Benefits & How to Use, 136-137
24 Carrot-Tini, 333

A

A "How-to" for Fish, 254-255
acai berry juice,
   Acai Blueberry Breakfast Shake, 19
Acai Blueberry Breakfast Shake, 19
acesulphamine potassium, 344
agave, 20
   blue, 36, 245, 301, 321, 338, 342, 360
   nectar, 69, 317, 344
   syrup, 204, 333
ale, 115
allspice, 175, 230, 246, 358
almond(s), 12
   butter, 325
   Chocolate Almond Cake, 325
   milk, 97
   real almond extract, 325
anchovy paste, 104, 211, 360
anise, 314, 326
annatto seeds, 246
apple, 23, 309
   cider,
      Hot Spiced Apple Cider, 326
   granny smith, 130
   Turkey Apple Breakfast Sausage, 58
   Puree of Parsnip, Celeriac and Apple Soup with Crispy Sage, 97
applesauce, 61, 322, 325
Argentinean Cowboy Steak with Grilled Onion Rings, Tomatoes and Chimichurri, 155
arrowroot, 338
   powder, 318, 341, 342, 350, 359, 360
artichoke hearts, 28, 44
   Creamy Artichoke Soup, 81
arugula, 136
   Beets, Blood Oranges and Arugula with Feta, 278
Asian fish sauce, 237
Asian Pear, Watercress, Pea Shoot and Blue Cheese Salad, 273
asparagus,
   baby,
      Roasted Red Potatoes, Asparagus, Frisee with Crispy Croutons, 187
      Smoked Salmon Asparagus Bundles, 52
   spears,
      Dover Sole Wrapped Asparagus with Dijon Blanc Sauce, 221
aspartame, 344
avocado(s), 15, 121, 144, 199, 215, 233
   Venice Beach Roasted Vegetable and Avocado Sub, 168
Aztec, 69

B

Baba Ghanoush, 125
Baby Yellow Potatoes with Parsley, 306
baguette,
   whole grain, 168, 195
   whole wheat, 293
Baked Chicken Tenders, 225
Baked Eggs with Tomatoes, Turkey Bacon, Chives and Toasted Breadcrumbs, 16

baking powder, 23, 28, 43, 51, 57, 61, 322, 325, 334
baking soda, 23, 28, 43, 322, 325
bamboo shoots, 184
banana(s), 27
   Super Moist Banana Walnut Bread, 51
basil, 129, 136, 148, 160, 164, 171, 175, 192, 226, 230, 238, 351
   leaves, 207, 250, 258, 351
      Basil Lemon Pesto, 126
Basil Lemon Pesto, 126, 172
bay leaf, 78, 82, 85, 89, 100, 111, 136, 156, 171, 253, 297, 359, 360
BBQ Chicken Chop Chop Salad, 215
BBQ Chicken Pizza, 163
BBQ Pork Ribs, 222
beans,
   baby lima, 93, 226
   black, 15, 112, 215
      Quinoa and Black Bean Lunch Bowl, 199
   garbanzo, 357
      flour, 176
      Orzo and Garbanzo Salad with Roasted Red Peppers and Dill, 277
      Persian Couscous and Garbanzos with Kumquats, 175
   kidney, 89, 112
   pinto, 112
   Three Bean Salad with Corn and Peppers, 112
   vanilla, 314
   white, 195
bee pollen, 19
beef,
   broth, 82, 222, 253, 294
   stock, 359
beer, 115
beet(s), 265
   Beets, Blood Oranges and Arugula with Feta, 278
   greens, 282
   red,
      Smooth and Hearty Borscht-Style Beet Soup, 78
   tops,
      German-Braised Beet Tops and Apples, 309
Beets, Blood Oranges and Arugula with Feta, 278
berries, fresh, 342
Berry Lemon Parfait, 341
beta carotene, 333
Blackened Sole, 238
blintz, 338
blue marlin steaks, Hawaiian,
   Grilled Blue Marlin with Strawberry Nectarine Salsa, 242
blueberries, 27, 341
   Acai Blueberry Breakfast Shake, 19
   Blueberry Blintzes, 338
   Hearty Blueberry Corn Cake, 23
Blueberry Blintzes, 338
boar shoulder, 246
bonito flakes, 353
borscht, 78
Braised Collard Greens, 297
braising, 297
brandy, 82
bread,
   baguette,
      whole grain, 168, 195
      whole wheat, 293
   breadcrumbs, 16, 245

French, 282, 353
   hoagie rolls, whole grain, 143
   hot dog buns, 192
   whole grain, 208, 230, 357
   whole grain dark rye, 65
   whole wheat flatbreads, 147
   whole wheat pizza dough, 163
breadcrumbs, 16, 245
broccoli,
   florets,
      Crustless Broccoli Quiche with Caramelized Onions and Blue Cheese, 66
   raab,
      Broccoli Raab (Rapini) with Sun Dried Tomatoes, 290
Broccoli Raab (Rapini) with Sun Dried Tomatoes, 290
broth,
   beef, 82, 222, 253, 294
   chicken, 44, 81, 97, 107, 111, 143, 151, 156, 245, 297, 302, 309, 350, 358
   mushroom, 103
   vegetable, 44, 78, 85, 89, 93, 97, 103, 107, 148, 183, 245, 297, 309, 350
Bruschetta with Ricotta, Beet Greens and Walnuts, 282
Brussels sprouts,
   Warm Brussels Sprouts Salad with Walnuts and Lemon, 270
buffalo,
   Buffalo Burger Dogs, 192
   Mediterranean Lamb & Buffalo Meatballs, 230
Buffalo Burger Dogs, 192
buns, hot dog, 192
buttermilk, 23, 43, 322, 325

C

cabbage,
   green, 86, 184, 302
      Mexicali Cabbage Patch Soup, 89
   purple and green, 301
cake,
   Chocolate Almond Cake, 325
   Hearty Blueberry Corn Cake, 23
   Plum Upside Down Cake, 322
   Whole Wheat Angel Food Cake with Fresh Strawberries, 321
calcium, 189
Campfire Salmon with Fire Roasted Peppers and Eggplant, 140
canapes,
   Fresh Fig Canapes with Mint and Balsamic Syrup, 200
   Prawn and Herbed Yogurt Cheese Canapes, 65
cantaloupe, Tuscan-style, 337
   Sweet 'N' Spicy Shrimp and Cantaloupe Salad, 152
capers, 360
Caramelized Crimini Mushrooms and Pearl Onions, 294
Cardini, Caesar, 211
carrot(s), 28, 78, 85, 86, 103, 176, 184, 196, 204, 218, 253, 265, 359
   juice,
      24 Carrot-Tini, 333
Cashew Miso Dressing, 262, 361

cashew(s), 12, 31, 237
    butter, 237
        Cashew Miso Dressing, 262, 361
Cava, 329
cayenne, 20, 44, 69, 118, 130, 152, 156, 159, 175, 176, 203, 225, 238, 266, 330, 357
celeriac,
    Celeriac and Fennel Salad with Pomegranate Seeds, 261
    Puree of Parsnip, Celeriac and Apple Soup with Crispy Sage, 97
Celeriac and Fennel Salad with Pomegranate Seeds, 261
celery, 85, 93, 103, 156, 176, 208, 265, 359
    celeriac, 97
        Celeriac and Fennel Salad with Pome-granate Seeds, 261
Champagne, brut, 329
cheddar,
    Irish cheddar, 302
    medium, 163
    sharp, 163
        Cheddar Jalapeno Corn Muffins, 57
Cheddar Jalapeno Corn Muffins, 57
cheese, 74-75
    blue,
        Asian Pear, Watercress, Pea Shoot and Blue Cheese Salad, 273
        French, 66
    cheddar,
        Irish cheddar, 302
        medium, 163
        sharp, 163
            Cheddar Jalapeno Corn Muffins, 57
    cotija, 211
    cottage, 75
    Danish, 66
    feta, 171, 277, 278
    goat, 75
    mozzarella balls, 258
    Neufchatel, 130
    Parmesan,
        Parmesan Croutons, 82, 353
        Roasted Vegetable Eggplant Parmesan, 180
    Parmigiano Reggiano, 75, 93, 126, 160, 183, 207, 298
    Pecorino Romano, 104, 207
    ricotta, 75, 160, 338
cherries, 100, 265
    bing, 274
        Cherry Protein Pop 'Ems, 31
    black cherry juice,
        White Peach and Black Cherry Bellissimo, 47
Cherry Protein Pop 'Ems, 31
chia seeds, 19, 28, 31, 35, 36
Chicken and Spinach Lasagna, 160
chicken,
    boneless skinless chicken breasts,
        Chicken and Spinach Lasagna, 160
Grilled Chicken Caesar Salad with Spicy Kefir Cae-sar Dressing and Grilled Mini Pita Bread, 211
    breast(s),
        BBQ Chicken Chop Chop Salad, 215
        BBQ Chicken Pizza, 163
    breast tenders,
        Baked Chicken Tenders, 225
    broth, 44, 81, 97, 107, 111, 143, 151, 156, 245, 297, 302, 309, 350, 358
    livers,
        Chicken Liver Pate, 130
    sausages, 115
        mild Italian chicken,
            Italian Sausage with Sloppy Peppers, 143
Chicken Liver Pate, 130

chile,
    chipotle powder, 144
    paste, 233, 237, 245
chiles,
    arbol, 118, 184
    guajillo, 118
    pasilla, 118
chili,
    paste, 301
    powder, 15, 89, 112, 115, 133, 179, 225, 298
    Chili Rubbed Grilled Ostrich Tenderloin, 249
Chili and Scrambled Egg Breakfast Tacos, 32
Chili Rubbed Grilled Ostrich Tenderloin, 249
Chimichurri, 155, 354
Chipotle Ranchero Sauce, 15, 350
chives, 16, 24, 28, 81, 136, 148, 208, 218, 351
chocolate, 69
    Chocolate Almond Cake, 325
Chocolate Almond Cake, 325
cholesterol, LDL, 69, 74
cilantro, 15, 136, 163, 179, 199, 215, 242, 301, 354, 355
cinnamon, 35, 61, 69, 175, 230, 249, 318, 330, 334, 358
    stick(s), 69, 314, 326
Citrus Salad with Mint, 40
Clean Chili, 32
Clean Cocktail Sauce, 70, 352
Clean Eating Cooking Spray, 348
Clean Marinara Sauce, 122, 160, 180, 230
cloves, 35, 249, 309, 330
    white, 326
club soda, 317, 329, 333
cocoa powder, 69, 325
coconut,
    butter, 12, 51, 61, 318, 322
    Coconut Shrimp with Spicy Orange Dipping Sauce, 241
    flakes, 12
    oil, 23, 334, 338
Coconut Shrimp with Spicy Orange Dipping Sauce, 241
coffee, 69, 325
Cognac, 82, 130, 317
Colcannon with Kale, 302
Cold Soba Noodle Salad with Cashew Miso Dressing, 262
collard greens,
    Braised Collard Greens, 297
cooking spray, Eat Clean, 15, 16, 23, 28, 31, 32, 43, 44, 48, 57, 61, 66, 100, 112, 115, 140, 144, 147, 155, 159, 160, 164, 168, 179, 187, 192, 211, 212, 215, 221, 225, 226, 234, 237, 238, 241, 242, 245, 249, 269, 325, 334, 338, 353, 357
coriander, 115, 136, 151, 179, 249
corn, 112, 215
    baby sweet, 184
    high fructose corn syrup, 344
    Smoky Slathered Corn on Cob, 298
    whole grain corn flour, 28, 225
cornmeal, 28, 43, 57, 225
    100% whole grain, 163
    Hearty Blueberry Corn Cake, 23
cornstarch, 43
couscous,
    Israeli Couscous Salad, 100
    Persian Couscous and Garbanzos with Kumquats, 175
crab, Dungeness, 70
Cranberry Pear Bellini, 329
cranberries, 269, 334
    juice,
        Cranberry Pear Bellini, 329
cream of tartar, 342
Creamy Artichoke Soup, 81
Creamy Guaca-De-Gallo, 121
Crispy Herb and Garlic Croutons, 357
Crunchy Baked Ginger Dill Salmon, 245

Crustless Broccoli Quiche with Caramelized Onions and Blue Cheese, 66
cucumber, 354
    Cucumber Mignonette, 70
    English, 94, 108, 121, 147, 204, 262
Cucumber Mignonette, 70
cumin, 15, 89, 112, 125, 144, 151, 152, 159, 175, 176, 179, 225, 246, 249, 266, 277, 350, 352, 357
currants, dried, 61, 100
curry powder, 130
    Curry Spiced Lentil Falafel with Tahini Sauce, 176
Curry Spiced Lentil Falafel with Tahini Sauce, 176
cyclamate, 344

D

Dashi, 86, 90, 353
dates, 23, 35, 61, 318
Dijon Blanc Sauce, 221, 358
dill, 65, 78, 107, 237, 277, 351
    Crunchy Baked Ginger Dill Salmon, 245
dolmas, 107
    Greek Brown Rice Dolmas, 107
Dover sole,
    Blackened Sole, 238
    Dover Sole Wrapped Asparagus with Dijon Blanc Sauce, 221
Dover Sole Wrapped Asparagus with Dijon Blanc Sauce, 221

E

Eat-Clean cooking spray, 15, 16, 23, 28, 31, 32, 43, 44, 48, 57, 61, 66, 100, 112, 115, 140, 144, 147, 155, 159, 160, 164, 168, 179, 187, 192, 211, 212, 215, 221, 225, 226, 234, 237, 238, 241, 242, 245, 249, 269, 325, 334, 338, 353, 357
Effervescent Dessert Fruit Soup, 337
Egg Drop Soup, 90
Egg Salad with a Twist, 208
eggplant, 125, 140, 168
    Roasted Vegetable Eggplant Parmesan, 180
egg(s), 24, 28, 43, 57, 66, 164, 187, 322, 334, 338
    Chili and Scrambled Egg Breakfast Tacos, 32
    Egg Drop Soup, 90
    Egg Salad with a Twist, 208
    ranch, 15
    white(s), 15, 23, 24, 28, 31, 32, 43, 44, 61, 66, 90, 160, 164, 187, 225, 241, 321, 322, 325, 334, 338, 342
        Baked Eggs with Tomatoes, Turkey Bacon, Chives and Toasted Breadcrumbs, 16
        Eggs Sardou with Warm Orange Vinaigrette, 44
Eggs Sardou with Warm Orange Vinaigrette, 44
endive, Belgian, 200
    Grilled Treviso and Endive with Cranberries and Pumpkin Seeds, 269
escarole, 261, 274
espresso, 69

F

falafels, 176
fava beans,
    Fresh Fava Beans with Lemon Anchovy Vinaigrette, 104
fennel,
    bulb, 265
        Celeriac and Fennel Salad with Pomegranate Seeds, 261
        Tomato Fennel Soup with Lima Beans, 93
    seeds, 143, 207
feta, 171, 277, 278
Fig Demi-Glace, 229, 359

figs,
    Fig Demi-Glace, 229, 359
    Fresh Fig Canapes with Mint and Balsamic
        Syrup, 200
filet mignon,
    Filet Mignon with Fig Demi-Glace, 229
Filet Mignon with Fig Demi-Glace, 229
fish, 254
flatbreads, whole wheat, 147
flaxseed, 12, 23, 27, 35, 51, 325
flour, 43
    corn, 43, 57
    pastry, 51, 322
    whole oat, 28
    whole wheat, 23, 28, 156, 163, 245, 253, 321,
        325, 334, 338
    whole wheat pastry, 57
French Green Lentil Salad with Easter Egg
    Radishes and Mache, 171
French Onion Soup with Parmesan Croutons, 82
Fresh Fava Beans with Lemon Anchovy
    Vinaigrette, 104
Fresh Fig Canapes with Mint and Balsamic
    Syrup, 200
frisee, head, 187
fructose, 344
fruit, dried, 12

G

Garden Veggie Stuffed Pita Pockets, 196
garlic,
    clove(s), 15, 24, 44, 58, 62, 73, 78, 81, 82, 85, 89,
        93, 94, 97, 104, 108, 111, 115, 118, 121, 122,
        125, 126, 129, 130, 133, 134, 143, 147, 148,
        151, 152, 156, 159, 160, 176, 183, 184, 192,
        207, 211, 215, 222, 226, 230, 237, 246, 250,
        253, 266, 270, 282, 285, 286, 289, 290, 293,
        294, 297, 302, 309, 350, 351, 352, 359, 360,
        361
        Crispy Herb and Garlic Croutons, 357
    minced, 351
    powder, 225, 238, 249, 358
    spears,
        Grilled Garlic Spears, 305
Gazpacho, 94
German-Braised Beet Tops and Apples, 309
gin, 333
ginger, 35, 249, 314, 361
    grated, 184, 204, 266, 301
    Crunchy Baked Ginger Dill Salmon, 245
granola, 12
grape leaves, 107
grapefruits, 40
Greek Brown Rice Dolmas, 107
Greek Lamb Flatbread Pizza, 147
Green Lentil and Vegetable Soup, 85
Grilled Blue Marlin with Strawberry Nectarine
    Salsa, 242
Grilled Chicken Caesar Salad with Spicy Kefir
    Caesar Dressing and Grilled Mini Pita
    Bread, 211
Grilled Fingerling Potatoes, 286
Grilled Garlic Spears, 305
Grilled Pineapple Salsa, 144, 355
Grilled Treviso and Endive with Cranberries and
    Pumpkin Seeds, 269
gumbo, 156

H

halibut filet,
    Halibut with Minted Lima Bean Puree, 226
Halibut with Minted Lima Bean Puree, 226
Hazelnut-Crusted Venison Medallions with Herb
    Roasted Carrots and Parsnips, 218

hazelnut(s),
    butter, 19
    Hazelnut-Crusted Venison Medallions with
        Herb Roasted Carrots and Parsnips, 218
Hearty Blueberry Corn Cake, 23
Herb and Garlic Croutons, 187
Herbed Yogurt Cheese, 65, 351
herbes de Provence, 66, 310
herbs, 136-137
    arugula, 136, 278
    basil, 129, 136, 148, 160, 164, 171, 175, 192, 226,
        230, 238, 351
        leaves, 207, 250, 258, 351
        Basil Lemon Pesto, 126
    bay leaf, 78, 82, 85, 89, 100, 111, 136, 156, 171,
        253, 297, 359, 360
    chives, 16, 24, 28, 81, 136, 148, 208, 218, 351
    cilantro, 15, 136, 163, 179, 199, 215, 242, 301, 355
    coriander, 115, 136, 151, 179, 249
    dill, 137
    fennel,
        bulb, 265
        Celeriac and Fennel Salad with
            Pomegranate Seeds, 261
        Tomato Fennel Soup with Lima
            Beans, 93
        seeds, 143, 207
    horseradish, 352
    How to Store Your Herbs, 137
    Italian, 28
    marjoram, 58
    mint, 40, 107, 108, 147, 148, 175, 200, 226, 230,
        242, 301, 337, 341, 351, 355
    oregano, 58, 137, 147, 160, 207
        leaves, 122
        Mexican, 89, 225
    parsley, 125, 137, 171, 176, 230, 261, 306,
        354, 360
        curly, 108
        flat leaf, 100, 234, 286
        stems, 359
    rosemary, 58, 85, 137, 183, 253, 294, 330, 357
        leaves, 159, 203
    sage, 58, 62, 97
        leaves, 97
    tarragon, 52, 104, 148
    thyme, 58, 62, 73, 81, 82, 85, 93, 97, 103, 137, 156,
        171, 183, 218, 250, 253, 286, 294, 357, 358,
        359, 360
hoagie rolls, whole grain, 143
honey, 12, 23, 69, 133, 204, 237, 261, 266, 273, 277,
    278, 314, 318, 322, 330, 341, 350, 352, 361
horseradish, 352
hot dogs, 192
hot sauce, 156
Hot Spiced Apple Cider, 326
How to Store Your Herbs, 137
Huevos Rancheros, 15

I

ice, 70
    cubes, 19
iodine, 189
iron, 189
Israeli Couscous Salad, 100
Italian herbs, 28
Italian Sausage with Sloppy Peppers, 143
Italian seasoning, 115

J

jalapeno(s),57, 112, 115, 121, 140, 355
    Cheddar Jalapeno Corn Muffins, 57
Jamaican Jerk Steak and Pineapple Lettuce
    Wraps, 212
Japanese Vegetable and Tofu Soup, 86
Jerk Seasoning, 212, 358
jicama, 355
Jump Start Granola, 12

K

kale, 302
katsuobushi, 353
kefir, low-fat, 19, 28, 57, 211
    Kefir Marinated Lamb Kebabs with
        Vegetables, 159
    Strawberry Peach Kefir Smoothie with
        Chia Seeds, 36
Kefir Marinated Lamb Kebabs with Vegetables, 159
kelp, 353
kenchenjiru, 86
kiwis, 342
kombucha, 47, 337
kumquats, 175

L

lamb,
    boneless leg of,
        Kefir Marinated Lamb Kebabs with
            Vegetables, 159
    chops, boneless loin,
        Greek Lamb Flatbread Pizza, 147
ground,
        Mediterranean Lamb & Buffalo
            Meatballs, 230
Las Ramblas, 195
leek(s), 81, 97
Leftover Pasta Pizza Pie, 164
lemon(s), 317, 326
    Basil Lemon Pesto, 126
    Berry Lemon Parfait, 341
    juice, 44, 81, 78, 97, 104, 107, 108, 125, 134, 147,
        148, 159, 171, 175, 187, 195, 199, 226, 250,
        258, 261, 266, 270, 273, 277, 282, 293, 305,
        318, 321, 330, 338, 350, 351, 352, 357, 360
    wedges, 52, 70, 238
    zest, 107, 148, 159, 175, 226, 250, 282, 329, 330,
        338, 342, 351, 360
lentils,
    brown,
        Curry Spiced Lentil Falafel with Tahini
            Sauce, 176
    French green,
        French Green Lentil Salad with Easter Egg
            Radishes and Mache, 171
        Green Lentil and Vegetable Soup, 85
    red, 78
lettuce, 192
    iceberg, 212
    romaine, 211, 215
    wraps, 212
lime, 140, 317
    juice, 20, 40, 112, 118, 121, 151, 211, 215, 242,
        245, 246, 301, 333, 337, 355
Long-Life Vegetable Stir-Fry, 184
Louisiana Creole, 44

M

Mache, 171
maple syrup, 100% pure, 58
Marionberry Crisp with Walnut Oat Topping, 318
marionberries,
    Marionberry Crisp with Walnut Oat
        Topping, 318
marjoram, 58
Mediterranean Lamb & Buffalo Meatballs, 230
meringue, 342
metabolism, 69
Mexicali Cabbage Patch Soup, 89
Mexican hot sauce, 32
Mexican Mocha Caliente, 69
mignon, 229
    filet,
        Filet Mignon with Fig
            Demi-Glace, 229

milk, 75, 81
   almond, 97
   buttermilk, 23, 43, 322, 325
   goat, 81
   low-fat, 28, 51, 61, 66, 69, 97, 225, 302, 338
   rice, 97
   skim, 57
   soy, 51, 97
millet, 31
mint, 40, 107, 108, 147, 148, 175, 200, 226, 230, 242, 301, 337, 341, 351, 355
   Halibut with Minted Lima Bean Puree, 226
miso, red,
   Cashew Miso Dressing, 262, 361
mixed greens, 152, 199, 237
molasses, 330
   blackstrap, 51, 133
   unsulfured, 62, 203, 322
"Morning Juice" blend, 333
mozzarella, 172, 180
   balls, 258
muffin(s), 61
   Cheddar Jalapeno Corn Muffins, 57
   English, 44
Multigrain Waffles with Raspberry Sauce, 43
mushroom(s), 196
   broth, 103
   crimini, 103, 183, 184
     Caramelized Crimini Mushrooms and Pearl Onions, 294
   morel,
     Sugar Snap Peas and Morels, 285
   Portobello, 86
     Pesto Stuffed Portobello Pizzas, 172
   white button, 24, 159, 184
mustard, 143, 225
   deli, 133
   Dijon, 44, 134, 208, 215, 274, 360
     Dijon Blanc Sauce, 358
   whole grain, 265
   yellow, 192

N

nectarines, 242
No Cook Fresh Tomato Sauce, 129
noodles, whole wheat lasagna, 160
nori, 204
nut butter, 27
nutmeg, 23, 58, 66, 318, 326, 358
nut(s),
   almond(s), 12
     butter, 325
       Chocolate Almond Cake, 325
     milk, 97
     real almond extract, 325
   butter, 27
   cashew(s), 12, 31, 237
     butter, 237
     Cashew Miso Dressing, 262, 361
   pine, 107, 126, 134, 290
   unsalted mixed,
     Vanishing Party Nuts, 203

O

oat(s), 19, 35
   bran, 27, 35
   flour, 61, 318
   groats,
     Oat Groat Risotto with Mushrooms, 103
     Oat Porridge with Holiday Spices, 35
   rolled, 12, 28, 31, 43, 318
     Oatmeal "Scuffins" with Currants and Dates, 61
   whole oat flour, 28
Oat Groat Risotto with Mushrooms, 103
Oat Porridge with Holiday Spices, 35

Oatmeal "Scuffins" with Currants and Dates, 61
oil,
   extra virgin olive, 15, 16, 24, 28, 44, 52, 58, 62, 66, 73, 81, 82, 85, 89, 93, 94, 97, 100, 103, 104, 107, 108, 111, 112, 122, 125, 126, 129, 134, 143, 147, 148, 152, 160, 171, 176, 180, 183, 187, 195, 207, 211, 215, 226, 258, 261, 265, 266, 269, 270, 273, 277, 278, 282, 285, 286, 289, 293, 297, 298, 302, 305, 306, 309, 310, 350, 351, 354, 357, 358, 360, 361
   olive, 78, 115, 130, 152, 156, 218, 253, 266, 294
     white truffle-infused, 208
   safflower, 43, 57, 133, 151, 184, 229, 359
   sesame, 86, 184, 233, 241, 301, 361
   walnut, 200, 274
okra, frozen or fresh, 156
Olive Tapenade, 234, 360
Olive Tapenade Stuffed Sole, 234
olives, 360
   green, 195
   kalamata, 147, 250
   Olive Tapenade, 234, 360
   Olive Tapenade Stuffed Sole, 234
omega-3 fatty acids, 189
onion(s), 66, 103, 156, 176, 233
   green, 107, 108, 212
   pearl,
     Caramelized Crimini Mushrooms and Pearl Onions, 294
   powder, 225, 238, 358
   red, 32, 107, 112, 121, 147, 155, 159, 163, 175, 192, 215, 242, 301, 350, 355
   sweet, 133
   white, 230
   yellow, 58, 73, 78, 85, 89, 93, 111, 115, 118, 122, 130, 143, 151, 179, 192, 207, 230, 253, 302, 309, 359
     French Onion Soup with Parmesan Croutons, 82
orange(s), 40, 317, 334
   bitters, 333
   blood orange juice,
     Beets, Blood Oranges and Arugula with Feta, 278
   juice, 27, 44, 100, 246, 314, 358
     Spicy Orange Dipping Sauce, 360
   mandarin,
     Sesame Mandarin Slaw, 301
   peel, 314
oregano, 58, 137, 147, 160, 207
   leaves, 122
   Mexican, 89, 225
Orzo and Garbanzo Salad with Roasted Red Peppers and Dill, 277
Orzo Frittata with Mushrooms, Peppers and Yellow Squash, 24
orzo pasta, whole wheat,
   Orzo and Garbanzo Salad with Roasted Red Peppers and Dill, 277
   Orzo Frittata with Mushrooms, Peppers and Yellow Squash, 24
ostrich tenderloin,
   Chili Rubbed Grilled Ostrich Tenderloin, 249
oysters, raw, 70

P

papaya,
   Papaya with a Kick, 20
Papaya with a Kick, 20
paprika, 238
   smoked, 115, 130, 133, 152, 155, 249, 297, 298
   sweet, 58, 133, 225
parchment, 255
Parmesan,
   Parmesan Croutons, 82, 353
   Roasted Vegetable Eggplant Parmesan, 180
Parmesan Croutons, 82, 353
Parmigiano Reggiano, 75, 93, 126, 160, 164

parsley, 125, 137, 171, 176, 230, 261, 306, 354, 360
   curly, 108
   flat leaf, 100, 234, 286
   stems, 359
parsnips, 218
   Puree of Parsnip, Celeriac and Apple Soup with Crispy Sage, 97
pasta, whole grain long strand,
   Leftover Pasta Pizza Pie, 164
Patty Pan Squash, 289
Pavlova with Fresh Summer Berries, 342
pea shoots,
   Asian Pear, Watercress, Pea Shoot and Blue Cheese Salad, 273
Peach and Heirloom Tomato Caprese Salad, 258
peach(es),
   Peach and Heirloom Tomato Caprese Salad, 258
   Strawberry Peach Kefir Smoothie with Chia Seeds, 36
   white,
     White Peach and Black Cherry Bellissimo, 47
     White Peach Sangria, 317
pear(s),
   Asian,
     Asian Pear, Watercress, Pea Shoot and Blue Cheese Salad, 273
   Bosc,
     Poached Pears, 314
   Cranberry Pear Bellini, 329
   puree, 329
peas, sugar snap,
   Sugar Snap Peas and Morels, 285
pepitas, 152
pepper(s),
   Anaheim, 179, 355
   cayenne, 20, 44, 69, 118, 130, 152, 156, 159, 175, 176, 203, 225, 238, 266, 330, 357
   chili, 242
   chipotle, 89, 133, 211
     Chipotle Ranchero Sauce, 15, 350
   Cubanell, 143
   green, 73, 94, 112, 115, 156, 171
   ground, 215
   habanero, 246
   Hungarian hot wax, 143
   Italian griller, 143
   jalapeno(s), 112, 115, 121, 140, 355
     Cheddar Jalapeno Corn Muffins, 57
   orange, 24, 115, 163
   pepperoncini,
     golden Greek, 163
     Sauteed Fresh Pepperoncini with Yogurt Cheese and Baguette, 293
   poblano, 89, 112
     Pulled Pork Poblano Verde, 151
   red, 24, 73, 94, 112, 140, 163, 179, 215, 262, 266, 277
   red bell, 143, 180, 184, 212, 350
   red chili, 115
   red pepper flakes, 93, 122, 207, 230, 290, 297, 360
   Scotch bonnet, 358
   serrano, 151
   white, 225, 238
   yellow, 115, 179, 215, 262
   yellow bell, 175, 180
peppercorns, black, 82, 238, 359
pepperoncini,
   golden Greek, 163
   Sauteed Fresh Pepperoncini with Yogurt Cheese and Baguette, 293
Persian Couscous and Garbanzos with Kumquats, 175
Pesto Stuffed Portobello Pizzas, 172
pickles, 192
pimentos, 195

pineapple, 40, 212, 337
  Grilled Pineapple Salsa, 144, 355
pistachios, 100
pita(s), whole wheat, 211
  Garden Veggie Stuffed Pita Pockets, 196
pizza,
  BBQ Chicken Pizza, 163
  Greek Lamb Flatbread Pizza, 147
  Leftover Pasta Pizza Pie, 164
  Pesto Stuffed Portobello Pizzas, 172
  whole wheat pizza dough, 163
Plum Upside Down Cake, 322
plums,
  dried, 35
  Plum Upside Down Cake, 322
pluots, 317
Poached Pears, 314
pomegranate, 261
pork,
  bone-in pork back ribs,
    BBQ Pork Ribs, 222
  shoulder,
    Pulled Pork Poblano Verde, 151
  tenderloin,
    Roasted Pork Tenderloin with Brown
      Sugar Sage Glaze, 62
potato(es),
  baby yellow,
    Baby Yellow Potatoes with Parsley, 306
  fingerling,
    Grilled Fingerling Potatoes, 286
  red, 302
    Roasted Red Potatoes, Asparagus, Frisee
      with Crispy Croutons, 187
  russet, 81
  sweet, 100, 266
    puree,
      Sweet Potato Custard with Spiced
        Walnut Clusters, 330
  Yukon gold, 86
    Potatoes O'Brien, 73
Potatoes O'Brien, 73
Prawn and Herbed Yogurt Cheese Canapes, 65
prawns, 70
  Prawn and Herbed Yogurt Cheese Canapes, 65
Prosecco, 329
protein, 16, 115, 188, 189
  plain, 19
  powder, 23, 27, 31, 36
  vanilla natural protein powder, 19
ptitim, 100
Puerco Pibil, 246
Pulled Pork Poblano Verde, 151
pumpkin seeds, 12, 269
Puree of Parsnip, Celeriac and Apple Soup with
  Crispy Sage, 97

Q
quinoa, 184
  Quinoa Risotto with Garlic Herb Criminis, 183
  Quinoa with Sausage and Peppers, 115
  white, 108
    Quinoa and Black Bean Lunch
      Bowl, 199
  whole grain traditional white, 148
Quinoa and Black Bean Lunch Bowl, 199
Quinoa Risotto with Garlic Herb
  Criminis, 183
Quinoa with Sausage and Peppers, 115

R
radicchio, 269, 274
radish(es), 196, 262
  daikon, 86, 204
  Easter egg, 171
rapini, 290
  Rapini Pesto, 134

Rapini Pesto, 134
raspberries, 27, 318
  Raspberry Sauce, 43, 350
Raspberry Sauce, 43, 350
red pepper flakes, 93, 122, 207, 230, 290, 297, 360
rhubarb,
  Rhubarb Walnut Dessert Torta, 334
Rhubarb Walnut Dessert Torta, 334
rice,
  brown,
    Greek Brown Rice Dolmas, 107
    Spanish Rice, 111
  brown calrose sushi, 204
  milk, 97
ricotta, 75, 160, 282
Roasted Delicata Squash, 310
Roasted Pork Tenderloin with Brown Sugar
  Sage Glaze, 62
Roasted Red Potatoes, Asparagus, Frisee with
  Crispy Croutons, 187
Roasted Vegetable Eggplant Parmesan, 180
Roasted Yam and Spinach Salad, 266
rosemary, 58, 85, 137, 183, 253, 294, 330, 357
  leaves, 159, 203
rotini, whole wheat, 207
  Spicy Italian Tempeh Sausage and Spinach
    with Rotini, 207
rum, dark, 326

S
saccharin, 344
sage, 58, 62, 97
  leaves, 97
salmon,
  filet(s), 250
    Crunchy Baked Ginger Dill Salmon, 245
    Salmon with Sun Dried Tomato Tapenade
      in Parchment, 250
  wild Sockeye,
    Campfire Salmon with Fire Roasted
      Peppers and Eggplant, 140
  smoked salmon lox,
    Smoked Salmon Asparagus Bundles, 52
  wild-caught, 204
Salmon with Sun Dried Tomato Tapenade in
  Parchment, 250
salsa, 199
Salsa Roja, 118, 179
salt,
  Celtic sea, 155
  Hawaiian, 233
  smoked, 62
sambal, 360
Sardou, Victorien, 44
sausages,
  andouille, 156
  chicken, 115
  mild Italian chicken,
    Italian Sausage with Sloppy
      Peppers, 143
  turkey, 115
saute, 285
Sauteed Fresh Pepperoncini with Yogurt Cheese
  and Baguette, 293
Sauteed Scallops with Four Herb Pesto and
  Quinoa, 148
Savory Vegetable Waffles, 28
scallion(s), 90, 100, 112, 184, 204, 233, 262
  Scallion Pistou, 48, 351
Scallion Pistou, 48, 351
scallops, large wild,
  Sauteed Scallops with Four Herb Pesto and
    Quinoa, 148
Scattered Sushi Bowl with Ginger Glazed
  Salmon, 204
scone, 61

scuffin, 61
  Oatmeal "Scuffins" with Currants and
    Dates, 61
Seafood Gumbo, 156
Seafood Platter of Crab, Prawns and Oysters on
  the Half Shell with Clean Cocktail Sauce and
  Cucumber Mignonette, 70
seasoning,
  Italian, 115
  Old Bay, 156
Sesame Mandarin Slaw, 301
sesame seeds, 184, 204, 262, 301
  black, 20, 273
  oil, 86, 184, 233, 241, 361
  Sesame Mandarin Slaw, 301
shake,
  Acai Blueberry Breakfast Shake, 19
shallot(s), 44, 183, 351, 354, 358
sherry, dry, 82
shrimp, 156
  Coconut Shrimp with Spicy Orange Dipping
    Sauce, 241
  large,
    Sweet 'N' Spicy Shrimp and Cantaloupe
      Salad, 152
  Shrimp Tacos with Grilled Pineapple Salsa, 144
Shrimp Tacos with Grilled Pineapple Salsa, 144
Smoked Salmon Asparagus Bundles, 52
Smoky Slathered Corn on Cob, 298
Smooth and Hearty Borscht-Style Beet Soup, 78
smoothie,
  Strawberry Peach Kefir Smoothie with
    Chia Seeds, 36
  Super Power Smoothie, 27
soba noodles, buckwheat,
  Cold Soba Noodle Salad with Cashew
    Miso Dressing, 262
sole filets,
  Olive Tapenade Stuffed Sole, 234
soy,
  milk, 51, 97
  sauce, 86, 184, 204, 233, 237, 273, 285, 289
Spanish Rice, 111
Spanish-Style Tuna Sandwich, 195
Spiced Walnut Clusters, 330
Spicy Ahi Poke with Avocado, 233
Spicy Clean BBQ Sauce, 133, 163, 215, 222
Spicy Italian Tempeh Sausage and Spinach
  with Rotini, 207
Spicy Orange Dipping Sauce, 360
spinach,
  baby, 44, 245
    Roasted Sweet Potato and Spinach
      Salad, 266
    Spicy Italian Tempeh Sausage and
      Spinach with Rotini, 207
  Chicken and Spinach Lasagna, 160
sprouts, deli, 196
squash,
  delicata squash,
    Roasted Delicata Squash, 310
  Patty Pan Squash, 289
  yellow, 24, 48
steak,
  beef flank,
    Jamaican Jerk Steak and Pineapple
      Lettuce Wraps, 212
  flat iron, 155
stevia, 344
strawberries, 242, 321, 337, 341
  Strawberry Peach Kefir Smoothie with
    Chia Seeds, 36
Strawberry Peach Kefir Smoothie with Chia
  Seeds, 36
sucralose, 344
sucrose, 344

sugar,
 brown, 12, 204, 297, 309, 318
 dark brown, 62
 turbinado, 28, 43, 51, 57, 61, 203, 321, 322, 325, 330, 334, 342, 358
 unrefined, 344
Sugar Snap Peas and Morels, 285
Summer Root Vegetable Salad with Fresh Cherries, 265
Summer Vegetable Platter with Baby Heirloom Tomatoes and Green Onion Pistou, 48
sunflower seed kernels, 12, 196
Super Moist Banana Walnut Bread, 51
Super Power Smoothie, 27
Sweet 'N' Spicy Shrimp and Cantaloupe Salad, 152
sweet potato,
 Roasted Sweet Potato and Spinach Salad, 266
Sweet Potato Custard with Spiced Walnut Clusters, 330
Sweet Potato Custard with Spiced Walnut Clusters, 330
Sweeteners, 344-345

T

Tabouli with Quinoa, 108
tacos,
 Chili and Scrambled Egg Breakfast Tacos, 32
 Shrimp Tacos with Grilled Pineapple Salsa, 144
tahini, 125, 273, 357
 Tahini Sauce, 176, 352
Tahini Sauce, 176, 352
tamari, 90, 301
tarragon, 52, 104, 148
tempeh,
 Spicy Italian Tempeh Sausage and Spinach with Rotini, 207
Three Bean Salad with Corn and Peppers, 112
thyme, 58, 62, 73, 81, 82, 85, 93, 97, 103, 137, 156, 171, 183, 218, 250, 253, 286, 294, 357, 358, 359, 360
Tobasco, 73, 352
tofu,
 Japanese Vegetable and Tofu Soup, 86
 Silken soft, 330, 341
 Tofu Fajitas with Peppers, 179
Tofu Fajitas with Peppers, 179
tomatillos, 151
Tomato Fennel Soup with Lima Beans, 93
tomato(es), 16, 89, 94, 108, 111, 115, 118, 121, 122, 143, 155, 208, 352
 baby heirloom cherry, 48
 campari, 172
 cherry, 147, 148, 159, 195
 grape, 148
 heirloom,
  Peach and Heirloom Tomato Caprese Salad, 258
 No Cook Fresh Tomato Sauce, 129
 paste, 122, 156, 192, 230, 253, 359
 pear, 48
 sauce, 122, 133, 350, 352
 slices, 168
 sun dried, 28, 164, 250, 290
 Tomato Fennel Soup with Lima Beans, 93
torta, 334
tortillas, 179
 whole grain corn, 15, 32, 144
treviso,
 Grilled Treviso and Endive with Cranberries and Pumpkin Seeds, 269
tuna,
 ahi,
  Spicy Ahi Poke with Avocado, 233
 albacore,
  Spanish-Style Tuna Sandwich, 195
 yellowfin,
  Yellowfin Tuna with Cashew Sauce, 237

turkey,
 ground,
  Turkey Apple Breakfast Sausage, 58
 low-fat turkey bacon, 16
 sausage, 115
Turkey Apple Breakfast Sausage, 58
turmeric, 159

U

V

vanilla, 12, 31, 36, 43, 321, 322, 330, 338, 341
 pure vanilla extract, 334
 real vanilla extract, 342
Vanishing Party Nuts, 203
vegetable,
 broth, 44, 78, 85, 89, 93, 97, 103, 107, 148, 183, 245, 297, 309, 350
 Garden Veggie Pita Pockets, 196
 Green Lentil and Vegetable Soup, 85
 Japanese Vegetable and Tofu Soup, 86
 juice, 94
 Long-Life Vegetable Stir-Fry, 184
 Savory Vegetable Waffles, 28
 stock, 207
 Summer Root Vegetable Salad with Fresh Cherries, 265
 Summer Vegetable Platter with Baby Heirloom Tomatoes and Green Onion Pistou, 48
Vegetarian Done Right, 188
vegetarianism, 188
Venice Beach Roasted Vegetable and Avocado Sub, 168
venison,
 shoulder, 253
  Venison Bourguignon, 253
 tenderloin,
  Hazelnut-Crusted Venison Medallions with Herb Roasted Carrots and Parsnips, 218
Venison Bourguignon, 253
vinegar,
 balsamic, 134, 200
 Champagne, 44, 278, 354
 cider, 62, 112, 133, 246, 297
 red wine, 94, 100, 215, 309, 351
 rice, 237
 rice wine, 184, 204, 361
 sherry, 82, 94, 152, 354
 white, 118, 342
 white balsamic, 171, 258, 265, 266, 269, 273, 274
 white wine, 82, 208, 358
vitamin B12, 189
vitamin D, 189
vodka, 333

W

waffles,
 Multigrain Waffles with Raspberry Sauce, 43
 Savory Vegetable Waffles, 28
wakame, 86, 90
walnut(s), 270, 282, 330
 oil, 200
 pieces, 148, 265, 274, 318, 351
 Rhubarb Walnut Dessert Torta, 334
 Super Moist Banana Walnut Bread, 51
Warm Brussels Sprouts Salad with Walnuts and Lemon, 270
Warm Orange Vinaigrette, 44
water, 85, 89, 100, 108, 148, 176, 204, 237, 314, 338, 353, 354
 cold, 321
 sparkling mineral, 47
water chestnuts, 184

watercress,
 Asian Pear, Watercress, Pea Shoot and Blue Cheese Salad, 273
watermelon, 40
wheat germ, 19, 31, 225
White Peach and Black Cherry Bellissimo, 47
White Peach Sangria, 317
Whole Wheat Angel Food Cake with Fresh Strawberries, 321
wine,
 dry red, 253, 359
 dry sparkling, 329
 dry white, 183
 red, 314
 sake rice, 90
 white, 103, 317
Winter Greens with Cherries and Walnuts, 274
Women's HealthSource Newsletter, 254
Worcestershire, 82
 sauce, 133, 352

X

Y

yeast, 302
Yellowfin Tuna with Cashew Sauce, 237
yogurt,
 Greek, 121, 179
 low-fat, 19, 27, 32, 78
Yogurt Cheese, 51, 121, 130, 147, 160, 168, 179, 196, 200, 208, 265, 293, 318, 338, 341, 342, 348, 351

Z

Zesty Hummus, 196, 199, 357
zinc, 189
zucchini, baby, 28, 48, 159, 168, 175, 180, 199, 215

PREVIEW ALL BOOKS IN THE EAT-CLEAN DIET® SERIES AT EATCLEANDIET.COM/BOOKS

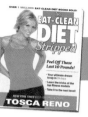

The Eat-Clean Diet Stripped

Tosca Reno shares the slim-down secrets of fitness models and celebrities, teaching you how to lose those last stubborn 10 pounds and keep them off. Includes 50 new recipes and a four-week meal plan.

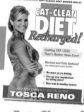

The Eat-Clean Diet Recharged!

Lose weight, feel happier, stay motivated and be more productive with Tosca Reno's no nonsense and no deprivation approach to weight loss and maintenance. Includes 50 new recipes and several meal plans.

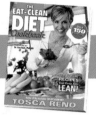

The Eat-Clean Diet Cookbook

Your go-to guide for Clean dishes, from soups to sauces to main courses and desserts. Info pages explain the Eat-Clean Principles, protein facts, sugar substitutes and more. Over 150 recipes!

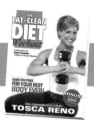

The Eat-Clean Diet Workout

Sculpt the body you want with Tosca's tried-and-true workout tips. Includes chapters devoted to each body part, equipment, training plans, nutrition and competition advice. Bonus 30-minute DVD!

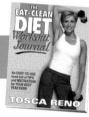

The Eat-Clean Diet Workout Journal

With daily journal space for reps, sets, weights, exercises, cardio and goal setting, along with motivational tips, quotes and photos, this workout journal is the perfect tool to help you track and reach your fitness goals.

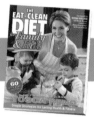

The Eat-Clean Diet for Family & Kids

Set the right example for your kids by eating healthy at home. With tons of tips, tricks and advice, in addition to 60 kid-friendly recipes, this book is a trusted resource for parents and families everywhere.

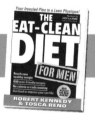

The Eat-Clean Diet for Men

Men can Eat Clean too! Tosca and her husband Robert show men they can sculpt a lean, muscular body, improve their health and have better sex all with a healthy diet – no rabbit food required. Includes 60 man-friendly recipes!

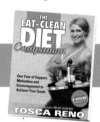

The Eat-Clean Diet Companion

Improve your chance of weight-loss success by journaling. This resource tool contains space to track meals and shopping lists, with inspirational quotes and photos, as well as food tips from Tosca herself.

RKP ROBERT KENNEDY PUBLISHING

RKPUBS.COM
TOSCARENO.COM